AGING AND CLINICAL PRACTICE: INFECTIOUS DISEASES

Diagnosis and Treatment

AGING AND CLINICAL PRACTICE: INFECTIOUS DISEASES

Diagnosis and Treatment

Thomas T. Yoshikawa, M.D.
Chief, Division of Geriatric Medicine; Medical Director, Nursing
Home Care Unit; and Clinical Director, Geriatric Research,
Education and Clinical Center (GRECC); Veterans Administration
Medical Center, West Los Angeles, Los Angeles, California.
Consultant, Infectious Diseases, Harbor-UCLA Medical Center,
Torrance, California.
Professor of Medicine, University of California at Los Angeles
(UCLA) School of Medicine, Los Angeles, California.
Dr. Yoshikawa is board certified in both internal medicine
and infectious diseases.

Dean C. Norman, M.D.
Associate Chief, Division of Geriatric Medicine; and Associate
Clinical Director, Geriatric Research, Education and Clinical
Center (GRECC); Veterans Administration Medical Center,
West Los Angeles, Los Angeles, California.
Consultant, Infectious Diseases, Harbor-UCLA Medical Center,
Torrance, California.
Assistant Professor of Medicine, University of California at
Los Angeles (UCLA) School of Medicine, Los Angeles, California.
Dr. Norman completed fellowships in both infectious diseases
and geriatric medicine and is board certified in internal medicine
and infectious diseases.

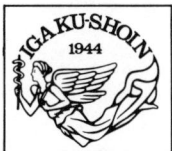

IGAKU-SHOIN   New York · Tokyo

Interior Design by Helen Iranyi
Cover Design by M 'N O Production Services, Inc.
Typesetting by Ampersand Inc.
Printing and Binding by Edwards Brothers

Published and distributed by

IGAKU-SHOIN Medical Publishers, Inc.
1140 Avenue of the Americas, New York, N.Y. 10036

IGAKU-SHOIN Ltd.,
5-24-3 Hongo, Bunkyo-ku, Tokyo

Library of Congress Cataloging-in-Publication Data

Yoshikawa, Thomas T.
  Infectious diseases.

  (Aging and clinical practice)
  Includes index.
  1. Communicable diseases.   2. Aged—Diseases.
3. Geriatrics.   I. Norman, Dean C.   II. Title.
III. Series.   [DNLM: 1. Communicable Diseases—in old
age. WC 100 Y65i]
RC112.Y67   1987   618.97'69   86-27354

ISBN: 0-89640-127-9 (New York)
ISBN: 4-260-14127-8 (Tokyo)

Printed and bound in U.S.A.

10 9 8 7 6 5 4 3 2 1

Preface

Geriatric medicine is a rapidly growing discipline. With more and more clinicians caring for the geriatric segment of our population, there is a greater demand for specialized knowledge and approach to care for the elderly. Caring for the elderly with infectious diseases is no exception.

Alhough there are several excellent textbooks on the broad aspects of infectious diseases, these fail to address the specialized problems that are encountered in the diagnosis and treatment of infections in the aged. Moreover, the few books that focus on infections in the elderly lack a primary emphasis on the geriatric aspects of infectious diseases. Rather, a broad description of an infectious disease problem is presented with only a relatively small portion of the discussion devoted to the management of the aging patient. Additionally, many, if not all, of these contributions are written by infectious disease specialists who are not practicing geriatricians.

This book attempts to rectify the above shortcomings. It is written by geriatricians with specialized interest, training, and experience in infectious diseases. Thus, infection in the aged is presented from a primary geriatrician's perspective. The book covers infections that are unique or clinically relevant to the elderly. The discussion focuses on important aspects in the diagnosis, treatment, and prevention of select infections and infectious disease problems as they may present in the elderly to the practicing clinician. The book is divided into three major parts: (*1*) characteristics and general management of infections; (*2*) specific infectious diseases; and (*3*) specific pathogens. Current references and a bibliography are provided at the end of each chapter.

This textbook should serve as valuable aid to clinicians on the management of geriatric patients with infections. Only through such efforts will we be able to improve the quality of life for a cherished and valued segment of the human population.

THOMAS T. YOSHIKAWA, M.D.
DEAN C. NORMAN, M.D.

*To our wives and children, who have
encouraged and supported us; and
To our parents Grace, Elaine, Amos, and
Owen, who taught us how to appreciate,
understand, and love the aging person.*

Acknowledgments

We are grateful to Jerry Sproul for his able assistance in typing the manuscript.

We are grateful to Takashi Makinodan, Ph.D., for his professional support, and to Mary Baker for her editorial assistance.

We are grateful to the VA Medical Center, West Los Angeles, for its commitment to the care of the elderly and training, education, and research in aging.

Lastly, we are forever grateful to the Veterans Administration for providing the resources, assistance, and guidance in implementing such pioneering programs as the Geriatric Research, Education and Clinical Centers, geriatric fellowships, and allied health traineeships, all of which serve to develop and establish better approaches to the care of the elderly.

Contents

Part 1

CHARACTERISTICS AND GENERAL MANAGEMENT OF INFECTIONS

Chapter 1

Epidemiology of Infectious Diseases

INCIDENCE AND PREVALENCE

Important Infections

Aging appears to place a person at greater risk for contracting an infectious disease. Although data are not available that substantiate the impression that the elderly are more susceptible to all infections, clinical and epidemiologic studies have confirmed that the incidence (the number of new cases identified during a given observation period) or prevalence (total number of new and old cases identified during a given observation period) of select infectious diseases rises or is the highest in the geriatric population (1). These particular infectious diseases and their associated problems are the focus of discussion for this textbook.

An example of the age-related incidence of infections is pneumonia. Pneumonia, especially bacterial pneumonia, has a predilection for the aged person, regardless of the setting. In a large municipal hospital, the mean age of 148 patients that were admitted with pneumonia was 51 years (2). Of 153 patients admitted to an intensive care unit for pneumonia, the mean ages of the patients were 58, 61, 70, and 71 years, depending on which of the four etiologic categories were analyzed (3). The attack rate of pneumonia during or following an influenza epidemic is the highest in the very young and very old, the incidence in the latter group being double to triple that of young adults (4). Alternatively, studies that describe pneumonia by etiologic pathogens frequently show the elderly to be at highest risk. In the classic investigation by Austrian and Gold (5) on pneumococcal pneumonia, one-third of the patients with pneumococcal bacteremia were 60 years and older. Similarly, of 325 cases of bacteremic pneumococcal pneumonia described by Mufson et al. (6), 41% of the patients were 50 years and over. Rose et al. showed that *Pseudomonas aeruginosa* pneumonia in adults may disproportionately occur in the geriatric population. In this study of 19 patients, 12 were 70 years or older.

Such compelling data as described for pneumonia are also available for the other important infectious diseases of the elderly. Those chapters devoted to each of these infectious disease problems discuss the association between aging and the increased frequency of infection.

Acute Hospitalization

Studies that have examined the causes for hospitalization of the elderly provide additional confirmatory data on the importance of infections in the health and well being of the aged. For example, in a large clinical investigation by Keating et al. (7), 1,202 ambulatory adults who came to an emergency room or clinic with an illness associated with fever (38.3°C or greater) were evaluated. The age distribution of the study patients ranged from 17 to over 80 years. However, 33% of the patients were 60 years and older. Moreover, in contrast to adults under the age of 40 in whom benign causes (pharyngitis, otitis media, or viral syndrome) of fever predominated, elderly patients with fever had serious and often life-threatening infections (over 90% of infections), such as, pneumonia, urinary tract infection, intraabdominal sepsis, or bacteremia (7).

Hospitalization either in an acute care facility or long-term care institution predisposes a patient to nosocomial infections. Elderly patients are at greater risk for nosocomial infections than are younger adults (8). In chronic care facilities, infectious diseases are a major problem in the elderly (9–11). Moreover, infections are frequently the most common reason to transfer patients from a long-term care facility to an acute care hospital. In a study by Gordon et al. (12), fever along with depression were the most frequent symptoms that resulted in hospitalization of elderly residents of a long-term care institution. Moreover, Irvine et al. (13) showed that of 128 nursing home residents who required acute hospitalization, 27% of the patients were admitted for infections, which was the leading primary diagnosis. Finally, approximately 17% (40 of 229 patients) in a chronic care facility required admission to an acute care hospital during a one-year period in a study by Tresch et al. (14). Infectious diseases were the most frequent reason given for hospitalization; they accounted for 30% of the admissions.

MORBIDITY AND MORTALITY

In addition to having an increased risk to many infectious diseases, the elderly with infections suffer higher rates of complications including death. Several factors contribute to this higher death rate: (1) limited reserve capacity to respond adequately to stress because of biologic changes of aging and/or underlying chronic diseases; (2) abnormalities in host defense mechanisms; (3) complications from other acute and chronic disorders; (4) higher prevalence of nosocomial infections; (5) delays in diagnosis and institution of treatment; (6) morbidity from invasive procedures; (7) poorer clinical response to treatment; and (8) higher frequency of adverse drug reactions.

A study by Keating et al. (7) examined the causes and outcomes of ambulatory adults seeking care at an emergency room or clinic for a febrile-associated illness. Table 1.1 summarizes the salient points of the study. Younger adults had more benign causes of fever, were hospitalized relatively infrequently, and uncommonly experienced life-threatening complications or death. With advancing age, elderly patients had almost exclusively more serious causes of fever, were hospitalized in the majority of instances, and suffered life-threatening morbidity or death four to five times more than did their younger cohorts.

Table 1.2 illustrates examples of differences in death rates from select infections in the elderly compared to young adults from clinical studies. It can be seen that regardless whether a bacterial infection occurred commonly in the aged or relatively infrequently, the mortality is still most

TABLE 1.1   Age, Causes of Fever, and Outcome

CAUSE OF FEVER OR OUTCOME	OCCURRENCE IN EACH AGE GROUP (%)			
	17–39	40–59	60–79	>80
Benign causes[a]	58	21	6	<1
Serious causes[b]	42	79	94	>99
Hospitalized[c]	26	56	69	76
Life-threatening[d]	3	11	17	13
Death	<1	3	5	7
Total cases[e]	459	164	244	126

SOURCE: Adapted from reference 7.
[a]Viral syndromes, otitis media, pharyngitis.
[b]Respiratory infections, urinary tract infection, cellulitis, intraabdominal infection and abscesses, drug reactions.
[c]Status not life-threatening.
[d]Intensive care unit admissions, respiratory failure, hypotension, bacteremia, mental status deterioration, intestinal perforation, abscesses.
[e]Number of cases studied in each age group.

TABLE 1.2 Comparative Mortality from
Select Infections in Young and Old Adults

| | MORTALITY | | |
INFECTION	OLD	YOUNG	REFERENCE
Gram-negative sepsis	70	26	15
Bacterial meningitis	41	13	16
Endocarditis	21	8.5	17
Acute appendicitis	2–14	<1–1.0	18
Acute cholecystitis	3–24	3	19
Acute pneumonia	39	8	20

severe with old age. Additionally, morbid events or complications from infections occur more frequently in the geriatric patient. For example, bacteremia secondary to urinary tract infections (pyelonephritis) may occur in nearly 50% of elderly women, but rarely in younger female patients (21), and the incidence of perforation of the appendix in the elderly is three times that of children and young adults (22).

CONCLUSION

Infections are common in the elderly and are associated with a disproportionately higher frequency of morbid events including death. Only through early and constant awareness that the elderly are at risk for a variety of infectious diseases can clinicians rapidly establish a diagnosis, institute proper treatment expeditiously and judiciously, and ultimately reduce the number of deaths and severe complications.

REFERENCES

1. Yoshikawa TT: Important infections in elderly persons. *West J Med* 135: 441–445, 1981.
2. Dorff GJ, Rytel MN, Farmer SG, et al: Etiologies and characteristic features of pneumonias in a municipal hospital. *Am J Med Sci* 266:349–358, 1973.
3. Stevens RM, Teres D, Skillman JJ, et al: Pneumonia in an intensive care unit. A 30-month experience. *Arch Intern Med* 134:106–111, 1974.
4. Foy AM, Cooney MK, Allen I, et al: Rates of pneumonia during influenza epidemics in Seattle, 1964 to 1975. *JAMA* 241:253–258, 1978.
5. Austrian R, Gold J: Pneumococcal bacteremia with especial reference to bacteremic pneumococcal pneumonia. *Ann Intern Med* 60:759–776, 1964.
6. Mufson MA, Kruss DM, Wasil RE, et al: Capsular types and outcome of bacteremic pneumococcal disease in the antibiotic era. *Arch Intern Med* 134:505–510, 1974.

7. Keating HJ III, Klimek JJ, Levine DS, et al: Effect of aging on the clinical significance of fever in ambulatory adult patients. *J Am Geriatr Soc* 32:282–287, 1984.

8. Freeman J, McGowan JE Jr: Risk factors for nosocomial infection. *J Infect Dis* 138:811–819, 1978.

9. Farber BF, Brennan C, Puntereri AJ, et al: A prospective study of nosocomial infections in a chronic care facility. *J Am Geriatr Soc* 32:499–502, 1984.

10. Nicolle LE, McIntyre M, Zacharias H, et al: Twelve-month surveillance of infection in institutionalized elderly men. *J Am Geriatr Soc* 32:513–519, 1984.

11. Finnegan TP, Austin TN, Cape RDT: A 12-month fever surveillance study in a Veterans' long-stay institution. *J Am Geriatr Soc* 33:590–594, 1985.

12. Gordon WZ, Kane RL, Rothenberg R: Acute hospitalization in a home for the aged. *J Am Geriatr Soc* 33:519–529, 1985.

13. Irvine PW, Van Buren N, Crossley K: Causes for hospitalization of nursing home residents: The role of infection. *J Am Geriatr Soc* 32:103–107, 1984.

14. Tresch DD, Simpson WM Jr, Burton JR: Relationship of long-term care and acute care facilities. The problem of patient transfer and continuity of care. *J Am Geriatr Soc* 33:819–826, 1985.

15. Hodgin UG, Sanford JP: Gram-negative rod bacteremia: An analysis of 100 patients. *Am J Med* 39:952–960, 1965.

16. Gorse GJ, Thrupp LD, Nudleman KL, et al: Bacterial meningitis in the elderly. *Arch Intern Med* 144:1603–1607, 1984.

17. Cantrell M, Yoshikawa TT: Aging and infective endocarditis. *J Am Geriatr Soc* 31:216–222, 1983.

18. Norman DC, Yoshikawa TT: Intraabdominal infection: Diagnosis and treatment in the elderly. *Gerontology* 30:327–338, 1984.

19. Fry DE, Cox RA, Harbrecht JB: Gangrene of the gallbladder. *South Med J* 74:666–668, 1981.

20. Sullivan RJ, Jr, Dowdle WR, Marine WM, et al: Adult pneumonia in a general hospital. *Arch Intern Med* 129:935–942, 1972.

21. Gleckman RA, Bradley PJ, Roth RM, et al: Bacteremic urosepsis: A phenomenon unique to elderly women. *J Urol* 133:174–175, 1985.

22. Peltokallio P, Jauhiainen K: Acute appendicitis in the aged patient. *Arch Surg* 100:140–143, 1970.

SUGGESTED READINGS

Yoshikawa TT, Norman DC, Grahn D: Infections in the aging population. *J Am Geriatr Soc* 33:496–503, 1985.

Yoshikawa T: Ageing and infectious diseases, in Pathy MSJ (ed): *Principles and Practice of Geriatric Medicine.* Chichester, John Wiley & Sons, Ltd, 1985, p 221.

Chapter 2

Predisposing Factors to Infection

Chapter 1 provided supportive epidemiologic data on the increased susceptibility of the elderly to many infectious diseases and on the impact of these infections on morbidity and mortality. In this chapter, the discussion focuses on those factors that appear to be associated with or directly play a role in predisposing the elderly to certain infectious diseases.

HOST PATHOGEN INTERACTION

For any infection to develop or be established, the microorganisms must be pathogenic or virulent to the host. Virulence of a microbe is dependent on (1) its ability to gain access to the host (e.g., attach to and penetrate mucocutaneous surfaces); (2) its ability to replicate in the host; (3) its success in avoiding or inhibiting host defense processes; and (4) its ability to induce damage or injury to the host (1). In addition to virulence, two other major factors influence the host's predisposition to infection. These factors are the quantity of organism(s) to which the host is exposed and the functional integrity of the host's defense mechanisms (1,2). This relationship between infection, virulence, quantity of organism (inoculum), and host defense mechanism (resistance) can be shown by this formula:

$$\text{Infection} = \frac{\text{Inoculum} \times \text{Virulence}}{\text{Host Resistance}}$$

Translated into clinical terms, this relationship states that the risk (or severity) of infection for an individual is *directly* influenced by the amount or number of microorganisms (inoculum) as well as by the type of pathogen (virulence) to which the host is exposed and is *inversely* affected by the functional integrity of host's defense mechanism (resistance). For example, in relatively healthy persons, serious infections can develop with exposure to sufficient numbers of such virulent pathogens as *Staphylococcus aureus* or *Pseudomonas aeruginosa*. However, low quantity of exposure to these organisms would not ordinarily cause infections in normal hosts. With individuals who have diminished host resistance, either low numbers of virulent microorganisms or high quantity of relatively avirulent microbes can cause devastating infections.

To evaluate the relationship of aging to increased susceptibility or risk to infections, it is then necessary to examine factors that might influence or directly impact on inoculum, virulence, and host resistance.

AGING AND RISK FACTORS TO INFECTION

Environmental Exposure

Hospitalization and chronic institutionalization place a patient at greater risk to serious infections. By the very nature of these facilities, that is, a setting for other infected patients, colonized or contaminated equipment, hospital beds and other supplies, and close contact or interaction with hospital personnel (who may be carriers or transmitters of pathogenic microbes), a patient has significant exposure to potential pathogenic organisms. The risk for acquiring a nosocomial infection in a hospital setting for the general population is approximately 5%. However, this risk increases with age, and is threefold higher in the elderly (3). Moreover, with increased longevity, which is associated with increased frequency of acute and chronic illness, the elderly are hospitalized more often and remain in the hospital, on the average, twice as long as younger adults (4). Similarly, nosocomial infections in chronic care facilities, which are occupied primarily by elderly patients, occur quite frequently, often at a rate exceeding the incidence of hospital infections (5,6). Thus, it is apparent that the aged inpatient is at greater risk of exposure to microorganisms.

Hospital-acquired infections in the elderly are predominantly urinary tract infections, pneumonia, surgical wound infections, and bacteremia (7). These are also common nosocomial infections in nursing homes and chronic care facilities (8). Unfortunately, most nosocomial infections are caused by aerobic or facultative anaerobic gram-negative bacilli; these bacteria notoriously cause serious infections in susceptible hosts, are often resistant to many antibiotics, and are associated with high death rates. Conversely, bacteremia caused by gram-negative bacilli occurs predominantly in a nosocomial setting with a disproportionate frequency occurring in the aged. Table 2.1 selectively summarizes data from three studies of bacteremia caused by three species of Enterobacteriaceae organisms, i.e., *Klebsiella, Enterobacter,* and *Citrobacter* (9–11). Similarly, *Pseudomonas aeruginosa* bacteremia is primarily a nosocomial disease (12).

Physiologic Changes of Aging on Host Defense Factors

It is well known that advancing age is associated with anatomic and functional changes in many of the tissues and organs of the body (13). These alterations may include diminished blood perfusion; degenerative processes; fibrosis and scarring; deposition of fat, pigments, or other material; calcification; loss of cells or tissue; increased or decreased permeability of vascular surfaces, and so on. These changes may compromise the ability of the host's tissue or organs to resist and control infectious agents. This disadvantage would be compounded by the presence of chronic underlying diseases. More importantly, the process of senescence may not only limit the host defense processes from being fully effective (e.g., decreased vascular perfusion to an organ will limit the number of polymorphonuclear leukocytes that can enter infected tissue), but also may cause changes in the functional integrity of various host defense mechanisms.

To better understand the potential impact of aging on the host defense mechanisms, a brief discussion is provided on the role of each of the major factors responsible for host resistance to infection.

OVERVIEW OF HOST DEFENSE MECHANISMS
The major factors in host resistance to infectious pathogens include the following. mucocutaneous surfaces, phagocytic cells, complement, humoral immunity, and cell-mediated immunity. Depending on the investigator, the classification of these factors may be varied and, at times, confusing. Mucocutaneous surfaces (skin and mucosal epithelial lining), phagocytic cells (mononuclear macrophages and polymorphonuclear

TABLE 2.1 Studies of Gram-Negative Bacillemia: Select Features

ORGANISM	PATIENTS >60 YEARS (%)	NOSOCOMIAL (%)	OVERALL MORTALITY (%)	REFERENCE
Klebsiella	60	77	25	9
Enterobacter	46	76	42	10
Citrobacter	65	77	48	11

neutrophils [PMN]), and complement have been called *nonspecific host factors, nonspecific immunity,* or *natural immunity.* Humoral and cell-mediated immunity has been termed *specific host factors, specific immunity,* or *acquired immunity.*

Figure 2.1 illustrates diagrammatically the role(s) and interrelationships of the various host defense mechanisms that follow exposure to and invasion by microorganisms. Although there is a sequential time course for many of these processes, often the activation of the various host responses occur concurrently or in a different order of events depending on the site of infection, type of organism, extent or severity of infection, previous exposure to the pathogen, functional integrity of the host defense mechanisms, and other unidentified factors.

The skin and mucous membrane are the first and most important barriers to infection. If nothing else, the mucocutaneous surface acts as a physical obstruction against the invasion of microbes. The physical dis-

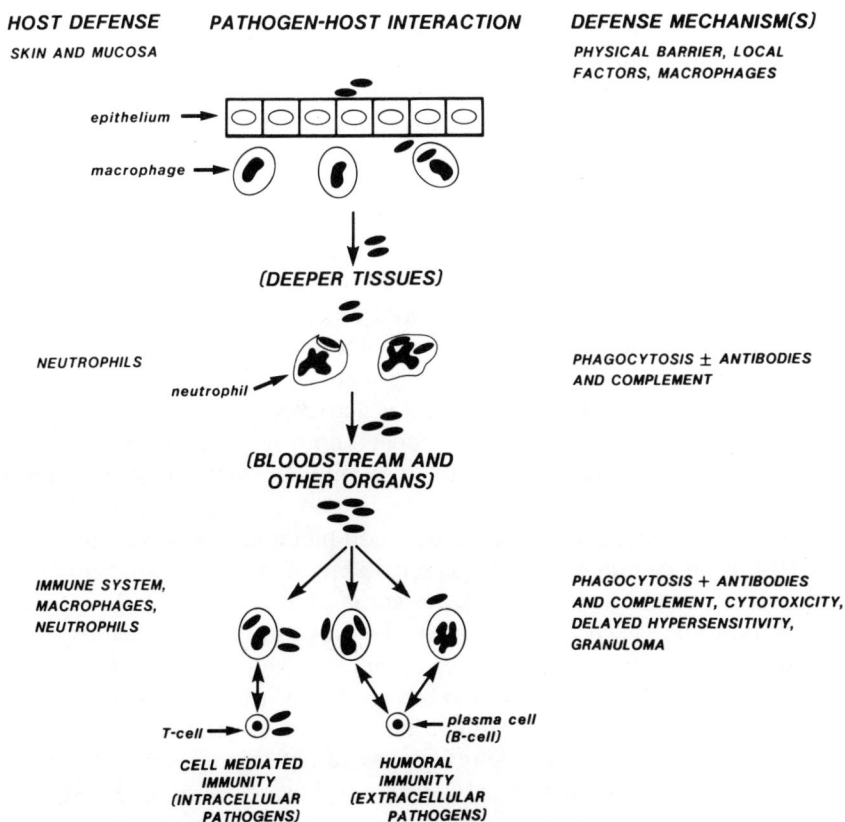

Figure 2.1. Host defense mechanisms against invasion of microorganisms.

ruption (trauma, burn, surgery, chemicals, disease, etc.) of these surfaces is the major means by which microbes can gain access to the host. Normal skin also has properties that tend to inhibit or minimize microbial replication; that is, it is relatively dry and mildly acidic; it produces secretions from glands that may have some microbicidal activity; and it has its own normal microflora that limits colonization by other more pathogenic organisms (14). Mucous membranes also aid in preventing microbial invasion by the action of cilia and by the secretion of mucus, which act to trap the pathogens; the microbes can then be removed by coughing (lungs), mechanical peristalsis (gastrointestinal tract), or secretions (nasopharynx).

Phagocytosis is the first line of defense once the invading microbe permeates or gains access through the mucocutaneous barrier. Two major cell types are important in phagocytosis. Tissue (mononuclear) macrophages that localize in different body sites (e.g., liver, spleen, lymph nodes) are derived from circulating monocytes that originate from bone marrow stem cells. Macrophages are the major defense system against blood stream invasion by microorganisms (e.g., bacteremia); they are also important in localization of tissue infection and are an active participant in the immune system. Polymorphonuclear neutrophils (PMN) are more important for preventing or limiting infection within tissues or organs. They respond quickly (in minutes) and their effectiveness depends on the functional integrity of numerous factors that include normal adherence, margination, movement (chemokinesis or chemotaxis), and microbial attachment, engulfment, and killing (15,16).

Complement is part of a system of 20 or more proteins that function through a series of cascading steps and are important in initiating cell chemotaxis, promoting opsonization (coating of microbes with complement or immunoglobulin to facilitate phagocytosis), and participating in cytoxicity reactions (16). Complement is activated by either the classic or alternate pathways. In nonimmune hosts (not previously exposed to the pathogen), early in the primary infection, the alternate pathway is more important (since it can be activated by bacterial components in the absence of immunoglobulin). The classic complement pathway is most important in the immune host who is rechallenged with a familiar microbe (since it is generally activated by antigen-antibody complexes) (15).

The immune system becomes activated only after previous exposure to a distinct antigen. However, natural killer cells, which are not typical of B lymphocytes or T lymphocytes, do not require prior exposure in order to reach their target cells. Therefore, in nonimmune hosts, the immune system does not play a major role in host resistance to infection early in the course of the disease. However, in immune hosts, an immune response may occur in concert with nonspecific host factors (e.g., phagocytosis and complement). Humoral immunity is derived from B lymphocytes, which ultimately transform into plasma cells. Plasma cells secrete immuno-globulins (A, D, E, G, and M) that function as antibodies with antigenic specificity (17). The primary antibody response (first exposure to an antigen) involves formation of IgM antigen-specific antibodies. A secondary antibody response follows with IgG antibodies. Most humoral (B cell) responses are regulated or modulated by other cells such as T helper or T suppressor cells. Antibodies assist in host defense by fixing complement, opsonizing or agglutinating organisms (permitting efficient phagocytosis), neutralizing toxins, and in some instances directly by lysing cells.

Cell-mediated immunity is dependent on thymus-derived (T) lymphocytes and their products. In the circulation, T cells make up 80 to 90% of the total lymphocytes. There are many types of T cells (T-cell subsets), and these T cells serve to fulfill the major functions of cellular immunity; for instance, they mediate delayed hypersensitivity reactions, cause cytolysis and provide memory (all of these functions by effector T cells), and regulate immune responses (T helper and T suppressor cells). Cell-mediated immunity starts with macrophage ingestion of microbes (or any antigen). The antigen is processed and presented by the macrophage to T-helper cells and effector T cells. Macrophages also synthesize and release a monokine called *interleukin 1* (also known as *lymphocyte-activating factor*), which activates the T-helper cells. Activated T-helper cells release a lymphokine, interleukin 2, which activates and stimulates other T cells to undergo cell division (clonal expansion) in response to the specific antigen. Whereas humoral immunity predominates in host defense against extracellular bacterial infection, cell-mediated immunity has a primary role in preventing and eliminating intracellular microbial pathogens like viruses, mycobacteria, and fungi. However, both systems frequently overlap in function with certain infections.

IMPACT OF AGING ON HOST DEFENSES

Mucocutaneous surfaces.   Advancing age results in many gross and histologic changes in the skin. Skin thickness decreases with loss of subcutaneous fat; vascular perfusion to the dermis may diminish; and skin structures including glands atrophy. Thus, the skin's physical barrier to microbes as well as some of its microbicidal properties are compromised in old age. In addition, the elderly are more prone to major and minor trauma, pressure sores, and certain skin diseases. All these factors predispose the elderly to more frequent and more severe skin and soft tissue infections. Similar age-related changes in the mucosal surfaces of the body cavities and organs most likely occur. These alterations could then compromise ciliary action, mucus secretion, and mechanical properties of these sites. Furthermore, such age-related disorders as chronic obstructive lung disease, atrophic gastritis, diverticulitis, ischemic bowel disease, inflammatory bowel disease, or colonic malignancy can damage mucosal surfaces and can predispose the elderly to infectious processes.

Phagocytosis. Although leukocyte function is most often assessed by the ability of leukocytes to perform phagocytosis, the integrity of white cells to defend against invading pathogens may also depend on a variety of other responses. Not only is the quantity or number of white blood cells important, but the ability of the leukocytes to reach the site of microorganisms (margination, adherence, chemotaxis), attack and engulf the pathogen (phagocytosis), and generate the metabolic reactions and products to kill the microbes is critical for successful elimination of infectious agents. Table 2.2 summarizes most of the studies that evaluate various components of leukocyte (primarily PMN) function in healthy elderly patients compared to a young adult control group (18–28). The results are quite heterogeneous depending on the investigator and particular parameters studied. Age does not appear to affect total leukocyte count or the relative number of PMN (18). Adherence of PMN (leukocytes must be able to stick to endothelial surfaces before they can leave the vascular compartment) is not impaired in the aged and frequently are better than controls (19,20,23,26). Chemotaxis may be normal (20,21) or depressed in the elderly (19,23,24,28). Similar inconsistencies are seen with phagocytosis (19–23), nitroblue tetrazolium test, and microbicidal capacity (18–25). It appears that leukocyte phagocytic activity can be normal in the elderly but also may show significant abnormalities. Whether these abnormalities contribute to the increased frequency or severity of infections in the elderly is not clear. Moreover, all of these studies (except a small subgroup of patients in study by Laharrague et al. [20]) were done in healthy elderly. It is unknown whether active infection in the elderly significantly alters leukocyte function.

Complement. There are only a limited number of investigations that assess the influence of old age on complement activity. These studies fail to show any significant negative effect of aging on the various components of complement (24,25). Others have demonstrated an increase in levels of CH50 (total complement activity), C1q, C4, C3, C5, and, C9 and a decrease in factor B in elderly persons (29).

Immune Function. Aging is associated with a decline in immune function, and this has been implicated as one major reason for the greater susceptibility of the elderly to infections (30). Those immunologic changes implicated in increasing risk of the elderly to infection include (*1*) decreased production of high-affinity antibody; (*2*) decreased primary antibody response; (*3*) decreased response to low-dose antigenic stimula

TABLE 2.2 Impact of Age on White Blood Cell Functions

NEUTROPHIL FUNCTION	RESULTS FROM STUDY (REFERENCE NO.)[a]										
	(18)	(19)	(20)	(21)	(22)	(23)	(24)	(25)	(26)	(27)	(28)
Total leukocyte count	N	—	—	—	—	—	—	—	—	—	—
Total PMN	N	—	—	—	—	—	—	—	—	—	—
Adherence (nylon fiber)	—	I	I	—	—	N	—	—	I	—	—
Capillary tube migration	—	N	D	N	—	—	—	—	—	—	—
Chemotaxis	—	D	N	N	D[b]	D[c]	D	—	—	—	D
Phagocytic activity	—	D	D	—	D[b]	D[c]	N	N	—	—	—
Microbicidal capacity	N	—	D	N	—	D	—	—	—	—	—
NBT test	N	D	D	—	D[b]	D	N	N	—	—	—
Superoxide production	D	—	—	—	—	—	—	—	—	—	—
Chemiluminescence	—	—	—	—	—	—	—	—	—	D	—

KEY: PMN, polymorphonuclear neutrophils; NBT, nitroblue tetrazolium.
[a]Results are expressed as no change (N), increase (I), or decrease (D) in elderly group when compared to younger controls. All results are for PMN except when indicated.
[b]Only monocytes studied.
[c]Both PMN and monocytes.

15

tion; (4) decreased response to microbial challenge; (5) increased frequency of monoclonal gammopathies; (6) increased frequency of autoantibodies; and (7) increased resistance to tolerance induction (30). The pathogenetic mechanisms for these abnormalities involve a variety of different cells, pathways, and functional sites. However, not all investigators have found similar abnormalities, and some have failed to confirm an age-related decline in immunity (31). These discrepancies only substantiate that the effect of aging on immune response may be variable and differ depending on the population studied, parameters used, and tests implemented. Table 2.3 summarizes the most consistent findings reported by investigators when various immunologic parameters were studied in an aging population (30,31). Little is known about the impact of aging on the function of secretory immunoglobulins, natural killer cells, and interferons.

Other Factors

UNDERLYING DISORDERS
Clearly aging is associated with the acquisition of more disease and illness. Moreover, many of these disorders are associated with a greater susceptibility to infectious diseases. This increased risk to infection is a result of the disorder (1) adversely affecting host defense mechanisms; (2) necessitating the patient to undergo diagnostic and/or therapeutic pro-

TABLE 2.3 Impact of Aging on Immune Function Parameters

PARAMETER	IMPACT OF AGE[a]		
	DECREASE	INCREASE	NO CHANGE
Number of total lymphocytes	+		+
Number of T helper cells	+		+
Number of T suppressor cells	+	+	+
Interleukin 1 activity	+		+
Interleukin 2 activity	+		
T-cell blastogenesis	+		
Delayed skin hypersensitivity	+		+
Number of B lymphocytes			+
Primary antibody response	+		+
Secondary antibody response	+		+
Immunoglobulin levels	+	+	+
Autoantibodies		+	
Monoclonal antibodies		+	
Natural killer cell activity[b]	+	+	+

[a]Results vary according to investigator.
[b]Limited data.

cedures that are associated with a high incidence of infection; (*3*) causing the patient to be hospitalized or institutionalized; or (*4*) requiring the patient to receive drugs that may adversely affect host resistance. Such illnesses or disorders that are associated with increased risk to infectious diseases and are also common to the elderly include cancers, certain leukemias, diabetes mellitus, chronic lung disease, certain collagen vascular diseases, obstructive uropathy, and cerebrovascular accidents.

NUTRITION
Poor nutrition and inadequate diets are common geriatric problems. Lack of optimal nutrients can place a host at greater risk to infection. Protein-energy malnutrition as well as deficiencies in specific nutrients can adversely affect virtually every component of the immune system as well as the nonspecific host factors (32,33). Such relationships between nutrition and immune competence has already been demonstrated in the elderly (34). More studies are needed to better define the precise nutrients and their effects on the elderly person's host resistance.

CONCLUSION

The elderly are predisposed to infectious diseases by the very nature of living longer. Longevity has resulted in physiologic changes of important host defense factors, chronic illnesses, and more and longer hospitalization. Additionally, factors such as poor nutrition may contribute to this susceptibility. We hope that information about risk factors will provide a better approach in the management and prevention of infectious diseases in the aged.

REFERENCES

1. McCloskey RV: Microbial virulence factors, in Mandell GL, Douglas GR Jr, Bennett JE (eds): *Principles and Practice of Infectious Diseases,* ed 1. New York, John Wiley & Sons, 1979, p 3.
2. Yoshikawa TT, Norman DC, Grahn D: Infections in the aging population. *J Am Geriatr Soc* 33:496–503, 1985.
3. Freeman J, McGowan JE, Jr: Risk factors for nosocomial infection. *J Infect Dis* 138:811–819, 1978.
4. Campion EW, Bang A, May MI: Why acute-care hospitals must undertake long-term care. *N Engl J Med* 308:71–75, 1983.
5. Garibaldi RA, Brodine S, Matsumiya S: Infections among patients in nursing homes: Policies, prevalence, and problems. *N Engl J Med* 305:731–735, 1981.
6. Magnussen MH, Robb SS: Nosocomial infections in a long-term care facility. *Am J Infect Control* 8:12–17, 1980.

7. Haley RW, Hooton TM, Culver DH, et al: Nosocomial infections in U.S. hospitals, 1975-1976. Estimated frequency of selected characteristics of patients. *Am J Med* 70:947-959, 1981.
8. Setia U, Serventi I, Lorenz P: Bacteremia in a long-term care facility. Spectrum and morbidity. *Arch Intern Med* 144:1633-1635, 1984.
9. De la Torre MG, Romero-Vivas J, Martinez-Beltrán J, et al: Klebsiella bacteremia: An analysis of 100 episodes. *Rev Infect Dis* 7:143-150, 1985.
10. Bouza E, de la Torre MG, Erice A et al: Enterobacter bacteremia. An analysis of 50 episodes. *Arch Intern Med* 145:1025-1027, 1985.
11. Drelichman V, Band JD: Bacteremia due to *Citrobacter diversus* and *Citrobacter freundii*. Incidence, risk factors and clinical outcomes. *Arch Intern Med* 145:1808-1810, 1985.
12. Bodey GP, Jadeja L, Elting L: Pseudomonas bacteremia: Retrospective analysis of 410 episodes. *Arch Intern Med* 145:1621-1629, 1985.
13. Goldman R: Decline in organ function with aging, in Rossman I: *Clinical Geriatrics,* ed 2. Philadelphia, J.B. Lippincott, 1979, p. 23.
14. Tramont ED: General or nonspecific host defense mechanisms, in Mandell GL, Douglas GR Jr, Bennett JE (eds): *Principles and Practice of Infectious Diseases,* ed 2, New York, John Wiley & Sons, 1985, p 25.
15. Cates KL: Host factors in bacteremia. *Am J Med* 15(1B):18-25, 1983.
16. Katz P: Clinical and laboratory evaluation of the immune system. *Med Clin North Am* 69:453-464, 1985.
17. Graziano FM, Bell CL: The normal immune response and what can go wrong: A classification of immunologic disorders. *Med Clin North Am* 69:439-452, 1985.
18. Nagel JE, Pyle PS, Chrest FJ, et al: Oxidative metabolism and bactericidal capacity of polymorphonuclear leukocytes from normal young and aged adults. *J Gerontol* 37:529-534, 1982.
19. Corberand J, Ngyen F, Laharrague P, et al: Polymorphonuclear functions and aging in humans. *J Am Geriatr Soc* 29:391-397, 1981.
20. Laharrague P, Corberand J, Fillola G, et al: Impairment of polymorphonuclear functions in hospital geriatric patients. *Gerontology* 29:325-331, 1983.
21. Gardner ID, Lim STK, Lawton JWM: Monocyte function in aging humans. *Mech Ageing Dev* 16:233-239, 1981.
22. Charpentier B, Fournier C, Fries D, et al: Immunological studies in human aging: I. *In vitro* functions of T cells and polymorphs. *J Clin Lab Immunol* 5:87-93, 1981.
23. Antonaci S, Jirillo E, Ventura MT, et al: Non-specific immunity in aging: Deficiency of monocyte and polymorphonuclear cell-mediated functions. *Mech Ageing Dev* 24:365-375, 1984.
24. Phair JP, Kauffman CA, Bjornson A, et al: Host defenses in the aged: Evaluation of components of the inflammatory and immune responses. *J Infect Dis* 138:67-73, 1978.
25. Palmblad J, Hand A: Ageing does not change blood granulocyte bactericidal capacity and levels of complement factors 3 and 4. *Gerontology* 24:381-385, 1978.

26. Silverman EM, Silverman AG: Granulocyte adherence in the elderly. *Am J Clin Pathol* 67:49–52, 1977.
27. Van Epps DE, Goodwin JS, Murphy S: Age-dependent variations in polymorphonuclear leukocyte chemiluminescence. *Infect Immunity* 22:57–61, 1978.
28. McLaughlin B, O'Malley K, Cotter TG: Age-related differences in granulocyte chemotaxis and degranulation. *Clin Sci* 70:59–62, 1986.
29. Nagaki K, Hiramatsu S, Inai S, et al: The effect of aging on complement protein levels. *J Clin Lab Immunol* 3:45–50, 1980.
30. Makinodan T, James SJ, Inamizu T, et al: Immunologic basis for susceptibility to infection in the aged. *Gerontology* 30:279–289, 1984.
31. Delafuente JC: Immunosenescence: Clinical and pharmacologic considerations. *Med Clin North Am* 69:475–486, 1985.
32. Corman LC: The relationship between nutrition, infection and immunity. *Med Clin North Am* 69:519–531, 1985.
33. Chandra RK: Nutrition, immunity and infection: Present knowledge and future direction. *Lancet* 1:688–691, 1983.
34. Chandra RK, Joshi R, Au B, et al: Nutrition and immunocompetence of the elderly. Effect of short-term nutritional supplementation on cell-mediated immunity and lymphocyte subsets. *Nutr Res* 2:223–232, 1982.

SUGGESTED READINGS

Felser JM, Raff MJ: Infectious diseases and aging. *J Am Geriatr Soc* 31:802–807, 1983.
Katz P: Clinical and laboratory evaluation of the immune system. *Med Clin North Am* 69:453–464, 1985.
Makinodan T, James SJ, Inamizu T, et al: Immunologic basis for susceptibility to infection in the aged. *Gerontology* 30:279–289, 1984.
Yoshikawa TT: Aging and infectious disease: State of the art. *Gerontology* 30:275–278, 1984.

Chapter 3

Clinical Features of Infection

FACTORS AFFECTING CLINICAL MANIFESTATIONS OF ILLNESSES

One of the more difficult, if not the most difficult, challenges encountered by clinicians caring for the elderly is the evaluation of these patients based on information solely derived from the patient history and physical examination. A variety of disabilities, illnesses, or diseases, including infection, are more likely to present in a nonclassic and often in a heterogeneous manner in the elderly (1). A number of factors may contribute to the unpredictability of clinical manifestations of acute and chronic disorders in the aged person. The following discussion briefly highlights some of these factors.

Underreporting of Symptoms

Many elderly patients fail to complain or report symptoms to a physician. Older adults may simply ascribe certain pains, discomforts, or physiologic irregularities to "old age" and assume that these changes are normal; thus, they may not report these symptoms to their physician. Moreover, cultural or ethnic factors may inhibit the aged from voicing complaints (e.g., certain elderly men may remain stoic and fail to seek medical care for a problem or illness because it may reflect weakness and lack of masculinity). Patients with dementia or other disorders that cause cognitive impairment or neuropsychiatric illness such as depression may fail to recognize, understand, and/or verbalize appropriately the changes in their health status. Finally, not uncommonly elderly patients have speech disorders (e.g., dysphasia or aphasia secondary to a stroke), or they may have an altered level of consciousness that impairs communication.

Altered Clinical Responses to and Expression of Illness

As a general rule, the majority of elderly patients with a specific disease or disease process manifest the usual and expected clinical features of that disorder. However, the elderly group most commonly exhibits atypical symptoms and signs for a given disorder or illness. One reason for this varied presentation is the difference in biologic expression of certain diseases in the aged. For example, hyperthyroidism classically manifests in the adult with clinical features of heat intolerance, weight loss, hyperactivity, hyperphagia, weakness, tachycardia, eye changes, and a goiter. However, in the elderly, evidence for hypermetabolism and hyperactivity may be limited or absent, and the presenting clinical manifestations may be congestive heart failure, cardiac arrhythmias, and apathy (so-called "apathetic hyperthyroidism") (2). These variations in biologic expression of diseases in geriatric patients must always be considered in their evaluation and assessment.

Alternatively, the elderly host response to a disease, disorder, or illness may be quite blunted, diverse, or nonspecific. The threshold for pain may be higher with old age for certain processes. For example, chest pain may not be the dominating feature for an acute myocardial infarction in an aging person, but congestive heart failure, altered mentation, falls, or sudden death may be the presenting clinical features. Or, abdominal pain or physical signs of tenderness and peritoneal inflammation may be minimal or absent in various causes of intraabdominal sepsis in the elderly (3). Finally, it should be emphasized that any illness can manifest with only nonspecific symptoms, such as weight loss, weakness, anorexia, nausea, or clinical features of cognitive impairment or dementia.

Coexisting Disabilities and Diseases

Aging brings on inevitable physiologic and anatomic changes that can confound the clinical expression of or the host response to a disease process. For example, chronic joint changes due to osteoarthritis may cause pain and discomfort in the elderly. These symptoms may mask the presence of another possibly acute process such as an infection in a joint, or they may cause both the patient and physician to assume that new joint complaints are attributable to the antecedent chronic disability rather than to a new or different problem. Similarly, correct or timely clinical diagnosis is a particular problem in the very old because of the frequent coexistence of one or more chronic underlying diseases and disabilities.

A few common examples of this problem are chronic lung disease, which may delay the diagnosis of pneumonia; dementia, which may mask an acute meningitis; rectal bleeding, which may be interpreted as being caused by preexisting diverticulosis rather than colorectal carcinoma; poor eating, which may be attributed to poor dentures; or a dysuric syndrome (frequency, urgency, and dysuria), which may be assumed to be caused by prostatic enlargement instead of a urinary tract infection. Finally, medications have more frequent and severe side effects in the elderly patient, and these adverse effects can also add confusion to the process of making a correct and precise diagnosis in these individuals.

There are no easy solutions or methods for clinicians to circumvent the problem of making a diagnosis in the presence of such confounding variables as biologic changes of aging, coexisting diseases and disabilities, and multiple medications. However, whenever an elderly patient elicits a history of a recent *change* in well being, independence, or previous chronic symptoms, a thorough assessment for a new illness or process is imperative despite the presence of multiple preexisting problems. Adhering to this recommendation will prevent the failure of diagnosing new and serious illnesses in the already severely debilitated elderly patient.

MANIFESTATIONS OF INFECTIONS

Fever

Fever, either by history or by physical examination, is a cardinal clinical feature of most infectious diseases. Generally, most older individuals who acquire an infection respond with a temperature elevation. Moreover, the presence of fever in an elderly patient most often augurs a serious illness, usually an infectious disease process. A study by Keating et al. (described in detail in Chapter 2) documented that fever in ambulatory elderly adults was associated with more serious, usually bacterial, infections when compared to younger adults with temperature elevations (who often had benign viral illnesses) (4). Moreover, prolonged fever of undetermined origin in the elderly is also generally associated with serious diseases, including infections (5). In a literature review by Esposito and Gleckman (6) of 111 cases of elderly patients with fever of unknown origin, infectious diseases accounted for 36% of the cases. The majority of infectious causes were confined to intraabdominal abscesses, infective endocarditis, and tuberculosis. Connective tissue disorders, notably giant cell arteritis (temporal arteritis; polymyalgia rheumatica), were responsible for 26% of fever of unknown origin cases; neoplasias (lymphomas and carcinomas) were associated with prolonged fever in 24% of patients.

Thus, the presence of fever in old individuals should never be assumed to be of benign origin until a careful and thorough evaluation has excluded potentially serious causes of fever.

However, it is also not uncommon to encounter sick elderly patients with proven infection who have no fever response. Obviously, the absence of a fever may dissuade the clinician from evaluating his/her ill elderly patient for a possible infectious disease. Finklestein et al. (6) reviewed their 187 cases of documented pneumococcal bacteremia in adults. Surprisingly, 29% of the elderly patients were afebrile, and they also had a lower mean temperature response and a lower mean peak temperature as compared to younger adults. Gleckman and Hibert (7) also described 25 elderly patients (mean age 81 years) who were afebrile in the presence of proven bacteremia. In addition to delays in diagnosis of an infection, low or absent fever responses in the presence of a serious infection (e.g., bacteremia) generally is associated with a poorer prognosis (8,9).

The mechanisms that explain the association of advanced aging and blunted temperature response have not been definitively elucidated. We recently reviewed this topic (10). Several postulates that may explain abnormal fever response with age include disturbances in thermal homeostasis (temperature perception, sudomotor responses, central nervous system regulation), qualitative and quantitative abnormalities in endogenous pyrogen (also called interleukin 1), diminished sensitivity of the hypothalamus to endogenous pyrogen, and failure to produce and conserve adequate body heat (10–12).

From this discussion, it should be evident that the *absence* of fever in the aged does not exclude the presence of an active infectious disease process. Fever, or its absence, in the elderly is only one clinical presentation that can be used to assist the clinician to suspecting a serious disease such as an infection.

Other Clinical Features

The clinical features of specific infections in the elderly are discussed in the succeeding chapters that focus on select infectious diseases.

Infections, like all other illnesses in the elderly, may occur with a variety of nonspecific or unusual manifestations (13). A loss of appetite, weakness, fatigue, altered mental status, or generalized pain may be caused by any infection, for example, pneumonia, urinary tract infection, intraabdominal abscess, infective endocarditis, and so on. Although diabetes mellitus out of control or that requires higher insulin doses is a clinical clue for infection in the elderly diabetic, occasionally unusual findings such as hypoglycemia may be a manifestation of sepsis in geriatric patients (14). With further clinical experience, other less common symptoms and signs of infection may be observed and reported.

Infections should be suspected in any elderly person who experiences a rather acute (in some instances subacute) change in well being, functional status, or independence in the presence or absence of typical clinical features of an infectious process.

CONCLUSION

Elderly patients with an infection generally can mount a fever response, and usually the presence of a temperature elevation indicates the presence of a serious illness, often an infectious disease. However, fever may be blunted or absent in the elderly with active infection. Furthermore, other clinical manifestations of an infection may range from typical features to nonspecific or unusual symptoms and signs. It thus behooves clinicians to always suspect an infectious disease process in an elderly person whose clinical status has inexplicably changed.

REFERENCES

1. Yoshikawa TT: Ageing and infectious diseases, in Pathy MS (ed): *Principles and Practice of Geriatric Medicine.* John Wiley & Sons, Ltd, Chichester, 1985, p 221.
2. Havard CWH: The thyroid and aging. *Clin Endocrinol Metabol* 10:163–178, 1981.
3. Norman DC, Yoshikawa TT: Intraabdominal infections in the elderly. *J Am Geriatr Soc* 31:677–684, 1983.
4. Keating HJ III, Klimek JJ, Levine DS, et al: Effect of aging in the clinical significance of fever in ambulatory adult patients. *J Am Geriatr Soc* 32:282–287, 1984.
5. Kauffman CA, Jones PG: Diagnosing fever of unknown origin in older patients. *Geriatrics* 39:46–51, 1984.
6. Finklestein MS, Petkun WM, Freedman ML, et al: Pneumococcal bacteremia in adults: Age-dependent differences in presentation and in outcome. *J Am Geriatr Soc* 31:19–27, 1983.
7. Gleckman R, Hibert D: Afebrile bacteremia: A phenomenon in geriatric patients. *JAMA* 248:1478–1481, 1981.
8. Weinstein MP, Murphy JR, Reller LB, et al: The clinical significance of positive blood cultures: A comprehensive analysis of 500 episodes of bacteremia and fungemia in adults. II. Clinical observations with special reference to factors influencing prognosis. *Rev Infect Dis* 5:54–70, 1983.
9. Bryant RE, Hood AF, Hood CE, et al: Factors affecting mortality of gram-negative rod bacteremia. *Arch Intern Med* 127:120–127, 1971.
10. Norman DC, Grahn D, Yoshikawa TT: Fever and aging. *J Am Geriatr Soc* 33:859–863, 1985.

11. Collins KJ, Exton-Smith AD: Thermal homeostasis in old age. *J Am Geriatr Soc* 31.519–524, 1983.
12. Jones PG, Kauffman CA, Bergman AG, et al: Fever in the elderly. Production of leukocytic pyrogen by monocytes from elderly persons. *Gerontology* 30:182–187, 1984.
13. Deal WB: Unusual manifestations of infectious diseases in the aging. *Geriatrics* 31:77–84, 1979.
14. Berkman P, Mirdler C, Yust I: Hypoglycemia as a manifestation of sepsis in an elderly patient. *J Am Geriatr Soc* 33:644–645, 1985.

SUGGESTED READINGS

Finklestein MS, Petkun WM, Freedman ML, et al: Pneumococcal bacteremia in adults: Age-dependent differences in presentation and in outcome. *J Am Geriatr Soc* 31:19–27, 1983.

Norman DC, Yoshikawa TT: Clinical presentation of infections in the elderly, in Cunha BA (ed): *Infectious Diseases of the Elderly.* John Wright-PSG Inc., New York, in press.

Norman DC, Grahn D, Yoshikawa TT: Fever and aging. *J Am Geriatr Soc* 33:859–863, 1985.

Chapter 4

Diagnostic Approach to Infections

GENERAL CONSIDERATIONS

We stated in the last chapter that most infections in the elderly have typical clinical findings. In these patients, the diagnostic approach is rather straightforward depending on the suspected infection. However, what about those older persons who have atypical or nonspecific symptoms and signs? Where does the clinician begin in the diagnostic evaluation of these patients? Obviously, every organ system cannot be examined with tests, and microbiologic studies cannot be done for every potential pathogen. Thus, every patient should be assessed on an individual basis in order to determine what and how many diagnostic tests and procedures should be implemented.

As a general guideline, the assessment of a patient with a potential infection should proceed when the following factors have been thoroughly considered: (*1*) What is the risk-benefit ratio for a test or procedure? (*2*) What is the cost versus benefit(s) of the test or procedure? and (*3*) Will the results of the test or procedure lead to a specific change in the patient's management? (1)

Risk Versus Benefits

There are a variety of tests that are useful in the diagnostic evaluation for an infection that generally are associated with low morbidity (risks) to the elderly patient. Usually, these are tests of the blood, urine, expectorated sputum, and feces, plain x-rays, imaging scans, and ultrasonography; and skin tests. However, at times, more invasive procedures may be required in order to achieve a precise infectious disease diagnosis. For example, expectorated sputum is often contaminated by the oropharygeal flora that may invalidate the interpretation of the culture results. To circumvent this problem, transtracheal aspiration has been performed (2), and some investigators recommend this procedure for elderly patients with presumptive pneumonia (3). However, the physician should exercise caution when using transtracheal aspiration because severe complications (including death) from this procedure have occurred in the elderly (4). Furthermore, much information is now available on the etiology of pneumonia in the aged (see Chapter 10 on pneumonia). Thus, in routine cases of pneumonia in the elderly, the risks of a transtracheal aspiration do not favor the elderly when assessed in terms of its potential benefits.

Since the elderly, especially the very old and frail, are generally at greater risk for complications from any invasive procedure, it is incumbent on the primary clinician to always carefully assess the benefits versus the risks.

Cost Versus Benefits

In the current practice of geriatric medicine, two opposing factors place the clinician in a difficult and unenviable position in the management of his/her elderly patients. On one side are pressures to use the most modern, and often expensive, high technology to diagnose or exclude serious diseases. The opposing factor is the enormous cost of medical care especially for the very old and the restrictions in reimbursement for health care of these individuals. With the limited medical payment provided by Medicare compounded by the advent of a DRG (Diagnosis Related Groups) system of reimbursement, clinicians must carefully weigh the benefits of a test in terms of its direct costs as well as additional cost encountered if complications from the test occur.

Effect on Management

Not infrequently, tests are ordered on a patient because they are considered to be a routine part of a workup and "standard of practice." However, in managing elderly patients, this attitude must be changed— tests should not be obtained simply for the sake of completeness of an evaluation or adhering to a preconceived standard of practice. In light of the concepts of risks-benefits and cost-benefits, tests should only be obtained if they will not only have a reasonable diagnostic yield, be low in risk, and be reasonable in cost, but also will improve patient management. If the results of a test or procedure, whether they are positive or negative, will not cause the physician to reassess his/her management strategy, then there is little justification for this laboratory examination.

Differential Diagnostic Considerations

Before any diagnostic evaluation of a suspected infection is initiated, the clinician should consider the most likely types of infections that occur in the elderly. This is extremely helpful in circumstances where the elderly patient is a poor historian, is unable to communicate, or has vague nonspecific complaints.

Elderly persons who are independent, living in the community, and relatively healthy are prone to respiratory infections (especially bacterial pneumonia), genitourinary infections (urinary tract infection, prostatic infection), and intraabdominal sepsis (cholecystitis, diverticulitis, appendicitis, and abscesses). Thus, if a thorough history and physical examination does not reveal an obvious source of infection, an initial evaluation for these specific infections is likely to be relatively quick, safe, and inexpensive with a high yield. Tests to be obtained initially should include a complete blood count, urinalysis with culture, blood cultures, chest x-ray, sputum examination (if patient has a cough and/or chest x-ray is abnormal), and tuberculin skin test. If this initial evaluation is nonrevealing, then liver function studies and abdominal ultrasonography should be obtained. Depending on these results, a radionuclide scan of the gallbladder or liver or a computed tomographic scan of the abdomen should be ordered. Failure to confirm the presence of any of the aforementioned infections should lead the physician to consider the possibility of infective endocarditis (if positive blood cultures are found), meningitis or brain abscess (if neurologic or mental status changes develop), septic arthritis (if joint complaints are established), or drug fever. Of course, such noninfectious illnesses as lymphoma, solid tumors, leukemia, and collagen vascular disorders may mimic an infectious disease, which eventually would have to be included in the evaluation if an infection could not be diagnosed.

Elderly patients in nursing homes or chronic care institutions frequently contract an infectious disease. The most common infections in this group are pneumonia, urinary tract infections, and skin and soft tissue infections (especially pressure sores). This triad can be easily remembered by the acronym *PUS*. Generally, appropriate tests for PUS result in defining the infection. However, if the initial assessment fails to show the infection to be in the lungs, urinary tract, or skin, the differential diagnosis should include disseminated tuberculosis, hepatitis, intraabdominal sepsis (including ischemic bowel disease), osteomyelitis, or drug reactions.

SPECIFIC DIAGNOSTIC TESTS

Clinical Assessment

A careful history and physical examination is still important in the assessment of an elderly patient with possible infection. A detailed mental status evaluation (e.g., Folstein test) should always be part of a geriatric assessment (5), as unexpected or subtle changes in mental status function may be the first clue to a possible active disease.

Blood and Body Fluids

Blood cultures are indispensable in the evaluation of any patient with suspected infection. They should also be obtained in any elderly patient who develops an undefined illness or change in health status. Generally two sets (one set having one bottle for facultative anaerobic bacteria and one bottle for obligate anaerobic organisms) of blood cultures obtained from separate venipuncture sites are adequate (6). If infective endocarditis or sepsis is suspected, additional blood cultures, three to four sets at different times in the day, are helpful.

Urinalysis with examination of the sediment for leukocytes and bacteria (Gram stain) is extremely cost effective, inexpensive, safe, and rewarding. Since urinary tract infection in the elderly may be associated with a paucity of genitourinary symptoms (7), routine examination of the urine is mandatory. In elderly men, the presence or absence of pyuria may have significant predictive value in excluding or diagnosing bacteriuria in the absence of genitourinary complaints (8). This may avoid unnecessary urine culture in men who are asymptomatic for genitourinary complaints, but who have other symptoms that are suggestive of an infectious process.

Body fluids that are important to examine and are generally obtained with low morbidity in the elderly are cerebrospinal, joint, and pleural fluids. These fluids should be immediately examined for leukocytes, protein, and glucose and should be stained for bacteria, mycobacteria, and fungi. Moreover, pleural fluid should always be cultured for both aerobic and anaerobic bacteria.

Sputum may have limited diagnostic value for a bacterial etiology if it is expectorated. However, expectorated sputum is reliable for diagnosing respiratory pathogens not normally found in the oropharynx, for example, mycobacteria and certain fungi (9).

Serologic studies have limited value in the early diagnosis of an infection. However, these tests should be done (when available) in the event a specific diagnosis may not be made for several days to weeks.

X-Rays and Scans

Plain film x-rays are diagnostically useful for assessing pleuropulmonary infections; osteomyelitis; septic arthritis; intestinal obstruction, free air in the abdomen, and large abdominal masses; and sinusitis. These procedures in the elderly are quick, safe, and inexpensive. Barium contrast studies of the gastrointestinal tract have limited yield in making a diagnosis of an intraabdominal infection. Moreover, a barium enema may be quite discomforting and stressful for the very old and frail. By comparison, an ultrasonographic scan is preferable over barium contrast studies for the evaluation of an intraabdominal abscess, as well as for biliary tract disease (10). This procedure is well tolerated by the elderly, is relatively quick and safe, and is cost effective.

Certain imaging scans such as computed tomography and magnetic resonance imaging are relatively sensitive diagnostic tools but are restricted by their high costs (11). Their use in the elderly should be limited to examination of the brain and abdomen (computed tomography). Radionuclide scans are less expensive and are useful for diagnosing bony lesions including osteomyelitis and liver-spleen defects (e.g., abscess) (12,13).

Invasive Procedures

Invasive procedures are generally more expensive, more hazardous, but are also more specific and accurate in diagnosing diseases including infections. These procedures include transbronchial biopsy and bronchial brushing, colonoscopy with biopsy, percutaneous needle aspirations and/ or biopsy (lung, liver, bone, and bone marrow), and open surgical procedures (thoracotomy, laparotomy). Careful assessment of all factors is imperative before recommending or denying such invasive procedures for diagnosis of an infectious process in the elderly.

CONCLUSION

The diagnostic approach to an infectious disease in the elderly patient should cover the most likely causes of infections in the elderly and then proceed with the safest, most rapid, least expensive, and most productive test available. These factors must be weighed before making decisions involving invasive diagnostic procedures in the elderly.

REFERENCES

1. Yoshikawa TT, Norman DC, Grahn D: Infections in the aging population. *J Am Geriatr Soc* 33:496–503, 1985.

2. Bartlett JG: Diagnostic accuracy of transtracheal aspiration bacteriologic studies. *Am Rev Respir Dis* 115:777–782, 1977.
3. Berk SL, Holtschaw MS, Kahn A, et al: Transtracheal aspiration in the severely ill elderly patient with bacterial pneumonia. *J Am Geriatr Soc* 29: 228–231, 1981.
4. Unger KM, Moser KM: Fatal complication of transtracheal aspiration. A report of two cases. *Arch Intern Med* 132:437–439, 1973.
5. Folstein MF, Folstein SE, McHugh PR: "Mini-Mental State." A practical method for grading the cognitive state of patients for the clinician. *Psychiatr Res* 12:189–198, 1975.
6. Washington JA II: Blood cultures. Principles and techniques. *Mayo Clin Proc* 50:91–98, 1975.
7. Yoshikawa TT: Unique aspects of urinary tract infection in the geriatric population. *Gerontology* 30:339–344, 1984.
8. Norman DC, Yamamura R, Yoshikawa TT: Pyuria: Its predictive value of asymptomatic bacteriuria in ambulatory elderly males. *J Urol* 135:520–522, 1986.
9. Irwin RS, Corrao WM: A perspective on sputum analyses in pneumonia. *Respir Care* 24:503–509, 1979.
10. Joseph AE: Imaging of abdominal abscesses. *Br Med J* 291:1446–1447, 1985.
11. Baker HL, Berquist TH, Kispert DB, et al: Magnetic resonance imaging in a routine clinical setting. *Mayo Clin Proc* 60:75–90, 1985.
12. Lentle BC, Russell HS, Percy JS, et al: Bone scintiscanning updated. *Ann Intern Med* 84:297–303, 1976.
13. Silva J Jr, Harvey WC: Detection of infections with gallium-67 and scintigraphic imaging. *J Infect Dis* 130:125–131, 1974.

SUGGESTED READINGS

Irwin RS, Corrao WM: A perspective in sputum analyses in pneumonia. *Respir Care* 24:503–509, 1979.
Joseph AE: Imaging of abdominal abscesses. *Br Med J* 291:1446–1447, 1985.
Washington JA II: Blood cultures: Principles and techniques. *Mayo Clin Proc* 50:91–98, 1975.

Chapter 5

Antimicrobial Therapy: Special Considerations

UNIQUE ASPECTS OF ANTIMICROBIAL AGENTS

The discovery of antimicrobial agents* has been one of the most significant advances in the history of medicine. Antimicrobial therapy, along with vaccination and the practice of antisepsis, has been responsible for saving countless lives since 1900 and, consequently, has played a major role in prolonging human life (1). Thus, we are now encountering a rapid growth in the aging population. Paradoxically, despite newer and more potent antimicrobial agents, infectious diseases still have an important impact on the health and well-being of mankind, particularly the elderly generation.

Although several antibiotics have the ability to kill organisms (microbicidal), they generally do not eliminate completely pathogens from body tissues or fluids. The salutary effect of antiinfective drugs is through halting microbial replication (reducing the inoculum or numbers of organisms) or possibly causing damage to the pathogen, making them less virulent. These actions permit the host's own defense mechanism to "catch up" and ultimately eradicate or eliminate the microbe.

Antimicrobial agents are a unique class of drugs. The target for the antibiotics is microorganisms, not the host's tissue or organs, which is the

---

*The terms *antibiotics* and *antiinfective agents or drugs* are used interchangeably with *antimicrobial agents*.

usual site of action for nonantimicrobial agents. Although most drugs have their primary pharmacologic action on one major organ or tissue, antiinfective drugs have the capacity for penetration and activity at many different organ sites or body cavities. Finally, in addition to the direct drug-related toxicities that are seen with most medications, antibiotics have the added side effects associated with superinfection or alteration of the host's natural indigenous microflora. Thus, appropriate and optimal antimicrobial therapy can only be administered to patients if the clinician is well versed in microbiology, clinical infectious disease, and pharmacology.

SPECIAL CONSIDERATIONS

Complexities of Diagnosis and Management

Earlier chapters have discussed differences in epidemiology, diagnosis, and clinical outcomes of infections in the elderly. Such differences have a major impact on the approach to antimicrobial therapy in the geriatric patient who is suspected of having an infectious disease process.

ETIOLOGIC CONSIDERATIONS
The most common infections in the elderly are respiratory infections (primarily bacterial pneumonia), urinary tract infections, soft tissue infections, and intraabdominal sepsis. Taken as a whole, the bacterial etiology of these infections varies considerably. Moreover, the etiologic pathogens for these (and other) infections in the elderly may differ from the microbes that cause the same type of infection in younger adults. Moreover, the etiology of many infections in the aged may be heterogeneous and often unpredictable for a given infected site in any single patient. Table 5.1 contrasts the etiologic differences for some important bacterial infections that occur in both young and old adults.

LIMITATIONS IN COLLECTION OF SPECIMENS
Chapter 4 emphasizes the potential increased risk of certain diagnostic procedures in the aged. This limits which body fluid or tissue can be obtained safely. Additionally, many frail and debilitated elderly patients are unable to cooperate fully in providing essential specimens for a microbiologic diagnosis (e.g., inability to cough and provide adequate sputum). Thus, the determination of a specific etiology for infection is frequently not possible in the geriatric patient.

MORBIDITY AND MORTALITY
It has been shown that the aged patient with a serious infection suffers a higher morbidity and mortality compared to his or her younger counter-

TABLE 5.1 Etiologic Differences of Bacterial Infections

INFECTION	USUAL PATHOGEN(S) IN YOUNG ADULTS	USUAL PATHOGEN(S) IN AGED ADULTS
Pneumonia (community acquired)	*Streptococcus pneumoniae* Anaerobic bacteria	*S. pneumoniae* Anaerobic bacteria *Hemophilus influenzae* Gram-negative bacilli *Legionella* sp. *Staphylococcus aureus*
Urinary tract infection (uncomplicated)	*Escherichia coli*	*E. coli* *Proteus* sp. *Klebsiella* sp. *Enterobacter* sp. Group D enterococci Coagulase-negative *Staphylococcus*
Meningitis	*S. pneumoniae* *Neisseria meningitidis*	*S. pneumoniae* *Listeria monocytogenes* *N. meningitidis* Gram-negative bacilli
Infective endocarditis	Viridans group streptococci *S. aureus*	Viridans group streptococci *Streptococcus bovis* Group D enterococci *S. aureus*
Septic arthritis	*Neisseria gonorrhoeae* *S. aureus*	*S. aureus* Gram-negative bacilli

part. The risk of these complications is further accelerated by delays in diagnosis that ultimately result in treatment delays. The varied clinical manifestations of infections in the old and the multiple coexisting underlying diseases that confound the signs and symptoms of an infection contribute to diagnostic delays. Therefore, if a potentially treatable infectious disease is considered in the differential diagnosis, administration of antibiotics should be implemented as soon as possible after appropriate (when feasible) diagnostic specimens and tests have been performed.

Thus, if infectious etiologies are quite varied in the elderly, specimen collection for a specific etiology may not be possible, and delays in treatment contribute to higher death rates, *empiric antimicrobial therapy is frequently necessary and justified in the elderly patient.* Moreover, empiric treatment usually requires *broad-spectrum antimicrobial drugs* either singly or in combinations.

PHARMACOKINETICS

Since this book does not provide an extensive review of the effect of aging on drug disposition, the reader is referred to several recent reviews on this topic (2–4). A brief discussion on the influence of important physiologic changes of aging or pharmacokinetics follows. These principles should be applied to antimicrobial drugs.

Absorption.   Although aging may be associated with reduced gastric pH, reduced gastric motility and emptying, decline in splancnic blood flow, and changes in intestinal absorptive surfaces, there is no conclusive evidence that drug absorption from the gastrointestinal tract is impaired in the elderly.

Distribution.   After a drug is absorbed from the gastrointestinal tract or is administered parenterally, it enters the circulation to be distributed to various body fluids and tissues. Aging causes a reduction in total body water and lean body mass and an increase in total body fat. Thus, it is possible to have greater changes in drug distribution (volume of distribution) in the elderly depending on physicochemical properties of the drug (water- versus fat-soluble). Serum albumin may decline by as much as 15 to 20% in the elderly. This change affects the ratio of bound to free drug available in the circulation (free drug is the active form). However, with the possible exception of a few antibiotics, age-related changes in volume of distribution and serum albumin have little impact clinically on antimicrobial therapy in the elderly.

Elimination.   Drug elimination may also involve drug metabolism, which usually occurs in the liver. The data on the effect of age on drug metabolism by the liver are extremely complex and often conflicting and inconclusive. In general, aging does appear to be associated with declines in certain phase I (preparative) reactions in the liver; there have been no definitive data on age-related changes in phase II (synthetic) reactions of the liver. In antimicrobial therapy, these potential changes with age have not been shown to influence antibiotic management in the aged.

Alternatively, renal function declines with age (5,6) and thus has an impact on antibiotic selection and dosage in the elderly patient. Glomerular filtration (or creatinine clearance) declines 0.5 to 1% per year after the age of 30 for the average person. However, there is considerable variability, and some elderly persons may still retain a completely normal creatinine clearance. Thus, it is important to measure regularly renal function in elderly patients who are receiving an antibiotic that (a) is excreted by the kidneys and (b) is potentially nephrotoxic. The use of the serum creatinine level as a measure of renal function is not reliable in the aged, as decreased muscle mass results in low serum creatinine values and may cause the clinician to assume erroneously that the patient has normal renal function.

Adverse Effects. Elderly patients experience more adverse drug effects than do younger subjects, since they receive more medications (increasing the likelihood of drug interactions), experience changes in drug disposition, and may be more sensitive to various drugs (3). Such factors influence antibiotic selection, dosing, and monitoring in the elderly.

COSTS

Ideally, all clinicians would prefer to make management decisions based on purely medical factors. However, the continued escalating costs of medical care of the aged has resulted in changes in reimbursement by Medicare. Instead of the previous fee-for-service form of payment, a prepayment format called DRG (Diagnosis Related Groups) has now been implemented by Medicare (7). Hospital costs as well as physician fees are predetermined by a special formula based on the nature of the illness, the age of the patient, complications, procedures, and so on. A lump sum is then paid to the health care facility. A financial profit or loss for the facility ultimately depends on how efficient they provide services and how soon the patient is discharged from the hospital. DRGs thus encourage early inpatient discharges (sometimes inappropriately) and a greater utilization of outpatient services and office practice.

These cost constraints and incentives for shorter hospital stays have an impact on antimicrobial drug therapy in elderly patients. The following factors need to be considered in the management of infectious diseases.

Specific Etiology and Narrow-Spectrum Drugs. Traditional teaching in infectious diseases taught clinicians to determine the specific etiologic organism of an infection and then to treat the patient with the most narrow-spectrum antibiotic that is effective against that pathogen. Moreover, if the patient then fails to improve clinically during a given observation period, the clinician would reevaluate the patient and possibly change therapy. This management approach, which still has great merits in general, suffers from the potential of prolonging the hospital stay of a patient (and increasing costs) if the initial therapeutic decision were incorrect. It has already been stated that the specific etiology of an infection in the elderly may be quite diverse and also often difficult to determine, particularly given the limitations in obtaining adequate clinical specimens. Thus, in the elderly, with a presumed infection, the following approach may be more appropriate:

1. Obtain, when possible, all appropriate clinical specimens for staining and culture before therapy.
2. The Gram stain (in the case of bacterial etiology) smear of a specimen should only be used to guide antibiotic therapy if (a) the specimen is obtained from a site that is not contaminated by the host's indigenous microflora, and (b) the smear shows typical morphology of a potential pathogen. Under these circumstances, therapy can be with a narrow-spectrum drug. However, if the patient is clinically unstable or appears toxic, a broad-spectrum antibiotic should be started initially regardless of the results of the Gram stain. When culture results are known, the antibiotic may be changed.
3. Since in the majority of cases the Gram stain is inconclusive, or the specimen is obtained from a site that is contaminated by the host's indigenous microflora (e.g., expectorated sputum), the initial antimicrobial regimen should consist of a broad-spectrum antibiotic that is effective against most of the potential etiologic pathogens for that infection. Only if culture results (which are also correlated with the Gram stain findings) indicate a specific pathogen should the antibiotic be changed to a narrow-spectrum drug.

Adverse Drug Reactions. The aged suffer more adverse drug effects. These complications prolong hospital stays and result in greater hospital costs. Therefore, antibiotics that have the greatest potential for causing serious adverse effects in the elderly should be avoided. For example, in the context of serious infections, especially those that involve gram-negative bacilli, a broad-spectrum antibiotic such as an aminoglycoside is frequently administered. However, these drugs produce the highest incidence of nephrotoxicity and ototoxicity. Aminoglycosides should be avoided in the elderly except under well-defined circumstances.

Drug Costs.   When drug costs are determined, it is important to include the cost of drug preparation and administration as well as expenses incurred from drug monitoring (e.g., drug levels). For example, if the purchasing wholesale cost of antibiotic A is more than antibiotic B, but it is administered on an every 12-hours drug regimen compared to an every 6-hours schedule for antibiotic B, then the total cost for antibiotic A may be significantly less than for antibiotic B. Moreover, if a drug has potentially serious side effects, frequent laboratory monitoring may be required (e.g., serum drug levels and renal function). This adds additional indirect costs to overall drug expenditures. In order to reduce costs, it is recommended that antibiotics selected for the elderly be drugs that (*1*) are relatively inexpensive (*2*) can be given with infrequent dosing, and (*3*) do not require laboratory monitoring.

SPECIFIC ANTIBACTERIAL DRUGS

Since the majority of important infections in the elderly are caused by bacteria, the specific antiinfective agents that are discussed are limited to antibacterial drugs.

Beta-Lactams

Beta-lactam antibiotics are especially useful for the treatment of bacterial infections in the elderly for the following reasons:

1. They have broad-spectrum activity that includes the common bacteria that infect the elderly.
2. Beta-lactams have a proven record of efficacy in a variety of infections. The number of studies involving elderly patients is limited but increasing.
3. These drugs are relatively safe and have minimal risk for renal, hepatic, or sensory organ damage, which is important in the case of the elderly.
4. Many beta-lactams may be conveniently administered on a once-, twice-, or three-times-a-day dosage regimen, which reduces administration costs.
5. Serum or body fluid levels need not be measured routinely for beta-lactam drugs.

Beta-lactam antibiotics, therefore, should be considered the drug of choice for most bacterial infections in the elderly. Moreover, in many instances beta-lactam antibiotics either singly or in combination with a second beta-lactam agent may be administered in place of an aminoglycoside (8,9).

The major disadvantage of some beta-lactam antibiotics is their relatively high purchasing costs. With the constant and rapid production of newer antibiotics by pharmaceutical companies, competition should eventually drive the price of most beta-lactam drugs to more acceptable levels. Also, beta-lactam drugs, with their broad spectrum, have the potential of selecting out resistant bacteria. So far, the impact of this potential has been relatively minor. However, with increased use of these agents, multiple resistant bacteria may become increasingly common, especially in hospitals and in chronic care facilities.

PENICILLINS

Penicillin G.   Penicillin G is the only naturally occurring penicillin. It is manufactured in a variety of forms including aqueous crystalline penicillin G (intravenous or intramuscular use), aqueous procaine penicillin G (intramuscular use only), benzathine penicillin G (long-acting; intramuscular use), and phenoxymethyl or phenoxyethyl penicillin (oral use) (10). Penicillin G is inexpensive, effective, and safe for the elderly. Since streptococcal infections are common in the elderly, penicillin G is the drug of choice for these infections. Meningitis in the aged caused by *Streptococcus pneumoniae, Listeria monocytogenes,* or *Neisseria meningitidis,* anaerobic infections (excluding *Bacteriodes fragilis*), and streptococcal endocarditis are effectively treated with this drug.

Ampicillin/Amoxicillin/Bacampicillin.   Ampicillin and amoxicillin (an analogue of ampicillin) have a similar antimicrobial spectrum. Amoxicillin has slightly better gastrointestinal absorption than does ampicillin and thus provides the convenience of an oral dosage regimen of three times per day rather than four doses a day (10,11). Most infections of the elderly that are treated with penicillin G may also be effectively managed with ampicillin or amoxicillin. However, these drugs have the added spectrum of activity against most *Hemophilus influenzae,* group D enterococcus, *Escherichia coli,* and indole-negative *Proteus mirabilis,* all of which are important pathogens in infections of the elderly. Ampicillin and amoxicillin are also relatively safe, although diarrhea, skin rashes, and occasionally antibiotic-associated colitis are potential side effects in all patients including the elderly. Bacampicillin is an ester form of ampicillin, which when given orally appears to have improved absorption and higher peak blood levels when compared to ampicillin. It has the advantage of a twice-a-day dose regimen, which improves compliance for the elderly (12).

Antistaphylococcal Penicillins. As we discuss in later chapters, staphylococci, both coagulase-positive and coagulase-negative species, are important pathogens in geriatric infections. Unfortunately, most staphylococci produce penicillinase, thus rendering such drugs as penicillin G, ampicillin, amoxicillin, and the antipseudomonas penicillins ineffective against these organisms. The semisynthetic penicillinase-resistant penicillins, such as methicillin, nafcillin, oxacillin, cloxacillin, dicloxacillin, and flucloxacillin are the drugs of choice for most staphylococcal infections. Antistaphylococcal penicillins have most of the spectrum of penicillin G except that they lack activity against *Neisseria* sp., group D enterococci, *Listeria monocytogenes,* and anaerobic bacteria. Of the parenteral forms, nafcillin or oxacillin is preferred over methicillin for the elderly, because the latter antibiotic has an increased risk of interstitial nephritis (13). However, oxacillin may be associated with hepatitis (14), and occasionally nafcillin causes neutropenia. Although nafcillin and oxacillin can be given by mouth, the major oral antistaphylococcal penicillins are cloxacillin, dicloxacillin, and flucloxacillin.

Antipseudomonas Penicillins. These penicillins have the broadest spectrum of activity, which includes many aerobic or facultative anaerobic bacteria as well as obligate anaerobes (15–17). Carbenicillin and ticarcillin were the earliest antipseudomonal agents with piperacillin, mezlocillin, and azlocillin becoming only recently available. Considered as a group, these antibiotics have all of the antibacterial spectrum of penicillin G but provide additional antimicrobial activity against *H. influenzae, E. coli, Proteus* sp. (indole-positive and indole-negative), *Morganella morganii, Providencia* sp., and *Pseudomonas aeruginosa.* Piperacillin, mezlocillin, and azlocillin (but not carbenicillin and ticarcillin) are also effective against most *Klebsiella* sp., *Enterobacter* sp., *Citrobacter* sp., and *Serratia marcescens.* All five of these antibiotics are quite effective against all anaerobes including *B. fragilis.* Therefore, the antipseudomonas penicillins should be considered seriously in the management of certain infections in the elderly. These agents are susceptible to penicillinase and are therefore ineffective against most staphylococci and penicillinase-producing strains of *H. influenzae, Neisseria,* anaerobes, or gram-negative bacilli. In the elderly, piperacillin, mezlocillin, or azlocillin are preferred because of their improved spectrum of activity and also because they have less sodium per gram of drug than carbenicillin and ticarcillin (which have 5 mEq of sodium per gram of drug). As a general recommendation, the antipseudomonas penicillins are infrequently administered alone because of the potential of resistant organisms developing. These agents are generally combined with another antibiotic, for example, an aminoglycoside.

Table 5.2 summarizes the spectrum of activity of the penicillins against pathogens that are relevant to geriatric infections. Doses for all penicillins in the elderly are the same as recommended for the general population. Dose reduction is recommended with moderate to severe renal dysfunction.

CEPHALOSPORINS
The cephalosporins are a family of beta-lactam drugs that include many types of antibiotics (18). Newer cephalosporins are continuously being produced and marketed. These agents are likely to become the most useful antibiotics for the treatment of bacterial infections in the elderly. The cephalosporins are classified according to their spectrum of activity: first, second, and third generation.

First-Generation Cephalosporins. This group is the oldest of the cephalosporins; cephalothin is the prototype drug. Other drugs in this class include cefazolin, cephapirin, cephradine, cephalexin, and cefadroxil. The first-generation cephalosporins are effective against *S. aureus, S. epidermidis, S. pneumoniae,* group A and B streptococci, viridans streptococci, *S. bovis, E. coli, P. mirabilis,* and *Klebsiella* sp., as well as anaerobic bacteria except *B. fragilis.* Pneumonia, soft tissue infection, osteomyelitis, endocarditis, and urinary tract infection in the elderly caused by one of the above susceptible organisms can be effectively treated by these antibiotics. However, meningitis should not be treated with first-generation cephalosporins, because these cephalosporins do not penetrate adequately into the cerebrospinal fluid. For parenteral therapy in the elderly, cefazolin is particularly useful because of its twice- or thrice-a-day dosage regimen and because it causes less pain than other cephalosporin preparations when given intramuscularly.

Second-Generation Cephalosporins. This class of cephalosporins has an increased gram-negative spectrum with some loss of gram-positive activity. Antibiotics in this group include cefamandole, cefuroxime, cefoxitin, ceforanide, cefonicid, and cefaclor. The antimicrobial activity of second-generation cephalosporins includes those of the first-generation cephalosporins (but with some loss of antistaphylococcal activity) and some improved spectrum against gram-negative bacilli and anaerobes depending on the drug. Cefoxitin has excellent activity against most anaerobes (except *Fusobacterium* sp. and some *Clostridium* sp.) including *B. fragilis* (the best of the currently available cephalosporins), as well as indole-positive and indole-negative *Proteus* sp., *Klebsiella* sp., and *Neisseria* sp. (19). Its high resistance to hydrolysis and degradation by beta-lactamases is responsible for its high activity. Cefamandole appears to be especially useful for infected elderly patients because of its good staphyl-

TABLE 5.2 Penicillins: Spectrum of Activity Against Important Bacteria

BACTERIA	PENICILLIN G	AMPICILLIN	ANTIPSEUDOMONAS[b]	ANTISTAPHYLOCOCCAL
S. aureus[a]	O	O	O	X
S. epidermidis[a]	O	O	O	X
Group A streptococcus	X	X	X	X
Group B streptococcus	X	X	X	X
Viridans streptococci	X	X	X	X
S. bovis	X	X	X	X
Enterococci	X[d]	X	X	O
N. meningitidis	X	X	X	O
L. monocytogenes	X	X	X	O
Anaerobic bacteria[c]	X	X	X	O
H. influenzae	O	X	X	O
E. coli	O	X	X	O
P. mirabilis	O	X	X	O
P. vulgaris	O	O	X	O
M. morganii	O	O	X	O
Providencia sp.	O	O	X	O
S. marcescens	O	O	X	O
P. aeruginosa	O	O	X	O
Citrobacter sp.	O	O	X	O
B. fragilis	O	O	X	O

KEY: X, generally active; O, generally inactive.
[a]Penicillinase-producing strain.
[b]Activities of Piperacillin, Mezlocillin, and Azlocillin only.
[c]Excluding B. fragilis.
[d]At high concentrations or combined with an aminoglycoside.

ococcal, streptococcal, *H. influenzae,* and gram-negative bacilli activity. However, cefuroxime may be preferred over cefamandole because it *does* penetrate the cerebrospinal fluid (the only first- or second-generation cephalosporin to cross the blood-brain barrier adequately), it can be given in a twice- or thrice-a-day dosage regimen and has essentially the same antimicrobial spectrum as cefamandole (20). Cefonicid may be useful for treating elderly patients because of its once- or twice-a-day regimen (21). Cefaclor and ceforanide have limited usefulness for the elderly patient.

Third-Generation Cephalosporins.   Table 5.3 lists the currently available third-generation cephalosporins as well as some of the newer cephalosporins that are under investigation. The major advantage of the third-generation cephalosporins is their greatly expanded activity against gram-negative bacilli (22). In addition, many of these drugs have excellent penetration into cerebrospinal fluid; they thus provide a safer and more effective antimicrobial treatment for gram-negative bacillary meningitis (which occurs in the aged) than did the previous therapy, which was with aminoglycosides. The spectrum of activity varies somewhat for each third-generation cephalosporin, and it is beyond the scope of this book to list this information. However, a few comments relevant to treating the aged are made for some of these antibiotics.

Ceftriaxone, ceftazidime, ceftizoxime, cefotaxime, and moxalactam penetrate well into the cerebrospinal fluid; cefoperazone has significantly less penetration across the blood-brain barrier (23). However, none of these agents are effective against *Listeria monocytogenes,* a significant meningopathogen in the elderly. Many of these drugs have diminished gram-positive activity compared to first- or second-generation cephalos-

TABLE 5.3   Third-Generation Cephalosporins and Investigational
              Cephalosporins

Currently available
  Cefotaxime
  Moxalactam
  Cefoperazone
  Ceftizoxime
  Ceftriaxone
  Ceftazidime
Under investigation
  Cefmenoxime
  Cefsulodin
  Cefperamide
  Ceftrizine
  Cefmetazole
  Cefroxadin

porins; therefore occasional failures can be expected with streptococcal or staphylococcal meningitis. Moxalactam's pharmacokinetics in the elderly has been studied with data indicating a diminished clearance in the aged because of impaired renal function (24). However, caution should be used in administering this drug to the elderly because of an associated coagulation disorder (25). Ceftriaxone is associated with mild decreased renal clearance corresponding to decreased creatinine clearance and requires no dose adjustment until the age of 75 years (26,27). This agent is quite useful for treating elderly patients because of its once- or twice-a-day dose regimen. Ceftazidime has the best activity against *Pseudomonas aeruginosa* of any currently available cephalosporin. It could be used safely for treating pseudomonas infections, including meningitis, in the elderly. Its pharmacokinetics in the elderly is similar to younger adults except for decreased renal clearance in patients with diminished creatinine clearance (28). Dose adjustment would ordinarily not be necessary for an elderly patient with normal renal function. Cefoperazone has been used extensively to treat a variety of infections (29). Its spectrum of activity, pharmacokinetics, and twice-a-day dose schedule are attractive for use in the aged. The drug is excreted predominantly through the bile (70–80%; hence, it is a good drug for biliary tract infection) and thus requires no dose adjustment in elderly patients who have mild to moderate renal dysfunction.

Adverse effects of third-generation cephalosporins are relatively infrequent (30). Hypersensitivity reactions (fever, rash, positive Coombs' test) (1–6%), phlebitis (1–5%), gastrointestinal effects (1–3%) including antibiotic-associated colitis (0–0.15%), thrombocytopenia (0.3–3.9%), leukopenia (0.3–2%), hemostatic abnormalities (0.5–6.7%) including clinical bleeding (0.1–0.5%), renal function tests abnormalities (0.5–2.1%), and superinfection (0.1–2.8%) have been the reported toxicities of these drugs. Thus, these antibiotics are relatively safe for elderly patients.

BETA-LACTAMASE INHIBITORS

Some of the penicillins lack extensive antimicrobial spectrum because of their susceptibility to beta-lactamase enzymes (penicillinase) produced by certain bacteria. Agents that irreversibly inhibit beta-lactamase may provide greater antimicrobial activity for these penicillins (including possibly cephalosporins). Sulbactam and clavulanic acid are agents that inhibit beta-lactamase (31,32). Currently, clavulanic acid has been marketed in combination with amoxicillin and ticarcillin. This combination has expanded amoxicillin's and ticarcillin's spectrum to include *S. aureus, Klebsiella* sp., and some other beta-lactamase-producing bacteria. Clavulanic acid is safe; therefore, these drug combinations have great appeal for use in the aged.

CARBAPENEMS

Carbapenems are one of the newest class of beta-lactam antibiotics. Imipenem, which is the generic name for N-formimidoyl thienamycin, is the first carbapenem to be developed and marketed. This antibiotic is administered in combination with cilastatin, a substance that inhibits an enzyme in the kidney that metabolizes imipenem. Imipenem is virtually active against most clinically relevant bacteria. It is active against all staphylococci, streptococci, *Listeria monocytogenes,* most gram-negative bacilli including *P. aeruginosa,* anaerobic bacteria including *B. fragilis, Neisseria* sp., and *Legionella* sp., as well as many other organisms that are not especially important to the elderly (33). Like other beta-lactam antibiotics, imipenem is relatively safe and should be considered for use in the elderly (34). Because of its high activity against most bacteria, imipenem may be appropriate as monotherapy for septic or extremely toxic elderly patients in whom the etiologic pathogen is unknown or is of mixed origin.

MONOBACTAMS

Monobactams are single-ringed beta-lactam antibiotics (penicillins, cephalosporins, and carbapenems have two rings in their basic structure) that are currently under investigation. Aztreonam is the first monobactam to be studied extensively. Monobactams are resistant to beta-lactamase, are active against gram-negative bacilli including *P. aeruginosa,* and have no activity against gram-positive or anaerobic bacteria (35). Thus agents like aztreonam have a spectrum similar to aminoglycosides but are not nephrotoxic. Aztreonam is excreted by the kidney (36) and has been shown to be as effective as gentamicin for treatment of serious urinary tract infections, even in elderly patients (37). It appears that aztreonam may be an agent that could be used to treat gram-negative infections in the elderly and thus possibly could supplant aminoglycosides. Other monobactams, such as carumonam, are also under investigation (38).

Table 5.4 summarizes the recommended doses for the major beta-lactam antibiotics that might be appropriate for the elderly. Dose adjustment is generally not required for these drugs in the elderly with normal renal function or mildly diminished creatinine clearance. The specific doses recommended for elderly (and all patients) varies considerably depending on the site and severity of infection and on the particular offending pathogen.

Vancomycin

Vancomycin is an important antibiotic to be considered in the therapeutic armamentarium for the elderly. It is a drug that is exceptionally ef-

TABLE 5.4 Dosage of Beta-Lactam Antibiotics Recommended for the Elderly

ANTIBIOTIC	ROUTE[a]	DOSAGE FOR 24 HOURS[b]
Penicillin G		
Aqueous crystalline	IV	4–20 mU in 4–6 doses
Procaine	IM	1.2–2.4 mU in 2–4 doses
Phenoxymethyl	PO	1–2 g in 4 doses
Ampicillin	PO	1–2 g in 4 doses
Ampicillin	IM, IV	6–12 g in 4–6 doses
Amoxicillin	PO	0.75–1.5 g in 3 doses
Bacampicillin	PO	1.6 g in 2 doses
Nafcillin or oxacillin	IM, IV	6–12 g in 4–6 doses
Cloxacillin	PO	2–4 g in 4 doses
Dicloxacillin	PO	1–2 g in 4 doses
Flucloxacillin	PO	1–2 g in 4 doses
Piperacillin, mezlocillin, or		
azlocillin	IM, IV	12–18 g in 4–6 doses
Cefazolin	IM, IV	1–4 g in 2–4 doses
Cefoxitin	IM, IV	4–12 g in 4–6 doses
Cefuroxime	IM, IV	2.25–4.5 g in 3 doses
Cefonicid	IM, IV	0.5–1.5 g in 1 dose
Cefoperazone	IM, IV	1–4 g in 2 doses
Ceftizoxime	IM, IV	1–6 g in 2–3 doses
Ceftriaxone	IM, IV	1–4 g in 1–2 doses
Ceftazidime	IM, IV	1–6 g in 2–3 doses
Amoxicillin/clavulanic acid	PO	0.75–1.5 g in 3 doses
Imipenem/Cilastatin	IV	2–4 g in 4 doses
Aztreonam	IV	1–2 g in 2–3 doses

[a]IV, intravenous; IM, intramuscular; PO, oral.
[b]mU, million units; g, grams; *doses* signifies equally divided doses.

fective against all strains of staphylococci (including beta-lactamase-producing strains and methicillin-resistant strains), all clinically relevant species of streptococci (including enterococci), diphtheroids (*Corynebacterium*), *Listeria,* and clostridia. Vancomycin has no activity against gram-negative bacilli or anaerobic bacteria. Its use in the elderly would be in those patients with serious infections caused by streptococci, staphylococci, or *Listeria* and have a significant penicillin allergy, in patients with methicillin-resistant *S. aureus* infection and in patients with *Clostridium difficile* colitis (39). The drug is excreted almost exclusively by the kidney and had been previously thought to have significant potential for renal dysfunction and ototoxicity. However, recent evidence suggests that vancomycin is quite safe (39). The pharmacokinetics of this drug in the elderly indicates that its clearance is reduced in this population (40). The recommended intravenous dose for vancomycin to reach a mean serum concentration of approximately 15–20 µg/ml is 30–40 mg/kg a day (or approximately 2 g a day) in two or four divided doses. In the elderly with normal renal function, a vancomycin dose of 500 mg every 8 hours or 750 mg every 12 hours may be adequate. A nomogram for vancomycin based on renal function is available (41). Serum peak and trough concentrations of this drug should be obtained in order to monitor properly its administration.

A new investigational glycopeptide, teicoplanin (also called teichomycin A2) is related to vancomycin and has a similar spectrum of activity. It has several advantages over vancomycin: (*1*) it is more active against streptococci, especially against enterococci; (*2*) it has a longer half-life (over 40 hours) and thus can be given once a day; and (*3*) it may be given intramuscularly (42). Thus, this drug might be an antibiotic of the future for the elderly.

Erythromycin

Erythromycin is a macrolide antibiotic that is very safe for all patients including the elderly. It may be taken orally or administered intravenously; intramuscular injections are to be avoided because of pain with injection and poor serum levels (43). Erythromycin is effective in treating most infections caused by such important geriatric pathogens as *S. pneumoniae* and other streptococci (not enterococci), *H. influenzae, Legionella* sp., and *Neisseria* sp. It may have activity against *L. monocytogenes* and anaerobic gram-positive cocci. This drug, however, does not penetrate into cerebrospinal fluid. The dose for elderly patients is the standard 2 g a day in four equally divided doses. For severe *Legionella* pneumonia, the dose may be increased to 4 g a day. Dose adjustment is not required for renal impairment. With high doses, gastrointestinal complaints occur (nausea, vomiting, diarrhea).

Clindamycin

Clindamycin is an important antibiotic for treating infections in the aged. Its aerobic gram-positive spectrum includes *S. pneumoniae* as well as other streptococci (except for enterococci) and most strains of *S. aureus* (44). Clindamycin has excellent antimicrobial activity against most anaerobic bacteria including *B. fragilis* (44). However, it is distinctly ineffective against *Clostridium difficile,* the causative pathogen of antibiotic-associated colitis. Clindamycin reaches most tissues except it does not enter cerebrospinal fluid. This drug, along with metronidazole, is most frequently used in the elderly for treating serious anaerobic infections, particularly if *B. fragilis* is involved. In elderly patients who are allergic to penicillin, clindamycin is an excellent alternative for most oral, sinopulmonary, skin, and soft tissue infections. The dose for clindamycin in the elderly is the same as for the general population, i.e., parenteral dose of 1,200–2,400 mg a day in three to four divided doses and oral dose of 450 mg in four divided doses. The major adverse effect is the potential for antibiotic-associated colitis.

Tetracyclines

The tetracyclines have been one of the most commonly prescribed antibiotics in the world, primarily because of their relatively broad spectrum of antibiotic activity and infrequent incidence of serious side effects. However, their use for treating common geriatric infections is relatively limited. Important pathogens in the elderly, such as streptococci, staphylococci, and gram-negative bacilli, have a relatively high frequency of resistance to tetracyclines. Currently, tetracyclines would only be recommended for the elderly as an alternative drug for *H. influenzae* respiratory infection, *Legionella* sp. infection, syphilis, and possibly *L. monocytogenes* infection (45). Of the available forms of tetracyclines, doxycycline would be preferred in the elderly because of its (*1*) longer half-life (and therefore, twice daily dosage regimen); (*2*) superior gastrointestinal absorption; and (*3*) low renal clearance (which permits standard dosage in the presence of renal dysfunction). Absorption of tetracycline in the gastrointestinal tract is decreased with dairy products, divalent and trivalent cations (aluminum, calcium, and magnesium—present in antacids), and iron-containing preparations (45). The recommended dose for doxycycline is 100–200 mg a day in two divided doses.

Trimethoprim-Sulfamethoxazole

The combination antibiotic trimethoprim-sulfamethoxazole (TMP-SMZ) is an extremely useful agent, either as a primary or secondary drug, for treating common infections in the geriatric population. TMP-SMZ has an extensive antibacterial spectrum including such important geriatric infectious pathogens as *S. pneumoniae* and other streptococci, *L. monocytogenes, Neisseria* sp., *H. influenzae,* and most Enterobacteriaceae gram-negative bacilli and non-aeruginosa *Pseudomonas* species (46). It has moderate activity against *S. aureus,* but is inactive against *P. aeruginosa* and anaerobic bacteria. The widespread popularity of TMP-SMZ in the general population is due to its aforementioned broad spectrum as well as to its antimicrobial activity against many sexually transmitted pathogens (*N. gonorrhoeae, Chlamydia* sp., and *Hemophilus ducreyi*), some agents of infectious diarrhea (*Salmonella, Shigella, E. coli*), and *Pneumocystis carinii*. The pharmacokinetics of TMP-SMZ make it a useful agent for the elderly. The drug is well absorbed orally; it distributes well into most tissues and body fluids (including cerebrospinal fluid, urine, and prostatic fluid), and it is relatively safe. TMP-SMZ is available in oral and parenteral forms. It is primarily used in the elderly for treating urinary tract infections, bacterial prostatitis, and some cases of bacterial bronchitis or pneumonia. TMP-SMZ should also be considered as a potential alternative agent for treating bacterial meningitis in the elderly caused by *S. pneumoniae, N. meningitidis, L. monocytogenes,* and select gram-negative bacilli (47). TMP-SMZ is commercially prepared as 80 mg TMP and 400 mg SMZ (or as a double-strength tablet). Depending on the site, type, and severity of infection, the daily oral dose for TMP-SMZ is 4–6 tablets in two or three divided doses. Dose adjustment should be made with moderate to severe renal impairment.

Metronidazole

Metronidazole is an antibiotic commonly used to treat giardiasis, trichomonal vaginitis, and invasive or extraintestinal amebiasis. However, its major use in the elderly would be in treating anaerobic bacterial infections, especially if *B. fragilis* is a potential pathogen (48). Metronidazole is bactericidal against most obligate anaerobes, but a few non-spore-forming anaerobic gram-positive cocci are resistant to this drug. It has minimal to no activity against aerobic gram-positive cocci (e.g., streptococci, staphylococci) or gram-negative bacilli. Metronidazole penetrates well into the brain and cerebrospinal fluid and is the drug of choice for anaerobic brain abscess (48). The recommended dose for metronidazole is 1.5–2 g a day in three or four divided doses, and dose adjustment is not required except for elderly patients with severe renal failure. It may be administered orally or parenterally.

Chloramphenicol

Chloramphenicol is an antiinfective agent that has potential but limited use in the elderly. Because of its potential for dose-related bone marrow suppression (usually erythrocytes) and for occasional, unpredictable idiosyncratic aplastic anemia (49), chloramphenicol must be used cautiously in any patient but especially the aged. In the elderly, it may be used to treat bacterial meningitis caused by *S. pneumoniae, N. meningitidis,* and *L. monocytogenes,* any *H. influenzae* infection, and anaerobic infections (including brain abscesses) (50). Chloramphenicol would generally be used as an alternative agent, when the primary drug of choice cannot be administered. The dose for chloramphenicol is 4 to 6 g a day in four divided doses. The drug is given intravenously (intramuscular route should be avoided because of unpredictable absorption); oral chloramphenicol is not recommended because of higher association of aplastic anemia (50).

Aminoglycosides

Aminoglycosides are excellent antibiotics for treating serious gram-negative bacillary infections including those caused by *P. aeruginosa* (51). Thus, these drugs are potentially useful for treating severely ill elderly paitents with gram-negative infections. However, aminoglycosides have the potential for causing nephrotoxicity (usually reversible) and eighth nerve damage (generally irreversible) (52)—adverse side effects that are particularly detrimental to the aged. The currently available amino-glycosides that are most commonly used in clinical practice are gentamicin, tobramycin, amikacin, and the newer agent called netilmicin. The following are indications under which aminoglycosides may be administered justifiably to an elderly patient.

1. Severe or life-threatening infection of unknown etiology in which the risk of death is greater than the risk of drug-induced ototoxicity or renal failure.
2. Serious *P. aeruginosa* infections (e.g., bacteremia, endocarditis, meningitis, pneumonia, osteomyelitis).
3. Infection caused by drug-resistant bacteria that are susceptible only to aminoglycosides.
4. Serious infection in which the addition of an aminoglycoside provides synergistic antimicrobial activity or provides bactericidal activity for tolerant organisms (bacteria are inhibited but are not killed by an antibiotic).

The pharmacokinetics of aminoglycosides in the elderly are similar to those of younger patients, and generally dose adjustment is not necessary for older persons with normal renal function (53–55). However, there is considerable interpatient variation in dose requirements for geriatric patients (56). Therefore, frequent monitoring of serum drug levels as well as assessment of renal and eighth nerve function are essential when administering aminoglycosides to the aged. Table 5.5 gives information on the recommended doses, desirable serum concentrations, and toxic serum levels for the aminoglycosides (57).

Fluoroquinolones

Fluoroquinolones are a new group of antibiotics that in the future may have great utility in the elderly. These drugs are similar structurally to nalidixic acid; they include norfloxacin, pefloxacin, ofloxacin, amifloxacin, enoxacin, and ciprofloxacin. They are highly active (and bactericidal) against most aerobic gram-negative bacilli including *P. aeruginosa* as well as staphylococci, streptococci (including enterococci), *H. influenzae,* and some anaerobes (58). These drugs can be given orally, on a two- or three-daily dose schedule and appear to be relatively safe (59).

TABLE 5.5 Aminoglycoside Dosages and Serum Concentrations

DRUG	DAILY DOSE	THERAPEUTIC SERUM CONCENTRATION (µg/ml)		TOXIC SERUM CONCENTRATION (µg/ml)	
		PEAK	TROUGH	PEAK	TROUGH
Gentamicin	5 mg/kg in 3 divided doses	6–10	1–2	>12	>2
Tobramycin	5 mg/kg in 3 divided doses	6–10	1–2	>12	>2
Amikacin	15 mg/kg in 2 divided doses	20–30	5–10	>35	>10
Netilmicin	6.5 mg/kg in 3 divided doses	10–14	2–4	>16	>4

Preliminary pharmacokinetic studies in relatively healthy elderly subjects show that ciprofloxacin elimination half-life is nearly twice as long in the aged compared to younger subjects (60). This was apparently due to diminished renal as well as non-renal clearance of the drug in the elderly. The potential advantage of the fluoroquinolones for the elderly is that they are oral agents with a low toxicity and an extended bacterial spectrum. Currently, ciprofloxacin is the most promising agent in limited clinical trials (61–62).

REFERENCES

1. Yoshikawa TT: Ageing and infectious disease, in Pathy MSJ (ed): *Principles and Practice of Geriatric Medicine.* London, John Wiley & Sons Ltd., Chichester 1985, p 221.
2. Yoshikawa TT: Physiology of aging. Impact on pharmacology. *Semin Anesthesia* 5:8-13, 1986.
3. Schmucker DL: Aging and drug disposition: An update. *Pharmacol Rev* 37: 133-148, 1985.
4. Greenblatt D, Sellers EM, Shader RI: Drug disposition in old age. *N Engl J Med* 306:1081-1083, 1982.
5. Brown WW, Davis BB, Spry LA, et al: Aging and the kidney. *Arch Intern Med* 146:1790-1796, 1986.
6. Anderson S, Brenner BM: Effects of aging on the renal glomerulus. *Am J Med* 80:435-442, 1986.
7. Jencks SF, Dobson A: Strategies for reforming Medicare's physician payments: Physician Diagnosis-Related Groups and other approaches. *N Engl J Med* 312:1492-1499, 1985.
8. Dejace P, Klastersky J: Comparative review of combination therapy: Two beta-lactams versus beta-lactam plus aminoglycosides. *Am J Med* 80(Suppl 6B)29-38, 1986.

9. Moellering RC Jr: Have the new beta-lactams rendered the aminoglycosides obsolete for the treatment of serious nosocomial infections? *Am J Med* 80(Suppl 6B):44–47, 1986.
10. Yoshikawa TT: Antimicrobial drugs, in Yoshikawa TT, Chow AW, Guze LB (eds): *Infectious Diseases: Diagnosis and Management.* New York, John Wiley & Sons, 1980, p 673.
11. Neu HC: Amoxicillin. *Ann Intern Med* 80:356–360, 1982.
12. Finegold SM, Gentry LO, Mogabgab W, et al: Controlled trial of bacampicillin and amoxicillin in therapy of bacterial infections of the lower respiratory tract. *Rev Infect Dis* 3:150–153, 1981.
13. Ditlove J, Weidmann P, Bernstein M, et al: Methicillin nephritis. *Medicine* 56:483–491, 1977.
14. Taylor C, Corrigan K, Steen S, et al: Oxacillin and hepatitis. *Ann Intern Med* 90:857–858, 1979.
15. Parry MF, Pancoast SJ: Antipseudomonal penicillins, in Ristuccia AM, Cunha BA (eds): *Antimicrobial Therapy.* New York, Raven Press, 1984, p 197.
16. Fu KP, Neu HC: Azlocillin and mezlocillin: New ureido penicillins. *Antimicrob Agents Chemother* 13:930–938, 1978.
17. Pancoast S, Prince AS, Francke EL, et al: Clinical evaluation of piperacillin therapy for infection. *Arch Intern Med* 141:1447–1450, 1981.
18. Fried JS, Hinthorn DR: The cephalosporins. *Disease-a-Month* 31:7–60, 1985.
19. Sanders CV, Greenberg RN, Marier RL: Cefamandole and cefoxitin. *Ann Intern Med* 103:70–78, 1985.
20. Neu HC, Fu KP: Cefuroxime, a beta-lactamase-resistant cephalosporin with a broad spectrum of gram-positive and -negative activity. *Antimicrob Agents Chemother* 13:657–664, 1978.
21. Pontzer RE, Kreiger RE, Boscia JA, et al: Single-dose cefonicid therapy for urinary tract infections. *Antimicrob Agents Chemother* 23:814–816, 1983.
22. Thornsberry C: Review of in vitro activity of third-generation cephalosporins and other newer beta-lactam antibiotics against clinically important bacteria. *Am J Med* 79(suppl 2A):14–20, 1985.
23. Norrby SR: Role of cephalosporins in the treatment of bacterial meningitis in adults. Overview with special emphasis on ceftazidime. *Am J Med* 79(suppl 2A):56–61, 1985.
24. Andritz MH, Smith RP, Baltch A, et al: Pharmacokinetics of moxalactam in elderly subjects. *Antimicrob Agents Chemother* 25:33–36, 1984.
25. Weitekamp MR, Aber RC: Prolonged bleeding times and bleeding diathesis associated with moxalactam administration. *JAMA* 249:69–71, 1983.
26. Luderer JR, Patel IH, Durkin J, et al: Age and ceftriaxone kinetics. *Clin Pharmacol Ther* 35:19–25, 1984.
27. Hayton WL, Stoeckel K: Age-associated changes in ceftriaxone pharmacokinetics. *Clin Pharmacokinet* 11:76–86, 1986.
28. LeBel M, Barbeau G, Vallee F, et al: Pharmacokinetics of ceftazidime in elderly volunteers. *Antimicrob Agents Chemother* 28:713–715, 1985.
29. Brogden RN, Carmine A, Heel RC, et al: Cefoperazone: A review of its *in vitro* antimicrobial activity, pharmacological properties and therapeutic efficacy. *Drugs* 22:423–460, 1981.

30. Meyers BR: Comparative toxicities of third-generation cephalosporins. *Am J Med* 79(suppl 2A):96–103, 1985.
31. English AR, Retsema JA, Girard AE, et al: CP-45,899, a beta-lactamase inhibitor that extends the antibacterial spectrum of beta-lactams. Initial bacteriological characterization. *Antimicrob Agents Chemother* 14:414–419, 1978.
32. Neu HC (editor): Proceedings of a symposium. Beta-lactamase inhibitors: therapeutic advances. *Am J Med* 79(5B):1–196, 1985.
33. Barza M: Imipenem: First of a new class of beta-lactam antibiotics. *Ann Intern Med* 103:552–560, 1985.
34. Colandra GB, Brown KR, Grad LC, et al: Review of adverse experiences and tolerability in the first 2,516 patients treated with imipenem/cilastatin. *Am J Med* 78(suppl 6A):73–78, 1985.
35. Neu HC: Use of the newer agents for antibiotic resistant infection. *Geriatrics* 40:100–106, 1985.
36. Mattie H, Matze-van der Lans A: Pharmacokinetics of aztreonam in infected patients. *J Antimicrob Chemother* 17:215–219, 1986.
37. Sattler FR, Schramm M, Moyer JE, et al: Aztreonam compared with gentamicin for treatment of serious urinary tract infection. *Lancet* 1:1315-1318, 1984.
38. Horber F, Egger H-J, Weidekamm E, et al: Pharmacokinetics of carumonam in patients with renal insufficiency. *Antimicrob Agents Chemother* 29:116–121, 1986.
39. Cunha BA, Ristuccia PA: Vancomycin, in Ristuccia PA, Cunha BA (eds): *Antimicrobial Therapy.* New York, Raven Press, 1984. p. 265.
40. Cutler NR, Narang PK, Lesko LJ, et al: Vancomycin disposition: The importance of age. *Clin Pharmacol Ther* 36:803–810, 1984.
41. Matzke GR, McGory RW, Halstenson CE, et al: Pharmacokinetics of vancomycin in patients with various degrees of renal function. *Antimicrob Agents Chemother* 25:433–437, 1984.
42. Glupczynski Y, Lagast H, Van Der Auwera P, et al: Clinical evaluation of teichoplanin for therapy of severe infections caused by gram-positive bacteria. *Antimicrob Agents Chemother* 29:52–57, 1986.
43. Washington JA II, Wilson WR: Erythromycin: A microbial and clinical perspective after 30 years of clinical use. *Mayo Clin Proc* 60:189–203, 271–278, 1985.
44. Dhawan VK, Thadepalli H: Clindamycin: A review of fifteen years experience. *Rev Infect Dis* 4:1133–1153, 1982.
45. Jonas M, Comer JB, Cunha BA: Tetracyclines, in Ristuccia AM, Cunha BA (eds): *Antimicrobial Therapy.* New York, Raven Press, 1984, p 219.
46. Salter AJ: Trimethoprim-sulfamethoxazole: an assessment of more than 12 years of use. *Rev Infect Dis* 4:196–236, 1982.
47. Levitz RE, Quintiliani R: Trimethoprim-sulfamethoxazole for bacterial meningitis. *Ann Intern Med* 100:881–890, 1984.
48. Finegold SM, George WL, Rolfe RD (eds): *First United States Metronidazole Conference. Proceedings from a Symposium. Tarpon Springs, Florida, February 19–20, 1982.* New York, Biomedical Information Corporation, 1982.
49. Baumelou E, Najean Y: Why still prescribe chloramphenicol in 1983? Comparison of the clinical and biological hematologic effects of chloramphenicol and thiamphenicol. *Blut* 47:317–320, 1983.

50. Shalit I, Marks MI: Chloramphenicol in the 1980s. *Drugs* 28:281–291, 1984.
51. Siegenthaler WE, Bonetti A, Luthy R: Aminoglycoside antibiotics in infectious diseases. *Am J Med* 80(Suppl 6B):2–14, 1986.
52. Meyer RD: Risk factors and comparisons of clinical nephrotoxicity of aminoglycosides. *Am J Med* 80(Suppl 6B):119–125, 1986.
53. Bauer LA, Blouin RA: Influence of age on tobramycin pharmacokinetics in patients with normal renal function. *Antimicrob Agents Chemother* 20: 587–589, 1981.
54. Bauer LA, Blouin RA: Gentamicin pharmacokinetics: Effect of aging in patients with normal renal function. *J Am Geriatr Soc* 30:309–311, 1982.
55. Yasuhara H, Kobayashi S, Sakamoto K, et al: Pharmacokinetics of amikacin and cephalothin in bedridden elderly patients. *J Clin Pharmacol* 22: 403–409, 1982.
56. Zaske DE, Irvine P, Strand LM, et al: Wide interpatient variations in gentamicin dose requirements for geriatric patients. *JAMA* 248:3122–3126, 1982.
57. Ristuccia AM: Aminoglycosides, in Ristuccia AM, Cuhna BA (eds): *Antimicrobial Therapy*. New York, Raven Press, 1984, p 305.
58. Wolfson JS, Hooper DC: The fluoroquinolones: structure, mechanisms of action and resistance, and spectra of activity in vitro. *Antimicrob Agents Chemother* 28:581–586, 1985.
59. Hooper DC, Wolfson JS: The fluoroquinolones: Pharmacology, clinical uses, and toxicities in humans. *Antimicrob Agents Chemother* 28:716–721, 1985.
60. LeBel M, Barbeau G, Bergeron MG, et al: Pharmacokinetics of ciprofloxacin in elderly subjects. *Pharmacotherapy* 6:87–91, 1986.
61. Ramirez CA, Bran JL, Mejia CR, et al: Open, prospective study of clinical efficacy of ciprofloxacin. *Antimicrob Agent Chemother* 28:128–132, 1985.
62. Ball AP: Overview of clinical experience with ciprofloxacin. *Eur J Clin Microbiol* 5:214–219, 1986.

SUGGESTED READINGS

Fried JS, Hinthorn DR: The cephalosporins. *Disease-a-Month* 31:7–60, 1985.
Ristuccia AM, Cunha BA: *Antimicrobial Therapy*. New York, Raven Press, 1984.
Schmucker DL: Aging and drug disposition: An update. *Pharmacol Rev* 37:133–148, 1985.

Chapter 6

Prevention of Infections

Prevention of infections is the most rational and perhaps the most cost-effective approach to reducing or possibly eliminating the morbidity, mortality, and expense of infectious diseases in the elderly. Unequivocally, prevention has proven to be an effective method of managing serious infections. The prevalence of such diseases as poliomyelitis, diphtheria, tetanus, smallpox, measles, rubella, and pertussis has been drastically reduced in children and the general adult population through preventive measures such as vaccination (1,2). Likewise, diarrheal scourges such as cholera have been eliminated in countries that practice public health, for example, by purifying drinking water. To a large degree, these advances in prevention have contributed to increased longevity in humans, particularly through a reduction in infant mortality. This has resulted in a drastic rise in the geriatric population. With the increase in the aging population has come the reemergence of infectious disease as a major factor in the quality and quantity of life (1).

In this chapter, the discussion focuses on aspects of infection prevention in the elderly.

ANTIMICROBIAL CHEMOPROPHYLAXIS

Antimicrobial chemoprophylaxis involves the administration of antibiotics to prevent infections. It may be applied to three distinct situations: (*1*) to prevent the acquisition of an exogenous organism that is not part of the normal microflora; (*2*) to prevent organisms normally present in one area of the body from gaining access to another site that is nor-

55

mally sterile; and (3) to prevent organisms already present in a normally sterile site from causing infections (3).

To justify the administration of antibiotics for purposes of antimicrobial chemoprophylaxis, several principles should be considered carefully (4):

1. The risk-benefit and cost-benefit ratios should be in favor of the patient. (Risks include adverse drug reactions, superinfections, and emergence of drug resistance, all which possibly result in morbidity, prolonged hospitalization, and excessive costs.)
2. The microorganism(s) should be exquisitely susceptible to the antibiotic(s), and there should be valid data that substantiate the value of chemoprophylaxis against this infection.
3. Antibiotics should be administered before exposure to or tissue contamination by the organism. However, in some cases, the period from organism invasion to active infection may be delayed or indolent; therefore, antibiotics still may be effective in preventing the infection despite being administered after microbial exposure.
4. The antibiotics should be administered for only the duration of organism exposure. In some instances, however, the duration of prophylaxis may be several months.

Medical Prophylaxis

Most of the accepted forms of medical prophylaxis are listed in Table 6.1 (3,4). However, the discussion in this chapter is limited to only those conditions that are especially important or relevant to the elderly.

INFECTIVE ENDOCARDITIS

Since infective endocarditis is an important disease in the elderly (see Chapter 12 on infective endocarditis), preventive measures against this infection are part of the overall management. Cardiac conditions that

TABLE 6.1 Medical Conditions that Warrant Antimicrobial Chemoprophylaxis

Rheumatic fever
Infective endocarditis
Meningococcal disease
Recurrent urinary tract infection
Malaria
Influenza A
Gonorrhea
Syphilis
Tuberculosis

warrant antibiotic prophylaxis include prosthetic heart valves (including bioprosthetic types), congenital cardiac malformations (except isolated secundum atrial septal defect and corrected patent ductus arteriosus), surgically constructed systemic-pulmonary shunts, rheumatic and other acquired valvular disease (e.g., syphilitic, degenerative), idiopathic hypertrophic subaortic stenosis, mitral valve prolapse, and a previous history of infective endocarditis (5).

There are many procedures that are associated with high-grade bacteremia (6), and these high-risk procedures should be preceded by antibiotics for all of the above-mentioned cardiac conditions. These procedures are listed in Table 6.2. However, because prosthetic cardiac valves and surgically constructed systemic-pulmonary shunts are at especially high risk for infection, it is probably prudent to administer prophylactic antibiotics for even low-risk procedures (5).

Table 6.3 summarizes the recommended antibiotic regimens for the prevention of endocarditis in patients who are undergoing oral or respiratory tract manipulation or surgery (5). The recommendations are divided according to native (natural) valve dysfunction (congenital and acquired disorders) and prosthetic valve and shunts. Regimens are designed to prevent infection from streptococci that include viridans streptococci, enterococci, and in some cases pneumococci.

For genitourinary and gastrointestinal procedures, ampicillin 2 g IV or IM plus gentamicin 1.5 mg/kg IV or IM is administered 30 to 60 minutes before the procedure. A repeat dose of both drugs is given 8 hours later. However, elderly patients with renal dysfunction should have the repeat gentamicin dose adjusted by either decreasing the dose at 8 hours or maintaining the same dose of 1.5 mg/kg but administering it at greater than 8 hours. Penicillin-allergic patients should have ampicillin replaced with vancomycin 1 g IV (given over 1 hour) administered 60 minutes before the procedure. A repeat dose of vancomycin is given 8 to 12 hours later (or adjusted with renal dysfunction). With these procedures abnor-

TABLE 6.2 High-Risk Procedures that Require Antibiotic Prophylaxis to Prevent Endocarditis

---

Dental work that is likely to produce gingival bleeding
Tonsillectomy and/or adenoidectomy
Surgical intervention or biopsy of respiratory mucosa
Bronchoscopy with a rigid bronchoscope
Incision and drainage of infected tissue
Genitourinary procedures (cystoscopy, prostatic surgery, urethral dilatation, urinary tract surgery, vaginal hysterectomy)
Gastrointestinal procedures (gallbladder surgery, colonic surgery, esophageal dilatation, sclerotherapy for esophageal varices, colonoscopy, upper gastrointestinal endoscopy with biopsy, or proctosigmoidoscopy with biopsy)

TABLE 6.3 Antibiotic Prophylaxis Regimens Against
Endocarditis in Oral and Respiratory Tract Procedures

CARDIAC CONDITION	ANTIBIOTIC REGIMEN
Native or natural valve damage (congenital and acquired disorders)	Phenoxymethyl penicillin, 2 g orally 1 hour before procedure. Then 1 g 6 hours later. OR Aqueous crystalline penicillin G, 2 million units IV or IM 30–60 minutes before procedure. Then 1 million units 6 hours later. OR For penicillin-allergic patients, erythromycin 1 g orally 1 hour before procedure. Then 500 mg 6 hours later. OR For penicillin-allergic patients, vancomycin 1 g IV (infused over 1 hour) 1 hour before procedure. No repeat dose necessary.
Prosthetic valve or shunts	Ampicillin 1–2 g IV or IM *plus* gentamicin 1.5 mg/kg IV or IM, 30 minutes before procedure. Repeat with dose 8 hours later or with oral penicillin 1 g, 6 hours later. OR For penicillin-allergic patients, vancomycin 1 g IV (infused over 1 hour) 1 hour before procedure. No repeat dose.

mal cardiac valves are at risk to infection from enterococci, thus an aminoglycoside is added for synergistic activity with ampicillin. Though aminoglycosides are ototoxic and nephrotoxic, the risk-benefit ratio favors their use in patients with artificial valves. Furthermore, patients with prosthetic devices are also at risk to gram-negative bacilli. Although not formally recommended by the American Heart Association, we suggest that elderly patients with prosthetic heart valves or systemic-pulmonary shunts receive the above prophylactic regimen for less invasive procedures or procedures with low-level bacteremia such as proctosigmoidoscopy without biopsy, liver biopsy, and barium enema as intravascular infections in this situation are a difficult management problem and may require extensive surgery for their resolution.

Endocarditis prophylaxis for cardiac surgery are discussed with surgical prophylaxis.

RECURRENT URINARY TRACT INFECTION
Recurrent urinary tract infection management is discussed in Chapter 14 on urinary tract infection. Nevertheless, it should be stated here that pro-

phylactic antibiotics generally have no role in urinary tract infections caused by chronic indwelling bladder catheters, major genitourinary tract anatomic and functional abnormalities, or nephrolithiasis or urolithiasis.

INFLUENZA A
The administration of amantadine for prophylaxis against influenza A is discussed in this chapter in the immunoprophylaxis section under influenza vaccine.

TUBERCULOSIS
Chemoprophylaxis against tuberculosis is discussed in Chapter 11 on tuberculosis.

Surgical Prophylaxis

Table 6.4 lists the surgical procedures in which antimicrobial chemoprophylaxis has generally been accepted as effective or appropriate (7). Most, if not all, of these surgical procedures are important to the elderly.

In order to understand the relative importance and effectiveness of antibiotic prophylaxis for surgical procedures, a statement should be made regarding surgical wound classification. Besides preventing wound infections, antimicrobial chemoprophylaxis is directed toward preventing (1) infections in and around the operative site, (2) bacteremia, and (3) nonoperative related infections (e.g., urinary tract infections). Table 6.5 illustrates the National Research Council classification of surgical wounds (3,8,9). Generally, wounds classified as *contaminated* or *dirty* have infec-

---

TABLE 6.4 Surgical Procedures that Warrant Antimicrobial Chemoprophylaxis

Colorectal surgery
Vaginal hysterectomy
Laryngeal and oropharyngeal resection for carcinoma
Gastroduodenal surgery[a]
Biliary tract surgery[a]
Cardiac surgery
Vascular surgery
Orthopedic surgery[b]
Urologic procedures[c]
Penetrating abdominal injury[d]

---

[a]For select high-risk patients only.
[b]Uncomplicated hip fractures, total hip replacement, insertion of other prostheses.
[c]Controversial
[d]Primarily intestinal injury. May consider this treatment rather than prophylaxis.

TABLE 6.5 Classification of Surgical Wounds

| CATEGORY | SURGICAL CONDITIONS | ANTICIPATED INFECTION RATE (%) | |
		NO ANTIBIOTICS	ANTIBIOTICS
Clean	Elective; primary closure; no drains; no entry into respiratory, gastrointestinal, or genitourinary tract; wound is nontraumatic; no inflammation of surgical site (*Example:* thyroidectomy)	1–2	NI[a]
Clean-contaminated	Intact sterile technique, but respiratory, gastrointestinal, or genitourinary tract is entered; no inflammation of surgical site (*Example:* vaginal hysterectomy)	10–20	7
Contaminated	Fresh trauma; major breaks in sterile techniques; gross spillage from gastrointestinal tract; entry into infected or inflamed biliary or urinary tracts; incisions into acute inflammation without pus (*Example:* cholecystectomy for acute cholecystitis)	20–35	10–15
Dirty	Perforated viscera; traumatic wounds with devitalized tissue; gross fecal spillage; foreign body contamination; presence of pus (*Example:* ruptured appendix)	25–50	15–35

SOURCE: Adapted from references 3, 8, and 9.
[a]NI, not indicated except for defined situations (see text).

tion; therefore antibiotics are not truly prophylactic but are therapeutic (3). The duration of antibiotics may then be more appropriate for a period beyond that of prophylaxis. Wounds classified as *clean* generally have a low infection rate and usually do not require prophylactic antibiotics. However, under select circumstances, i.e., insertion of prosthesis such as cardiac valve, vascular grafts, and arterial grafts, even though the infection rate is low, infection is likely to be catastrophic. Therefore, as was noted above in the case of prosthetic cardiac valves, antibiotic prophylaxis has been recommended. The clean-contaminated wounds are those in which the administration of antibiotics appears to be the most rational for true prophylaxis.

COLORECTAL SURGERY
The clinical data is overwhelming for the value of antimicrobial chemoprophylaxis for preventing infections that are associated with colorectal surgery (7,10). For elderly patients who undergo elective colorectal surgery with no other infectious risk factors, antimicrobial prophylaxis can simply be with preoperative oral antibiotics. These regimens include (4): (*1*) neomycin, 1 g, plus nonabsorbable erythromycin base 1 g, which is taken orally three times during the day and night before surgery; (*2*) neomycin as in (*1*) plus metronidazole, 1 g orally 24 hours before surgery followed by 200 mg orally every 8 hours until surgery; and (*3*) neomycin as in (*1*) and (*2*) plus tetracycline 250 mg orally every 8 hours which is begun 24 hours before surgery.

In high-risk or debilitated elderly patients; in patients who cannot take oral medications (or who are allergic to these agents); or in patients with bowel obstruction, active inflammation, or infection, parenteral antibiotics should be administered. Since the fecal flora is a mixture of aerobic and anaerobic bacteria, a broad-spectrum agent would be indicated. In the elderly, agents such as cefoxitin or one of the third-generation cephalosporins (see Chapter 5 on antimicrobial therapy: special considerations) would be effective and safe. A preoperative intravenous dose of 1 to 2 g followed by doses 24 to 48 hours postoperatively would be appropriate.

VAGINAL HYSTERECTOMY
Although vaginal hysterectomy is performed more commonly in younger or middle-aged women, elderly women do have this procedure performed, often for uterine prolapse (11). Most studies indicate that preoperative antibiotics reduce postoperative pelvic and wound infections (7). Although no controlled studies have been done in an elderly population, fever or documented infection does occur in 30% of aged women who undergo vaginal hysterectomy without prophylactic antibiotics (11). A single preoperative dose (1–2 g) with a long-acting cephalosporin, for

example, cefazolin, cefonicid, cefoperazone, or ceftriaxone, most likely would be effective and safe in elderly women.

LARYNGEAL AND PHARYNGEAL CARCINOMA RESECTION

Serious postoperative wound infections with aerobic gram-positive and gram-negative bacteria as well as anaerobes may occur in 80 to 90% of patients who undergo resection for laryngeal or pharyngeal carcinoma but receive no antibiotics (12,13). The prophylactic combination of clindamycin plus gentamicin has been shown to be superior to a first-generation cephalosporin (cefazolin) (14). However, as stated in Chapter 5, aminoglycoside antibiotics should be avoided in the elderly whenever possible. A third-generation cephalosporin has been effective and safe for head and neck cancer surgery (13). A regimen that could be used to obviate the problem of aminoglycosides would be cefoperazone 1 to 2 g IV preoperatively and continued for 24 hours postoperatively.

GASTRODUODENAL SURGERY

Patients with achlorhydria, gastrointestinal hemorrhage, or gastric obstruction are at higher risk for postoperative wound infection (15). The elderly thus fall into a high risk group. Preoperative antibiotic prophylaxis with a first-generation cephalosporin, for example, cefazolin 1 to 2 g is an effective regimen. Doses beyond the operative period are unnecessary (16).

BILIARY TRACT SURGERY

Postoperative infections following biliary tract surgery occur significantly more in the elderly; in patients with acute cholecystitis, common duct obstruction, cholangitis, or obstructive jaundice; in patients who undergo emergency cholecystectomy; and in diabetics (17). Numerous studies have shown the infection rates that follow gallbladder surgery in patients with and without prophylatic antibiotics were 0 to 9% and 5 to 28%, respectively (17,18). Thus, elderly patients who undergo elective biliary tract surgery should receive preoperative prophylactic antibiotics, since 10 to 18% of these patients will have positive bile cultures (19), and the presence of bacteria in bile significantly increases wound infection likelihood. A single preoperative intravenous dose of cefazolin 1 to 2 g, cefuroxime 1.5 g, or ceftriaxone 1 to 2 g would be effective, safe, and inexpensive (18–20).

CARDIAC SURGERY

Prophylactic antibiotics are recommended for patients undergoing open-heart surgery for placement of prosthetic heart valves or implantation of other prosthetic material (5,7). Prophylaxis is directed primarily against staphylococci. A preoperative dose with cefazolin (1–2 g) followed by no more than 2 days of drug administration is more than adequate. If methicillin-resistant strains of staphylococci occur with a high prevalence, vancomycin should be substituted (500 mg preoperatively followed by 1.5 to 2.0 g a day in two to four divided doses).

VASCULAR SURGERY

Since peripheral vascular surgery is performed commonly in the elderly, the risk of infection for these procedures is important. However, the incidence of infection varies with the site of surgery (7). Abdominal aorta and lower-extremity vascular surgery may benefit from prophylaxis with the same regimen as described for cardiac surgery. The high cost that results from infectious complications of an implanted vascular graft justifies consideration of antibiotic prophylaxis (21).

ORTHOPEDIC SURGERY

Elderly patients who undergo surgery for hip fracture (nail, plate, or prosthesis), total hip replacement, or insertion of other prosthetic devices should receive preoperative prophylactic antibiotics (22). A single preoperative dose with a semisynthetic penicillinase-resistant penicillin (oxacillin or nafcillin; 2 g) or a first-generation cephalosporin (cefazolin 1–2 g) continued for 48 hours postoperatively is effective prophylaxis.

UROLOGIC PROCEDURES

Controversy exists as to whether prophylactic antibiotics are warranted for urologic surgery and procedures. Careful reviews of multiple studies show that most reports had major flaws in experimental design (23). In addition, the end point for the studies varied, that is, bacteriuria, sepsis, or wound infection; the patients had indwelling bladder catheters for varying periods postoperatively; the urologic procedures that were investigated differed; and antibiotics were administered at different times (7,23). However, it should be emphasized that in patients with bacteriuria preprocedure antibiotics are given for *treatment* and *not* for prophylaxis and are mandatory to prevent bacteremia from manipulation of an infection in the genitourinary tract.

More recently, several investigations have been performed that used prophylactic antibiotics with the newer broad-spectrum beta-lactam drugs for both transurethral and open prostatectomies (24,25). Infection rates without antibiotics were 19 to 30% in contrast to an infection rate of 0 to 13% with preoperative antimicrobial prophylaxis (24). Based on this more current evidence, it is suggested that elderly men who undergo prostatectomy, either transurethral or open, receive a single preoperative dose (1–2 hours before surgery) of a broad-spectrum third-generation cephalosporin, for example, ceftriaxone, ceftazidime or cefoperazone.

Other urologic procedures in the elderly (or in the debilitated, diabetic, or immunocompromised) that warrant consideration for preoperative prophylactic antibiotics include invasive stone-removing procedures, nephrectomy, cystotomy, partial cystectomy, insertion of foreign body or prosthesis, or any bowel reconstructive procedure (e.g., ileal conduit) (24). Antibiotic prophylaxis is not necessary for routine cystoscopy, simple retrograde pyelography, orchiectomy, or varicocelectomy.

PENETRATING ABDOMINAL INJURY

Penetrating abdominal injury (usually gunshot or knife wounds) that result in major visceral injuries, especially the intestine, are associated with a high infection rate. These infections include acute peritonitis, intraabdominal abscess, sepsis, wound infections, and postoperative pneumonia and/or urinary tract infection. With intestinal damage, mixed infections with aerobic and anaerobic bacteria predominate. Under these circumstances, the category of surgery would be considered *dirty*. Preoperative antibiotics, although considered prophylactic, may be truly therapeutic. Numerous studies that have used a variety of single-drug regimens or multiple-drug combinations (with aerobic and anaerobic spectrum) have shown efficacy in reducing the infection rate to a level between 15 to 30% (26–29). The duration of antibiotic administration in these studies varied from 12 hours to 5 days.

For the elderly patient who suffers an intraabdominal injury to a major viscera, especially the intestine, antibiotic administration should begin immediately with intravenous cefoxitin 2 g every 4 to 6 hours and continued for 48 hours postoperatively. If fever, leukocytosis, or other evidence of infection develops, the antibiotic should be continued for a full course of treatment. Other antibiotics that could be used in the elderly include some of the third-generation cephalosporins with good anaerobic spectrum (e.g., ceftizoxime), imipenem, or a combination of clindamycin or metronidazole with a beta-lactam drug with good aerobic gram-negative bacilli antimicrobial activity (e.g., third-generation cephalosporins, aztreonam). Aminoglycoside antibiotics should be reserved for those who fail to respond to these regimens because of resistant bacteria.

IMMUNOPROPHYLAXIS

Influenza Vaccine

Influenza infection causes the greatest morbidity and mortality in the geriatric population. Between 1957 and 1985, 10,000 or more deaths occurred with 18 epidemics of influenza; 80 to 90% of the excessive deaths associated with influenza or pneumonia occur in persons 65 years or older (30). In closed institutions, such as a nursing home, influenza outbreaks are a major concern with attack rates of 30 to 35% in susceptible patients (31,32).

There are three major types of influenza virus—Type A, B, and C. The influenza virus is an orthomyxovirus that has two major surface glycoproteins, hemagglutinin (H) and neuraminidase (N). These glycoproteins are highly antigenic and serve to type and subtype the strain of influenza virus. There are five hemagglutinin types (H_0, H_1, H_2, H_3, and Sw) and two types of neuraminidase (N_1 and N_2). Standard nomenclature designates the virus strain by virus type, geographic origin, serial number (not always used), and year of occurrence (33). For example, in the 1985–1986 vaccine, strains included are A/Philippine/2/82 (H_3N_2); A/Chile/1/83 (H_1N_1); B/USSR/100/83. The vaccine for 1986–1987 is significantly different from that of 1985–1986. The newer vaccine will consist of the following: A/Mississippi/1/85 (H_3N_2); A/Chile/1/83 (H_1N_1); B/Ann Arbor/1/86 (34).

For immunization to be effective against influenza infection, the vaccine strains must contain the same antigens as the infecting wild strain virus. For influenza A, antibody that is directed against the H is the most important since it neutralizes infectivity, whereas antibody to N only limits the rate at which the infection spreads from cell to cell (33). When minor changes in H and N occur within a family of strains of virus, this is termed *antigenic drift*. However, major changes in H and N glycoproteins are called *antigenic shift*. Such a change may result in worldwide influenza pandemic.

Immunoprophylaxis with influenza vaccine should be administered with the highest priority to the following groups of individuals: (*1*) any person regardless of age with chronic cardiovascular or pulmonary disorders, and (*2*) residents of nursing homes and other chronic care facilities. The next priority groups for vaccination are health care professionals with extensive contact with patients in the highest priority group (see above); healthy persons 65 years and older; and any persons regardless of age with a chronic metabolic disorder (including diabetes mellitus), anemia, renal failure, asthma, or immunosuppression (30).

The efficacy of the influenza vaccine in preventing clinical disease in the elderly has been debated (35,36). Some studies documented poor antibody response to the vaccine in aged persons (37,38). However, other investigations showed no difference in antibody response to influenza vaccine amongst younger adults and the elderly (39,40). Moreover, even with poor serologic responses (41), influenza vaccination appeared to reduce the frequency of serious respiratory illness including pneumonia (41–43). When vaccine and wild virus antigens are immunologically closely related the vaccine efficacy is 70% (44). Most, but not all, studies of influenza vaccine showed an efficacy in nursing home settings in terms of a reduction in the clinical severity of the disease (45); efficacy in reduction of incidence of illness varied considerably. Therefore, it is recommended that influenza vaccine be given to elderly persons. The elderly should receive either the whole or split virus vaccine, which is given (0.5 ml) intramuscularly. The vaccine should be given annually; it may also be administered concurrently (but at different sites) with the pneumococcal vaccine. The vaccine should be avoided in persons with anaphylactic sensitivity to eggs or in persons with an acute febrile illness.

Recently, several Asian countries have reported influenza outbreaks caused by a A (H_1N_1) strain that is poorly inhibited by antibodies induced by the A/Chile/1/83 strain. Consequently, a supplemental monovalent vaccine with the A/Taiwan/1/86 (H_1N_1) antigen has been made available (46). It is recommended for persons under the age of 35 years. Thus, most elderly persons will not require this supplemental vaccine.

Amantadine hydrochloride is an antiviral agent that is specific for influenza A only. It interferes with viral replication and shedding. Amantadine is 70 to 90% effective in preventing influenza A illness (47). It may also reduce clinical symptoms in an infected person if given within 24 to 48 hours of onset of illness (30,48). Amantadine is recommended for the following patients (34): (1) patients in closed institutions during an influenza A outbreak; (2) unvaccinated staff who provide care to high-risk patients of chronic care institutions or hospitals that experience a presumed influenza A outbreak; (3) high-risk patients who receive the vaccine, but who require protection until antibodies develop (about 2 weeks); (4) persons who are unable to tolerate the vaccine (during influenza outbreak); (5) unvaccinated persons who provide care for high-risk persons in the home setting (e.g., family members, visiting nurses) when influenza A outbreaks occur in their communities; (6) immunodeficient persons or persons who are expected to have poor antibody responses to the vaccine; and (7) high-risk patients who are already ill (they must be given the drug within 48 hours of exposure). Although the standard dose of amantadine is 100 mg twice a day, taken orally, in the elderly, the dose should be 100 mg once a day (30,49). Elderly patients with creatinine clearances of 30–39 ml/min/1.73 m^3 (body surface), 20–29 ml/min/1.73 m^3, or 10–19 ml/min/1.73 m^2 should receive amantadine 200 mg twice weekly, 100 mg thrice weekly, or 200 mg alternated with 100 mg every 7 days, respectively (30). However, the drug may cause stimulation of the central nervous system, which would result in insomnia and agitation in the elderly. Amantadine is contraindicated in persons with severe renal failure or who have an active seizure disorder.

Pneumococcal Vaccine

Pneumococcal (*Streptococcus pneumoniae*) pneumonia is the most common cause of bacterial pneumonia in young and old adults. (See Chapter 10 on pneumonia) The elderly (1) are at greater risk for pneumococcal pneumonia (two or three times that of general population); (2) experience a higher rate of bacteremia (three times more often); and (*3*) suffer higher death rate than younger adults (50). Even with effective antimicrobial chemotherapy available, bacteremic pneumococcal disease has a mortality of approximately 20 to 25% in the general population largely due to overwhelming illness. Thus, prevention in high-risk persons to pneumococcal disease is essential.

Those illnesses or disorders that predispose a person to severe pneumococcal infection include chronic cardiopulmonary disease, splenic dysfunction, multiple myeloma, Hodgkin's disease, alcoholism, chronic liver disease, immunosuppression, renal failure, sickle cell disease, cerebrospinal fluid leak, and nephrosis. Old age is also a risk factor (51). However, it is not uniformly accepted that vaccinating the elderly with pneumococcal vaccine is effective in preventing pneumococcal infections.

The 14-valent pneumococcal vaccine (which contains 14 serotypes of pneumococcal polysaccharide) became commercially available in the late 1970s. Its efficacy in young adults was 80% (52). However, little data were available on the efficacy of this vaccine in the elderly. Moreover, in one study of institutionalized elderly who received the 14-valent vaccine, a significant reduction in pneumococcal pneumonia could not be demonstrated in this population (53). Additionally, serologic responses in the elderly to the vaccine appeared to be less than in younger adults (54).

More recent studies suggest that the efficacy of the 14-valent vaccine in preventing pneumonia or bronchitis in patients over the age of 55 years was no better than placebo (55). However, certain serotypes common to the elderly are not included in this vaccine (49). A newer 23-serotype vaccine, which includes serotypes that infect the aged, is now available. Its serotypes account for 85% of bacteremic pneumococcal pneumonias (51). Although its efficacy in the elderly is not well established, it is most likely near 65 to 70%.

Although incontrovertible data on the efficacy of pneumococcal vaccine in the elderly is not available, it is still recommended that healthy elderly persons 65 years and older receive this vaccine. (Elderly persons with the previously mentioned risk factors for pneumococcal disease should undoubtedly receive the vaccine.) A *single* 0.5 ml dose given subcutaneously or intramuscularly is administered. Repeat doses are not to be given. Side effects are mild, primarily local discomfort, redness, and induration. We await ongoing efficacy studies.

Tetanus Vaccine

Tetanus is an important disease of the elderly (see Chapter 17 on tetanus). In the United States from 1982 through 1984, 59% of the reported 253 cases of tetanus occurred in persons 60 years or older. The case-fatality rate was 52% for persons 60 years and older compared to 13% for persons under 60 years (56). The major factor for this high incidence in the elderly is waning immunity to tetanus.

Protective immunity to tetanus is present if there is a serum antitoxin level of 0.01 unit/ml or greater. Based on this criterion, it has been shown that at least 50% of persons 60 years or older lack protective levels of circulating antitoxin (57,58). Moreover, it appears that serum antitoxin level in response to tetanus toxoid may be less in the elderly as compared to younger adults (59). Therefore, adequate and up-to-date immunization against tetanus in the elderly is important.

If an elderly person has received the standard three primary doses of tetanus, a booster dose is only required every *10 years* after the last dose (5 years if the person suffers a wound that is tetanus prone, e.g., more than 6 hours old, devitalized tissue). For primary series, after the first dose, the second dose is given 4 to 8 weeks later, and the third dose is given 6 to 12 months after the second dose (60). The primary series in recommended for all elderly persons who have not been previously immunized or have an uncertain history of immunization (61). Elderly persons should receive the adult tetanus-diphtheria toxoid preparation (not pediatric preparation). (For wound management, see Chapter 17 on tetanus.)

REFERENCES

1. Yoshikawa TT: Geriatric infectious diseases: An emerging problem. *J Am Geriatr Soc* 31:34–39, 1983.
2. Sever JL: Infectious diseases and immunization. *Rev Infect Dis* 4:136–146, 1982.
3. Hirschmann JV, Inui TS: Antimicrobial prophylaxis: A critique of recent trials. *Rev Infect Dis* 2:1–23, 1980.
4. Oill PA: Antimicrobial chemoprophylaxis, in Yoshikawa TT, Chow AW, Guze LB (eds): *Infectious Diseases: Diagnosis and Management*. New York, John Wiley & Sons. 1980, p 777.
5. Shulman ST, Amren DP, Bisno AI, et al: Prevention of bacterial endocarditis: A statement for health professionals by the Committee on Rheumatic Fever and Infective Endocarditis of the Counsel on Cardiovascular Disease in the Young. *Circulation* 70:1123A–1127A, 1984.
6. Everett ED, Hirschmann JV: Transient bacteremia and endocarditis prophylaxis. A review. *Medicine* 56:61–77, 1977.
7. Guglielmo BJ, Hohn DC, Koo JJ, et al: Antibiotic prophylaxis in surgical procedures. *Arch Surg* 118:943–955, 1983.
8. National Academy of Sciences, National Research Council: Postoperative wound infections: The influence of ultraviolet irradiation of the operating room and various other factors. *Ann Surg* 160(suppl):1–192, 1964.
9. Polk HC, Jr, Simpson CJ, Simmons BP, et al: Guidelines for prevention of surgical wound infection. *Arch Surg* 118:1213–1217, 1983.

10. Peck JJ, Fuchs PC, Gustafson ME: Antimicrobial prophylaxis in elective colon surgery. Experience of 1,035 operations in a community hospital. *Am J Surg* 147:633-637, 1984.
11. Ellenbrogen A, Agranat A, Grunstein S: The role of vaginal hysterectomy in the aged woman. *J Am Geriatr Soc* 29:426-428, 1981.
12. Becker GD, Parell GJ: Cefazolin prophylaxis in head and neck cancer surgery. *Ann Otol Rhinol Laryngol* 88:183-186, 1979.
13. Johnson JT, Yu VL, Meyers EN, et al: Efficacy of two third-generation cephalosporins in prophylaxis for head and neck surgery. *Arch Otolaryngol* 110:224-227, 1984.
14. Johnson JT, Meyers EN, Thearle PB, et al: Antimicrobial prophylaxis for contaminated head and neck surgery. *Laryngoscope* 94:46-51, 1984.
15. Gatehouse D, Dimock F, Burden DW, et al: Prediction of wound sepsis following gastric operations. *Br J Surg* 65:551-554, 1978.
16. Stone HH, Haney BB, Kolb LD, et al: Prophylactic and preventive antibiotic therapy: Timing, duration and economics. *Ann Surg* 189:691-699, 1979.
17. Kaufman Z, Engelberg M, Eliashiv A, et al: Systemic prophylactic antibiotics in elective biliary surgery. *Arch Surg* 119:1002-1004, 1984.
18. Harnoss B-M, Hirner A, Krüselmann M, et al: Antibiotic infection prophylaxis in gallbladder surgery: A prospective randomized study. *Chemotherapy* 31:76-82, 1985.
19. Norman DC, Yoshikawa TT: Intraabdominal infection: Diagnosis and treatment in the elderly patient. *Gerontology* 30:327-338, 1984.
20. Thomas M, Browning AK, McFarland RJ: Excretion of cefuroxime in biliary disease. *Surg Gynecol Obstet* 158:272-274, 1984.
21. Kaiser AB, Roach AC, Mulherin JL, et al: The cost effectiveness of antimicrobial prophylaxis in clean vascular surgery. *J Infect Dis* 147:1103, 1983.
22. Norden CW: A critical review of antibiotic prophylaxis in orthopedic surgery. *Rev Infect Dis* 5:928-932, 1983.
23. Chodak GW, Plaut ME: Systemic antibiotics for prophylaxis in urologic surgery: A critical review. *J Urol* 121:695-699, 1979.
24. Childs SJ, Vaughan ED: Genitourinary surgical prophylaxis. *Infect Surg* 2:701-710, 1983.
25. Prokocimer P, Quazza M, Gebert C, et al: Short-term prophylactic antibiotics in patients undergoing prostatectomy: Report of a double-blind randomized trial with 2 intravenous doses of cefotaxime. *J Urol* 135:60-64, 1986.
26. Nichols RL, Smith JW, Klein DB, et al: Risk of infection after penetrating abdominal trauma. *N Engl J Med* 311:1065-1070, 1984.
27. Rowlands BJ, Ericsson CD: Comparative studies of antibiotic therapy after penetrating abdominal trauma. *Am J Surg* 148:791-795, 1984.
28. Gentry LO, Feliciano DV, Lea AS, et al: Perioperative antibiotic therapy for penetrating injuries of the abdomen. *Ann Surg* 200:564-566, 1984.
29. Dellinger EP, Wertz MJ, Lennard S, et al: Efficacy of short-course antibiotic prophylaxis after penetrating intestinal injury. A prospective randomized trial. *Arch Surg* 121:23-34, 1986.

30. Centers for Disease Control, Department of Health and Human Services: Recommendations for prevention and control of influenza: Recommendations of the Immunization Practices Advisory Committee. *Ann Intern Med* 105:399-404, 1986.
31. Hall WN, Goodman RA, Noble GR, et al: An outbreak of influenza B in an elderly population. *J Infect Dis* 144:297-302, 1981.
32. Van Voris LP, Belishe RB, Shaffer JL: Nosocomial influenza B virus infection in the elderly. *Ann Intern Med* 96:153-158, 1982.
33. Seneca H: Influenza: Epidemiology, etiology, immunization and management. *J Am Geriatr Soc* 28:241-250, 1980.
34. Immunization Practices Advisory Committee: Prevention and control of influenza. *MMWR* 35:317-331, 1986.
35. Ruben FL: Prevention of influenza in the elderly. *J Am Geriatr Soc* 30:577-580, 1982.
36. Horman JJ, Stetler HC, Israel E, et al: An outbreak of influenza A in a nursing home. *Am J Public Health* 76:501-504, 1986.
37. Phair J, Kauffman CA, Bjornson A, et al: Failure to respond to influenza vaccine in the aged: Correlation with B-cell numbers and function. *J Lab Clin Med* 92:822-828, 1978.
38. Brandriss MW, Schlesinger JJ, Douglas RG, Jr: Responses of elderly subjects to a new subunit influenza virus vaccine. *Rev Infect Dis* 145:277, 1982.
39. LaMontagne JR, Nobel GR, Quinnan GV, et al: Summary of clinical trials of inactivated influenza vaccine—1978. *Rev Infect Dis* 5:723-736, 1983.
40. Cate TR, Couch RB, Parker D, et al: Reactogenicity, immunogenicity, and antibody persistence in adults given inactivated influenza virus vaccines—1978. *Rev Infect Dis* 5:737-747, 1983.
41. Howells CHL, Jenkins-Vesselinova CK, Evans AD, et al: Influenza vaccination and mortality from bronchopneumonia in the elderly. *Lancet* 1:381-383, 1975.
42. Barker WH, Mullooly JP: Influenza vaccination of elderly persons. Reduction in pneumonia and influenza hospitalizations and deaths. *JAMA* 244:2547-2549, 1980.
43. Patriarca PA, Weber PA, Parker RA, et al: Efficacy of influenza vaccine in nursing homes: Reduction in illness and complications during an influenza A (H₃N₂) epidemic. *JAMA* 253:1136-1139, 1985.
44. Barker WH, Mullooly JP: Effectiveness of inactivated vaccine among noninstitutionalized elderly persons, in Kendall AP, Patriarca PA (eds): *Options for the Control of Influenza.* New York, Alan R. Liss, 1986, p 169.
45. Barker WH: Influenza and nursing homes. *Am J Public Health* 76:491-492, 1986.
46. Centers for Disease Control, Department of Health and Human Services: Monovalent influenza A (H₁N₁) vaccine, 1986-1987: Recommendations of the Immunization Practices Advisory Committee. *Ann Intern Med* 105:737-739, 1986.
47. Atkinson WL, Arden NH, Patriarca PA, et al:Amantadine prophylaxis during an institutional outbreak of type A(H₁N₁) influenza. *Arch Intern Med* 146:1751-1756, 1986.

48. Berk SL, Alvarez S: Vaccinating the elderly: Recommendations and rationale. *Geriatrics* 41:79–87, 1986.
49. Aoki FY, Sitar DS: Amantadine kinetics in healthy elderly men: Implications for influenza prevention. *Clin Pharmacol Ther* 37:137–144, 1985.
50. Fedson DS: Improving the use of pneumococcal vaccine through a strategy of hospital-based immunization: A review of its rationale and implications. *J Am Geriatr Soc* 33:142–150, 1985.
51. Health and Public Policy Committee, American College of Physicians: Pneumococcal vaccine. *Ann Intern Med* 104:118–120, 1986.
52. Smit P, Oberholzer D, Koornhof HJ, et al: Protective efficacy of pneumococcal polysaccharide vaccines. *JAMA* 238:2613–2616, 1977.
53. Bentley DW, Ha K, Mamot K, et al: Pneumococcal vaccine in the institutionalized elderly: Design of a nonrandomized trial and preliminary results. *Rev Infect Dis* 3(suppl):S71–S81, 1981.
54. Ammann AJ, Schiffman G, Austrian R: The antibody responses to pneumococcal capsular polysaccharides in aged individuals. *Proc Soc Exp Biol Med* 164:312–316, 1980.
55. Simberkoff MS, Cross AP, Al-Ibrahim M, et al: Efficacy of pneumococcal vaccine in high-risk patients: Results of a Veterans Administration cooperative study. *N Engl J Med* 315:1318–1327, 1986.
56. Division of Immunogenetics, Centers for Disease Control: Tetanus—United States, 1982–1984. *MMWR* 34:602–611, 1985.
57. Ruben FL, Nagel J, Fireman P: Antitoxin responses in the elderly to tetanus-diphtheria (TD) immunization. *Am J Epidemiol* 108:145–149, 1978.
58. Weiss BP, Strassburg MA, Feeley JC: Tetanus and diphtheria immunity in an elderly population in Los Angeles County. *Am J Public Health* 73:802–804, 1983.
59. Carbon PY, Tremolieres F, Gibert C: Serum levels of antibody to toxoid during tetanus and after specific immunization of patients with tetanus. *J Infect Dis* 145:278, 1982.
60. Immunization Practices Advisory Committee: Diphtheria, tetanus, and pertussis: Guidelines for vaccine prophylaxis and other preventive measures. *MMWR* 34:405–426, 1985.
61. Adams SL: Tetanus immunization for nursing home residents. *JAMA* 256:526, 1986.

SUGGESTED READINGS

Centers for Disease Control, Department of Health and Human Services: Recommendations for prevention and control of influenza. Recommendations of the Immunization Practices Advisory Committee. *Ann Intern Med* 105:399–404, 1986.
Division of Immunogenetics, Centers for Disease Control: Tetanus—United States, 1982–1984. *MMWR* 34:602–611, 1985.
Guglielmo BJ, Hohn DC, Koo PJ, et al: Antibiotic prophylaxis in surgical procedures. *Arch Surg* 118:943–955, 1983.

Health and Public Policy Committee, American College of Physicians: Pneumococcal vaccine. *Ann Intern Med* 104:118–120, 1986.

Immunization Practices Advisory Committee: Diphtheria, tetanus, and pertussis: Guidelines for vaccine prophylaxis and other preventive measures. *MMWR* 34:405–426, 1985.

Shulman ST, Amren DP, Bisno AI, et al: Prevention of bacterial endocarditis. A statement for health professionals by the Committee on Rheumatic Fever and Infective Endocarditis of the Counsel on Cardiovascular Disease in the Young. *Circulation* 70:1123A–1127A, 1984.

Chapter 7

Infections in the Nursing Home Population

GENERAL CONSIDERATIONS

In Chapter 1, it was stated that infections are a major problem or complication in nursing home residents or patients (hereafter also referred to as *nursing home population*). Additionally, the most common reason for hospitalization of the nursing home patient is an acute infectious disease process (1–3). However, precise data on the frequency, nature, and characteristics of infections in the nursing home population are not readily available, and existing studies are difficult to interpret. In large part, the confusion in interpretation of studies of infections in the nursing home population is due to differences in study design, methodology, and data analysis.

Study Design, Methodology, and Data Analysis

The majority of studies of nosocomial infections have been in acute care settings. The limited number of investigations done in long-term care institutions, such as a nursing home, have been predominantly at Veterans Administration facilities (4–8). Of course, this results in data collection on a predominantly male population, which is in contrast to the usual sex dominance of women in most community and private nursing homes and long-term care facilities.

Direct comparison of the studies is difficult because of the variability in data collection methods. Studies may be prospective or retrospective. Data collection may be based solely on chart reviews or may be obtained from investigators who examined the patients directly. Moreover, surveillance periods vary from study to study, which may be for 1 day (9,10), 1 month (8), 2 months (4), 6 months (10) or 1 year (5–7). Thus, the frequency and type of infection vary depending on the time of the year and duration of surveillance. For example, seasonal illnesses (e.g., influenza) and epidemic outbreaks of infection may or may not be included as part of the data, depending on the time and duration of the surveillance period.

Most acute hospital nosocomial studies record incidence rates per 100 discharges. This method has little application in the study of infections in long-term care facilities in which patients' average length of stay may be several years. Consequently, alternative methods have been used for data reporting of infection rates in nursing homes and chronic care institutions. Nevertheless, there remains a lack of consistency or uniformity in methodology. Methods used to report infection rates in long-stay facilities include infections per 100 patients at risk (4,9), infections per 100 patient care days (5), infections per 100 patient years (6), fevers (infections) per 24 patient months (7), infections per 100 resident months (10) and infections per 1,000 resident days (8). Thus, for clinicians (and investigators too!) marked differences in study design make analysis and comparison of study results difficult.

In Chapter 1, we defined the difference between incidence and prevalence. Most studies report incidence data but others may use prevalence data. Since incidence of infections records only the *new* infections that occurr in the surveillance period, this is a more accurate reflection of the infection rate. Prevalence of infection records all infections, new and old, during the observation period. Thus, such chronic infections as decubitus ulcers or catheter-related bacteriuria are overemphasized and yield an inaccurate pattern of infectious disease (7). Moreover, the criteria used to define an infection are also important in interpreting infection rate. For example, distinguishing between asymptomatic bacteriuria versus true symptomatic urinary tract infection is critical, as chronically catheterized bacteriuric elderly patients may be afebrile and may have no genitourinary complaints, and thus may be labeled as having *asymptomatic bacteriuria.* Yet, they may have true clinically relevant urinary tract infection that is manifested by such nonspecific symptoms as altered mentation, anorexia, weakness, and so on (see Chapter 3 on clinical features of infection). Also, criteria used to define fever may vary from investigator to investigator (5–7); infection may occur without fever in the elderly, leading to underestimation of the infection rate if its presence is used as a necessary criterion for infection.

Table 7.1 summarizes the study design and results of several recent reports on infections in long-term care facilities.

TYPES OF INFECTIONS

Despite the shortcomings of studies that survey the infection rates and types in the nursing home population, it can be seen from Table 7.1 that certain infections clearly occur with greater frequency, such as pneumonia, urinary tract infection, and skin/soft tissue infections. This trend is confirmed in a study of Setia et al., who surveyed the frequency of bacteremia in long-term care facilities (see Table 7.2 for a summary of this study) (11). A total of 100 cases of bacteremia were identified over a 24-month period of surveillance in 460 patients (342 women and 118 men) who resided in a long-term care facility. Of the 100 bacteremic cases, 56, 14, and 10 cases were caused by urinary tract infection, skin and soft tissue infection, and respiratory tract infection, respectively. The overall mortality was 35%. Nearly 70% of all bacteremia was caused by aerobic or facultative anaerobic gram-negative bacilli with 25% of bacteremic episodes due to gram-positive cocci; the remaining cases were mixed organisms and anaerobes.

The following discussion provides the brief and salient features of some of the important infections in the nursing home population. More detailed comments as well as management recommendations should be reviewed in the individual chapters that discuss some of these infections.

Pneumonia

Bacterial pneumonia is the most common lower respiratory tract infection in nursing home patients and is caused primarily by aspiration. Because colonization of the pharynx by gram-negative bacilli is a common occurrence in residents of nursing homes (12), aspiration pneumonia is associated with a relatively high number of cases of gram-negative bacillary pneumonia in this population. In nursing home patients in whom bacteriologic data could be obtained, *Streptococcus pneumoniae;* gram-negative bacilli, especially *Klebsiella* sp.; *Hemophilus influenzae; Staphylococcus aureus,* and anaerobes were found to be the dominant etiologic pathogens (6,7,11,13). Unfortunately, in almost half of the nursing home patients with clinical and radiologic evidence of pneumonia, sputum for culture is not obtainable (6,7). Thus, in nursing home patients with evidence of pneumonia in whom reliable sputum cannot be obtained, blood cultures should be drawn and patients should receive empiric antimicrobial therapy with such broad-spectrum antibiotics as cefuroxime or one of the third-generation cephalosporins. Patients should be treated in an acute care hospital unless the chronic

TABLE 7.1 Studies of Infections in Long-Stay Facilities

PARAMETER	STUDIES BY REFERENCE NUMBER					
	4	5	6	7	8	9
Type of facility	VA[a]	VA	VA	VA	VA	Com[b]
Prospective (P) or retrospective (R)	P	P	P	P	R	P
Prevalence (Pr) or incidence (In)	In	In	In	In	Pr	Pr
Duration of surveillance (months)	2	12	12	12	1	1/30 (1 day)
Infection rate: number of infections per	100 pt[c] at risk	100 pt care days	100 pt years	24 pt months	1000 pt days	100 pt at risk
Total number of patients infected	72	111	68	86	22	86
Mean or median age (years)	71	68	79	77	78	81
Total number of infections	72	127	111	114[d]	22	97
Pneumonia/Bronchitis	11/0	29/0	29/6	33/3	5/0	11/0
Urinary tract infection	58	34	3	26	11	14
Skin or soft tissue infection	9	2	21	2	5	32
Primary bacteremia	2	2	0	4	0	NS[e]
Gastroenteritis	NS	10	19	NS	0	7
Upper respiratory infection	NS	28	3	NS	1	8
Conjunctivitis	NS	15	NS	NS	0	18
Other infections	1	9	2	NS	0	7
Unknown	NS	NS	25	40	0	NS

[a]Veterans Administration.
[b]Community.
[c]Patients.
[d]Total fever episodes.
[e]Not stated.

TABLE 7.2 Bacteremia in a Long-Term Care Facility

PARAMETER	RESULTS
Total patients studied	460
Females	342
Males	118
Median age (range)	77 (20–100) years
Number of patients with positive blood cultures	100
Females	64
Males	36
Median age (range)	79 (20–100) years
Source of bacteremia	
Urinary tract	56
Skin/soft tissue	14
Respiratory tract	10
Gastrointestinal tract	6
Endocardium	4
Miscellaneous	3
Unknown	7
Pathogens isolated (all sites)	
Escherichia coli	33
Klebsiella sp.	15
Proteus sp.	14
Other gram-negative bacilli	10
Staphylococcus aureus	14
Streptococcus pneumoniae	1
Group D enterococcus	5
Other streptococci	7
Anaerobes	2
Polymicrobial causes	9

SOURCE: Adapted from reference 10.

care facility has (*1*) adequate 24-hour nursing for careful observation of patients; (*2*) ready access to such tests as arterial blood gas, microbiologic studies, x-rays, complete blood count and chemistry panel (electrolytes, renal function); (*3*) sufficient oxygen source and well-stocked pharmacy; and (*4*) a physician who is willing and capable of daily evaluation of the patient.

Urinary Tract Infection

The prevalence of urinary tract infection (UTI) in the elderly varies considerably depending on nature of the underlying disease(s), presence or absence of genitourinary abnormalities, and functional and residential status of the patient (14). In long-stay facilities, the prevalence of UTI has been reported to be 17 to 50% (14). Although elderly patients in nursing homes who are continent of urine do develop UTI, clearly incontinent patients, particularly those with chronic indwelling bladder catheters, have the highest frequency of developing bacteriuria (15,16). Therefore, the major concern and sources for UTI in the nursing home population is catheter-associated bacteriuria. Several important comments on catheter-related bacteriuria deserve emphasis:

1. Virtually all patients with chronic indwelling bladder catheters (i.e., over 30 days) have bacteriuria (9,17). Most patients are asymptomatic and do not require therapy.
2. Antibiotic therapy should be reserved for only those patients who develop clinical symptoms or a change in health status that is assumed to be due to UTI. Chronic administration of antibiotics does not permanently eliminate bacteriuria but only allows re-colonization of urine by organisms with multiple resistance (to antibiotics) (18,19).
3. Routine surveillance cultures of the urine have no value in pre-dicting the etiology of subsequent symptomatic UTI or urosepsis, because the bacterial flora rapidly changes, as early as 1 week to 1 month (20,21).
4. Culture of urine for microbiology from patients with chronic in-dwelling catheters should be performed *after* removal of the old catheter and insertion of a new catheter. Catheters in place for weeks to months become heavily colonized with multiple organisms, and these microorganisms may not be representative of the microflora in the bladder (22–24).
5. The microflora of catheter-associated bacteriuria is frequently polymicrobial with multiple species of gram-negative bacilli (*Escherichia coli, Klebsiella* sp., *Proteus* sp., *Enterobacter* sp., *Serratia marcescens, Pseudomonas* sp.), and enterococci. Under circumstances in which empiric antibiotic therapy is indicated, drugs with broad spectrum against gram-negative bacilli as well as enterococci are recommended (e.g., ampicillin plus an aminoglycoside or a third-generation cephalosporin).

Tuberculosis

Tuberculosis is now a disease primarily of the geriatric age group (25). Although reactivation of primary or previous tuberculous infection appears to be the major pathogenetic mechanism for most cases of tuberculosis in the elderly, new or primary infection does occur in the aged, especially those who live in nursing homes (26). In one nursing home study, 17% of the residents who became infected with mycobacteria (based on skin test conversion) developed primary pulmonary tuberculosis (27).

This infection can spread from an index case to other susceptible residents in the nursing home (27). Therefore, in the nursing home population, the following recommendations should be considered:

1. Routine tuberculin skin testing should be performed on all new patients who are admitted to a nursing home. Negative skin test results should be repeated along with control dermal antigens to exclude the booster effect and cutaneous anergy.
2. In patients who develop an insidious change in health status or well being, active tuberculosis must be excluded.
3. Chemoprophylaxis against tuberculosis should be considered for nursing home residents who are susceptible to active disease (see Chapter 11 on tuberculosis) (28).
4. Elderly patients who receive isoniazid for either treatment or chemoprophylaxis should have periodic monitoring of liver function tests.

Gastroenteritis

Any of the common causes of infectious diarrhea can occur in nursing home residents via person-to-person transmission or food contamination (29). Food poisoning secondary to *Staphylococcus aureus* and *Clostridium perfringens* are the most common types and should be considered as a cause for diarrhea in institutionalized elderly. Infections caused by *Shigella* sp., although not commonly reported in nursing homes, can be devastating because of the relatively low inoculum (10^{1}–10^{2} bacteria) required to cause infection (29). Rotavirus has been frequently reported as a cause of diarrhea in patients who reside in nursing homes (30,31). The attack rate in geriatric patients in long-term facilities may be between 35 to 50% (32). The disease is usually self-limiting, with 1–3 days of diarrhea and occasional vomiting, but it can cause death in the elderly (up to 10% affected), primarily from complications of dehydration.

In nursing home patients who develop diarrhea with or without vomiting, it should be determined immediately whether the patient is (*1*) septic (with fever), (*2*) adequately hydrated, and (*3*) able to take oral fluids. It should also be ascertained whether other patients have suffered similar types of symptoms. If the patient is clinically stable, then stool cultures for enteric pathogens (*Salmonella* sp., *Shigella* sp., *Campylobacter* sp., *Vibrio parahaemolyticus,* and *Yersinia enterocolitica*) should be taken, and the patient should be managed with oral fluids. Therapy is dictated by stool culture results. Sicker patients should be sent to an acute care facility. If rotavirus is suspected, serologic studies or special stool examination is necessary to confirm the diagnosis.

Hepatitis

Viral hepatitis can occur in the elderly. Hepatitis B infection in closed institutions for the aged does occur with significant frequency (33,34). Diagnosis is made by serologic studies and by liver function tests. Patients suspected of viral hepatitis (either A or B) should be temporarily kept in isolation with health care personnel practicing careful hygiene and precautions in handling of needles and stools. Elderly patients with viral hepatitis can be managed in the nursing home if (1) the patient is clinically stable and able to eat; (2) proper isolation techniques can be observed; and (3) laboratory tests to monitor liver function are available.

REFERENCES

1. Irvine PW, Van Buren N, Krossley K: Causes for hospitalization of nursing home residents: The role of infection. *J Am Geriatr Soc* 32:103–107, 1984.
2. Gordon WZ, Kane RL, Rothenberg R: Acute hospitalization in a home for the aged. *J Am Geriatr Soc* 33:519–523, 1985.
3. Tresch DD, Simpson WM, Burton JR: Relationship of long-term and acute-care facilities. The problem of patient transfer and continuity of care. *J Am Geriatr Soc* 33:819–826, 1985.
4. Magnussen MH, Robb SS: Nosocomial infections in a long-term care facility. *Am J Infect Control* 8:12–17, 1980.
5. Farber BF, Brennen C, Puntereri AJ, et al: A prospective study of nosocomial infections in a chronic care facility. *J Am Geriatr Soc* 32:499–502, 1984.
6. Nicolle LE, McIntyre M, Zacharias H, et al: Twelve-month surveillance of infections in institutionalized elderly men. *J Am Geriatr Soc* 32:513–519, 1984.
7. Finnegan TP, Austin TW, Cape RDT: A 12-month fever surveillance study in a Veterans' long-stay institution. *J Am Geriatr Soc* 33:590–594, 1985.
8. Franson TR, Duthe EH, Jr, Cooper JE, et al: Prevalence survey of infections and their predisposing factors at a hospital-based nursing home care unit. *J Am Geriatr Soc* 34:95–100, 1986.
9. Garibaldi RA, Brodine S, Matsumiya S: Infections among patients in nursing homes. *N Engl J Med* 305:731–735, 1981.
10. Scheckler WE, Peterson PJ: Infection and infection control among residents of eight rural Wisconsin nursing homes. *Arch Intern Med* 146:1981–1984, 1986.
11. Setia U, Serventi I, Lorenz P: Bacteremia in a long-term care facility. Spectrum and mortality. *Arch Intern Med* 144:1633–1635, 1984.
12. Valenti WM, Trudell RG, Bentley DW: Factors predisposing to oropharyngeal colonization with gram-negative bacilli in the aged. *N Engl J Med* 298:1108–1111, 1978.
13. Garb JL, Brown RB, Garb JR, et al: Difference in etiology of pneumonia in nursing home and community patients. *JAMA* 240:2169–2172, 1978.

14. Yoshikawa TT: Unique aspects of urinary tract infection in the geriatric population. *Gerontology* 30:339–344, 1984.
15. Ouslander JG, Kane RL, Abrass IB: Urinary incontinence in elderly nursing home patients. *JAMA* 248:1194–1198, 1982.
16. Sherman FT, Tucci V, Libow LS, et al: Nosocomial urinary-tract infections in a skilled nursing facility. *J Am Geriatr Soc* 28:456–461, 1980.
17. MacFarlane DE: Prevention and treatment of catheter-associated urinary tract infections. *J Infect* 10:96–106, 1985.
18. Bjork DT, Pelletier LL, Tight RR: Urinary tract infections with antibiotic resistant organisms in catheterized nursing home patients. *Infect Control* 5:173–176, 1984.
19. Gaynes RP, Weinstein RA, Chamberlin W, et al: Antibiotic-resistant flora in nursing home patients admitted to the hospital. *Arch Intern Med* 145: 1804–1807, 1985.
20. Alling B, Brandberg A, Seeberg S, et al: Aerobic and anaerobic microflora of the urinary tract of geriatric patients during long-term care. *J Infect Dis* 127:34–39, 1973.
21. Breitenbucher RB: Bacterial changes in the urine samples of patients with long-term indwelling catheters. *Arch Intern Med* 144:1585–1588, 1984.
22. Rubin M, Berger SA, Zodda FN, Jr, et al: Effect of catheter replacement on bacterial counts in urine aspirated from indwelling catheters. *J Infect Dis* 142:291, 1980.
23. Jones RF, Young PS, Marosszeky JE: Treatment of infection in the presence of indwelling urethral catheter. *Br J Urol* 54:316–319, 1982.
24. Grahn D, Norman DC, White ML, et al: Validity of urinary catheter specimen for diagnosis of urinary tract infections in the elderly. *Arch Intern Med* 145:1858–1860, 1985.
25. Nagami PH, Yoshikawa TT: Tuberculosis in the geriatric patient. *J Am Geriatr Soc* 31:356–363, 1983.
26. Stead WW, Lofgren JP, Warren E, et al: Tuberculosis as an endemic and nosocomial infection among the elderly in nursing homes. *N Engl J Med* 312:1483–1487, 1985.
27. Stead WW: Tuberculosis among elderly persons: An outbreak in a nursing home. *Ann Intern Med* 94:606–610, 1981.
28. Cooper JK: Decision analysis for tuberculosis preventive treatment in nursing homes. *J Am Geriatr Soc* 34:814–817, 1986.
29. Plotkin GR, Kluge RM, Waldman RH: Gastroenteritis: etiology, pathophysiology and clinical manifestations. *Medicine* 58:95–114, 1979.
30. Halvorsrud J, Orstavik I: An epidemic of rotavirus-associated gastroenteritis in a nursing home for the elderly. *Scand J Infect Dis* 12:161–164, 1980.
31. Cubitt WD, Hozel H: An outbreak of rotavirus infection in a long-stay ward of a geriatric hospital. *J Clin Pathol* 33:306–308, 1980.
32. Marrie TJ, Lee SHS, Faulkner RS, et al: Rotavirus infection in a geriatric population. *Arch Intern Med* 142:313–316, 1982.
33. Chiaramonte M, Floreani A, Naccarato R: Hepatitis B virus infection in homes for the aged. *J Med Virol* 9:247–255, 1982.
34. Feng CS: Prevalence of hepatitis B in an adult psychiatric hospital. *J Am Geriatr Soc* 30:326–328, 1982.

SUGGESTED READINGS

Finnegan TP, Austin TW, Cape RDT: A 12-month fever surveillance study in a Veterans' long-stay institution. *J Am Geriatr Soc* 30:590–594, 1985.

Garibaldi RA, Brodine S, Matsumiya S: Infections among patients in nursing homes. *N Engl J Med* 305:731–735, 1981.

Irvine PW, Van Buren N, Krossley K: Causes for hospitalization of nursing home residents: The role of infection. *J Am Geriatr Soc* 32:103–107, 1984.

Setia U, Serventi I, Lorenz P: Bacteremia in a long-term care facility. Spectrum and mortality. *Arch Intern Med* 144:1633–1635, 1984.

Part 2

SPECIFIC INFECTIOUS DISEASES

Chapter 8

Pericranial Infections

In this chapter, only infections that have a special predilection for the elderly or that are particularly severe in elderly persons are reviewed.

LUDWIG'S ANGINA

General Considerations

Ludwig's angina is a rapidly spreading, life-threatening infection that involves the submandibular, submaxillary, and sublingual spaces. Most cases are odontogenic in origin (50–90%), although tooth extraction, lacerations of the mouth, and peritonsillar abscess can predispose a person to this infection (1–4).

Etiology

As with other odontogenic infections, Ludwig's angina is caused by the oral microflora that are common to persons with poor oral hygiene (e.g., peridontal disease). This flora includes aerobic and anaerobic bacteria, with streptococci being the leading aerobic isolates and with *Bacteroides, Peptococcus,* and *Fusobacterium* species being the leading anaerobic isolates found in patients with odontogenic orofacial infections (3).

Clinical Manifestations

Patients usually appear toxic and classically have bilateral brawny non-pitting edema in the submandibular spaces (3). Elevation of the floor of the mouth occurs, and the tongue may obstruct the airway and impair swallowing. With progression of the infection, swelling of the face and neck may ensue and further compromise the airway.

Diagnostic Approach

Diagnosis is made on clinical grounds and should be considered in patients with painful swelling of the face and neck who complain of drooling, difficulty swallowing, or dyspnea (4).

Treatment

The airway must be carefully and quickly assessed in an intensive care setting. Tracheotomy, which in this case is safer than endotracheal intubation, may be necessary to preserve the airway.

Parenteral antibiotics should be begun shortly after blood cultures are obtained. Initially, chemotherapy should be initiated with a drug with effective activity against anaerobic bacteria (e.g., penicillin G [10–12 million units a day], clindamycin [1,200–2,400 mg a day], cefoxitin [8–12 g a day], metronidazole [1.5–2.0 g a day]). In patients who acquire the infection in a hospital or institutional setting, antibiotics that are effective against staphylococci (e.g., nafcillin, 8–12 g a day) and aerobic gram-negative bacilli (e.g., gentamicin, 5 mg/kg a day) should be added to the initial empiric regimen until culture data return.

If an abscess or fluctuance is present, needle aspiration or surgical drainage may be necessary (4). The fluid should be smeared by Gram stain and appropriately cultured for aerobic and anaerobic bacteria.

SUPPURATIVE PAROTITIS

Suppurative parotitis is seen predominantly in elderly patients with dehydration and/or sialolithiasis. Patients with this disease usually have fever and acute painful and tender swelling of the parotid gland. Staphylococci have been the most commonly isolated bacteria, and antimicrobial agents directed against this pathogen should be used (e.g., nafcillin [8–12 g a day], oxacillin [8–12 g a day], cefazolin [2–4 g a day]) (1,5). Surgical drainage and decompression of the gland may be required. As in the case of Ludwig's angina, progression of the infection may cause involvement of the deep tissues of the neck; therefore, patients with acute suppurative parotitis need to be monitored carefully for this complication.

BLEPHARITIS

Blepharitis is the term used to indicate inflammation of eyelid margins. Bacterial infection is the most common cause of this problem, and both *Staphylococcus aureus* and coagulase-negative staphylococci are the predominant pathogens.

Blepharitis may be acute or chronic and manifests as hyperemia and small ulcerations of the lid margins with crusted scaly exudate at bases of the eyelashes (6,7). Obstruction and suppuration of the meibomian glands may be present along with conjunctivitis (7).

Treatment is with topical antibiotics active against staphylococci (e.g., bacitracin) and lid scrubs with diluted shampoo. Occasionally, oral or parenteral antimicrobial therapy may be necessary. Cultures should be taken before initiation of therapy.

Ophthalmologic consultation should be obtained in most cases.

MALIGNANT EXTERNAL OTITIS

General Considerations

Malignant external otitis (MEO) is a rare but potentially fatal disease of the external ear canal that occurrs in elderly diabetics or debilitated patients (8–10). Mortality is high, ranging from 23 to 53% (8,10). The term *malignant* stems from the relentless, invasive nature of this disease (9), which often extends to involve important structures that are anatomically situated close to the external ear canal (e.g., temporal bone, cranial nerves, internal jugular vein, and carotid artery).

Etiology

Pseudomonas aeruginosa is isolated in virtually all cases, usually in pure culture. This pathogen is thought to be a "secondary invader" that replaces other bacterial flora that have colonized the skin of the external canal that has been damaged by trauma (10). Poor vascularity and propensity of *P. aeruginosa* to invade tissue and blood vessels as well as diminished host defenses in this population allows persistence and spread of infection (10).

Clinical Manifestations

MEO should be suspected in elderly diabetic patients with persistent otitis externa despite topical therapy. Symptoms and signs of MEO depend on whether or not extension of infection to adjacent structures has occurred. For example, involvement of the VII cranial nerve causes facial paralysis on the affected side. However, characteristic local symptoms and findings include ear pain with persistent drainage. Tender swelling of the auricle and periauricular tissues are usually present (8,10). Granulation tissue is seen on examination of the external ear canal, and probing may reveal diseased cartilage and pus (10). Of note, patients may be afebrile and appear nontoxic (8).

Diagnostic Approach

The diagnosis of MEO is made on clinical grounds. Culture of external ear canal tissue or exudate yields *P. aeruginosa* (see above).

Computed tomography and radionuclide bone scans as well as plain x-ray film tomography are useful in delineating bony destruction and soft tissue masses (10).

Treatment

MEO is best managed by a combination of parenteral antibiotic therapy and surgical débridement (11). Antimicrobial therapy should consist of an antipseudomonal penicillin, (azlocillin, piperacillin, or mezlocillin [all of these at 12–18 g a day]) that is combined with an aminoglycoside (e.g., tobramycin, 5 mg/kg a day). Other agents that are nonnephrotoxic but have good activity against *P. aeruginosa* include ceftazidime (4–6 g a day) and aztreonam (1–2 g a day) (11). In theory, these agents may be used alone in serious *P. aeruginosa* infections. However, susceptibility data that establish their in vitro effectiveness against the clinical isolate must be obtained before their use. In all patients who receive aminoglycosides, serial audiograms and renal function tests should be obtained, and serum peak and trough aminoglycoside levels should be carefully monitored to adjust optimally the aminoglycoside dosage.

REFERENCES

1. Chow AW: Infections of the oral cavity, neck and head, in Mandell GL, Douglas RG, Bennett JE, (eds): *Principles and Practice of Infectious Diseases.* New York, John Wiley & Sons, 1985, p 375.
2. Finegold SM, George WL, Mulligan ME: Anaerobic infections. Part I. *Disease-a-Month* 31:1–77, 1985.
3. Chow AW, Roger SM, Brady FA: Orofacial odontogenic infections. *Ann Intern Med* 88:392–402, 1978.
4. Corcoran JC, Axline SG: Infectious diseases in the geriatric patient. *Otolaryngol Clin North Am* 15(2):421–438, 1982.

5. Carpenter JL, Artenstein MS: Use of diagnostic microbiologic facilities in the diagnosis of head and neck infections. *Otolaryngol Clin North Am* 9(3): 611–629, 1976.
6. Hirst LW, Thomas JV, Green WR: Periocular infections, in Mandell GL, Douglas RG, Bennett JE, (eds): *Principles and Practice of Infectious Diseases.* New York, John Wiley & Sons, 1985, p. 767–771.
7. Smolin G, Okomoto M: Staphylococcal blepharitis. *Arch Ophthamol* 95: 812–816, 1977.
8. Zaky DA, Bentley DW, Lowy K, et al: Malignant external otitis: A severe form of otitis in diabetic patients. *Am J Med* 61:298–302, 1976.
9. Dawson DA: Malignant otitis externa. *J Laryngol Otol* 92:803–810, 1978.
10. Anon JB, Miller GW: Malignant external otitis. *South Med J* 77:1541–1544, 1984.
11. Neu HC: Contemporary antibiotic therapy in otolaryngology. *Otolaryngol Clin North Am* 17(4):745–760, 1984.

SUGGESTED READINGS

Anon JB, Miller GW: Malignant external otitis. *South Med J* 77:1541–1544, 1984.
Chow AW, Roger SM, Brady FA: Orofacial odontogenic infections. *Ann Intern Med* 88:392–402, 1978.
Neu HC: Contemporary antibiotic therapy in otolaryngology. *Otolaryngol Clin North Am* 17(4):745–760, 1984.

Chapter 9

Central Nervous System Infections

Central nervous system (CNS) infections in the elderly are relatively infrequent when compared to young children. However, in the adult population, certain CNS infections increase in frequency with advancing age. More importantly, CNS infections in the elderly (*1*) are associated with a high morbidity and mortality; (*2*) may not be diagnosed because of low clinical suspicion and atypical clinical features; and (*3*) may have etiologies that differ from those of younger adults.

In this chapter, the discussion focuses only on CNS infections that are especially relevant to the elderly and that may be encountered in clinical practice.

MENINGITIS

Whenever meningitis is diagnosed in an elderly patient, a bacterial or mycobacterial (tuberculous) pathogen should be considered as the most likely etiology. Although viral meningitis can occur in the older patient, its frequency is distinctly low. Therefore, clinicians should diagnose "aseptic" (viral) meningitis (which generally requires no chemotherapy) in the aged only after all other potentially treatable causes of CNS infections have been excluded. Table 9.1 summarizes the frequency of bacterial, tuberculous, and aseptic meningitis by age groups based on retro-

TABLE 9.1 Etiology of Meningitis by Age

AGE CATEGORY (YEARS)	NUMBER OF PATIENTS CLASSIFIED BY ETIOLOGY OF MENINGITIS		
	BACTERIAL	TUBERCULOUS	ASEPTIC
10–30	7	3	94
31–50	9	4	12
51–70	18	3	3
70+	9	1	0

SOURCE: Adapted from reference 1.

spective analysis of infectious meningitis (excluding a few cases of fungal causes) that occurred at a university referral hospital (1).

Bacterial Meningitis

GENERAL CONSIDERATIONS
Bacterial meningitis appears to be diagnosed more frequently in the geriatric population than in previous years. It is not clear whether this reflects a higher incidence or simply a greater diagnostic acumen by clinicians (2). In the general population, this infection has over a 90% mortality if untreated or if treated inappropriately, but with early appropriate therapy the death rate may be reduced to 10 to 20% (3). In the elderly mortality rates range from 40 to 80% despite appropriate antimicrobial therapy (4,5). Factors that contribute to the high mortality include delays in diagnosis and therefore delays in treatment, presence of underlying diseases, and etiologic pathogens that are difficult to eradicate (6).

ETIOLOGY
In neonates, streptococci (especially group B), aerobic gram-negative bacilli (especially *Escherichia coli*), and *Listeria monocytogenes* are the most common causes of bacterial meningitis. As children get older, *Hemophilis influenzae, Neisseria meningitidis,* and *Streptococcus pneumoniae* dominate as meningopathogens. In healthy adults *N. meningitidis* and *S. pneumoniae* are the primary causes of meningitis (7). However, in the elderly, the bacterial etiology of meningitis closely resembles that of neonates and children such as *S. pneumoniae,* aerobic gram-negative bacilli, *Listeria monocytogenes, N. meningitidis,* and occasionally *H. influenzae* (4,6,8). Moreover, *L. monocytogenes, E. coli,* and *Klebsiella* sp. meningitis (nontraumatic) occur almost exclusively in neonates, the el-

derly, and immunosuppressed hosts and are associated with exceedingly high mortality (9,10). It would appear that defects in host defense mechanisms may be a common predisposing factor in all three groups (see Chapter 2 on predisposing factors to infection).

CLINICAL MANIFESTATIONS
Presentation. Most patients with bacterial meningitis, including the elderly, develop abrupt onset of fever, headache, altered mental status, and nuchal rigidity (2). However, in a small but significant number of old patients with meningitis, these typical manifestations of meningitis may be absent or minimal. Symptoms may be insidious, as long as 42 days (4); fever may be low grade without headache or nuchal rigidity, particularly in cases of gram-negative bacillary meningitis (11,12). Furthermore, unexplained mental status change or seizures may be the only finding (12). To further confuse matters, nuchal rigidity is frequently found in elderly patients without meningitis because of such common disorders as cerebrovascular accident and cervical spine disease among others (13).

Source of Infection. Meningitis may result from other focal infections. Moreover, the site of infection may provide clues to the etiology of bacterial meningitis. Table 9.2 shows the common meningopathogens that cause meningitis in the elderly and the common probable source for these organisms. The presence of one of these primary infections should alert the physician to the possibility of a secondary bacterial meningitis in the elderly, especially if the patient's clinical and/or mental status does not improve with therapy of the primary infection.

DIAGNOSTIC APPROACH
Differential Diagnosis. The other diagnostic considerations include nonbacterial causes of meningitis, brain abscess, sepsis, stroke, or subdural hematoma.

Lumbar Puncture. The diagnosis of bacterial meningitis is only confirmed by examination of the cerebrospinal fluid (CSF). However, a lumbar puncture should be postponed in patients in whom a CNS mass lesion or intracranial hypertension is suspected, that is, in patients with focal neurologic findings, rapid obtundation, or papilledema. In these elderly patients, a computed tomography (CT) scan should be done immediately. If the CT scan does not show evidence of a mass effect or intracranial hypertension, a lumbar puncture should then be performed. The CSF findings of bacterial meningitis in the elderly are the same as

TABLE 9.2 Meningopathogens in the Elderly
and Their Primary Source of Infection

MENINGOPATHOGEN	PRIMARY SOURCE OF INFECTION
Streptococcus pneumoniae	Lungs, middle ear, mastoid, skull fracture
Gram-negative bacilli	Urinary tract, cranial surgery or trauma, pressure sore, bone, lungs
Listeria monocytogenes	Unknown. Possibly from contaminated foods or animal contact
Neisseria meningitidis	Pharynx (asymptomatic carrier)
Hemophilus influenzae	Lungs

those for younger patients. The opening pressure is often elevated, the total white blood cell count is generally over 500/mm^3 with a differential count showing more than 90% polymorphonuclear white blood cells (PMN); the protein concentration is high, usually above 100 mg/dl; there is hypoglycorrhachia (low CSF glucose—40 mg/dl or less) with the CSF glucose less than 40% of a simultaneous peripheral blood glucose; and a positive Gram stain in 60 to 80% of cases. The CSF should be sent immediately for culture. If the CSF Gram stain is negative, the specimen should be processed for the following: (*1*) counterimmunoelectrophoresis (or latex agglutination) for bacterial antigens (*N. meningitidis, H. influenzae, S. pneumoniae, E. coli*); (*2*) limulus lysate assay for endotoxin (for gram-negative bacilli as well as *H. influenzae* and *N. meningitidis*); (*3*) India ink preparation; (*4*) acid-fast bacilli smear; (*5*) serology for cryptococcal antigen and coccidioidal complement fixation tests (in western and southwestern U.S.); and (*6*) culture for mycobacteria and fungi. Although fungal and mycobacterial meningitis typically have a lymphocytic predominance in the CSF white cell count, these infections on occasion can present early in their course with a predominance of PMNs.

Other Tests. All elderly patients should have blood cultures obtained. A chest x-ray, urinalysis with culture, blood glucose, and complete blood count are essential. Ordering of other microbiologic studies as well as diagnostic x-rays or scans are dependent on clinical findings and evidence of other sites of infection.

TREATMENT
If clinical evidence of sepsis with unstable hemodynamic parameters is present, this is the first priority in management (see Chapter 18 on sepsis for details).

Bacterial meningitis is only effectively treated with high-dose intravenous antibiotics. Treatment must be initiated as soon as the diagnosis is suspected and after appropriate diagnostic studies have been obtained. Based on the Gram stain findings, a reasonably accurate guess of the potential meningopathogen can be made, and then appropriate antibiotics can be started before CSF or blood culture data return. Table 9.3 provides suggestions for antibiotic treatment based on CSF Gram stain findings.

In elderly patients in whom the CSF Gram stain findings are negative but bacterial meningitis is still suspected, empiric antimicrobial therapy is recommended. In the absence of any identifiable predisposing factors or other primary site of infection, the antibiotic of choice would be penicillin G, 20 million units a day, (or ampicillin 12 g a day) plus an aminoglycoside (e.g., amikacin 15 mg/kg a day). Other alternative regimens could be (1) chloramphenicol 4–6 g a day plus an aminoglycoside; (2) trimethoprim-sulfamethoxazole (10–15 mg/kg a day of trimethoprim and 50–75 mg/kg a day of sulfamethoxazole) plus an aminoglycoside; or (3) ampicillin plus a third-generation cephalosporin.

A special comment should be made regarding gram-negative bacillary meningitis. These infections have a high mortality and are difficult to treat. In suspected cases (based on CSF Gram stain, limulus lysate test, or presence of gram-negative infection at another site), empiric treatment should be with a third-generation cephalosporin (ceftizoxime, ceftriaxone, cefotaxime, or ceftazidime) combined with an aminoglycoside. When CSF culture results confirm a specific gram-negative bacilli, then the aminoglycoside may be discontinued if the organism is susceptible to one of the third-generation cephalosporins. However, in some patients, the organism may only be susceptible to an aminoglycoside, and in such cases, daily supplemental intrathecal aminoglycoside may be required in addition to intravenous doses.

Elderly patients should be treated for a minimum of 14 days. Other complications should be aggressively managed (e.g., seizures, cerebral edema, syndrome of inappropriate antidiuretic hormone [SIADH], aspiration, etc.).

PREVENTION

With the exception of a few organisms, prevention of bacterial meningitis for close contacts to an index case is not a concern. For contacts of a patient with *N. meningitidis* (meningococcal) meningitis, chemoprophylaxis with rifampin is indicated for (1) members of the same household; (2) persons who have had close contact with index case for 4 or more hours a day during the week before onset of the meningitis; and (3) hospital personnel who have had intimate contact with infected patients' respiratory secretions (14). Adults should receive rifampin in an oral dose of 600 mg every 12 hours for 2 days; children 1 month to 12 years should receive 10 mg per kilogram body weight every 12 hours for 2 days with one-half this dose given to children under 1 month of age. If the *N. meningitidis* is a type A, C, Y, or W-135 strain, vaccines for these strains are available and should be administered to all close contacts (as indicated above) (14).

Occasionally, *H. influenzae* may cause meningitis in an elderly person. Close contacts (as defined above for meningococcal meningitis), especially children, should receive rifampin prophylaxis. Adults also require chemoprophylaxis to eliminate colonization from all contacts. Rifampin for adults is given orally in a dose of 600 mg once a day for 4 days; children 1 month to 12 years of age should receive 20 mg per kilogram body weight once a day for 4 days and those younger than 1 month should receive half this dose (14).

Tuberculous Meningitis

GENERAL CONSIDERATIONS

Tuberculosis is now a disease primarily of the elderly (see Chapter 11 on tuberculosis) (15). Thus, it is not surprising that older persons may contract extrapulmonary tuberculosis, including tuberculous meningitis. The pathogenesis of tuberculous meningitis occurs in two stages. Initially, a primary tuberculosis infection (usually lung) or, less commonly, chronic pulmonary or extrapulmonary tuberculosis causes hematogenous spread of the mycobacteria organisms to the brain or meninges. Occasionally, this may result in meningitis, but usually a caseous focus develops. At some later time, the caseous focus discharges tuberculous organisms or antigens into the subarachnoid space that result in meningitis (16).

Earlier studies of tuberculous meningitis indicated only a 4 to 15% incidence in persons 60 years and older (17,18). However, in a more recent study approximately 40% of the 21 cases of tuberculous meningitis were in this age group (19). More importantly, in this investigation, five of six patients over 65 years died. Elderly survivors were all left with serious neurologic sequelae, that is, hemiplegia or hydrocephalus. Thus, like bacterial meningitis, tuberculosis of the CNS is a devastating infection in the geriatric patient.

ETIOLOGY

Most cases of tuberculous meningitis in the elderly are caused by *Mycobacterium tuberculosis*. Rarely, there may be an occasional elderly patient with nontuberculous mycobacterial meningitis (19).

TABLE 9.3 Empiric Antibiotic Therapy for Meningitis in the Elderly

GRAM STAIN FINDINGS	POTENTIAL ORGANISM(S)	TREATMENT OF CHOICE	ALTERNATE DRUGS
Gram-positive cocci	Streptococcus pneumoniae Staphyloeoccus aureus	Penicillin G[a] (or Ampicillin[b]) PLUS Nafcillin[c] (or Oxacillin[c])	Vancomycin[d]
Gram-positive diplococci	S. pneumoniae	Penicillin G OR Ampicillin	Chloramphenicol[e] OR Trimethoprim-sulfamethoxazole (TMP-SMZ)[f] OR Vancomycin
Gram-positive bacilli	Listeria monocytogenes	Penicillin G OR Ampicillin	TMP-SMZ OR ?Chloramphenicol OR ?Vancomycin OR ?Imipenem[g]

Organism		
Gram-negative cocci	*Neisseria meningitidis*	Penicillin G OR Ampicillin	Chloramphenicol OR TMP-SMZ OR Ceftriaxone[g]
Gram-negative bacilli	*Escherichia coli* *Klebsiella* sp.	Ceftriaxone[h] PLUS aminoglycoside[i]	Piperacillin[j] PLUS aminoglycoside OR TMP-SMZ PLUS aminoglycoside

NOTE: The following doses are for normal renal function.
[a] 20 million units/day in 6 divided doses.
[b] 12 g/day in 6 divided doses.
[c] 12 g/day in 6 divided doses.
[d] 1.5–2.0 g/day in 2 or 4 divided doses.
[e] 4–6 g/day in 4 divided doses.
[f] 10–15 mg/kg/day TMP and 50–75 mg/kg/day SMZ in 3–4 divided doses.
[g] 4 g/day in 4 divided doses (efficacy not proven).
[h] 4 g/day in 2 divided doses; ceftizoxime, cefotaxime, or ceftazidime may be equally effective. If *Pseudomonas* is considered, ceftazidime (6 g/day in 3 divided doses) should be used.
[i] Amikacin 15 mg/kg in 2 divided doses is preferred.
[j] 18 g/day in 6 divided doses.

CLINICAL MANIFESTATIONS

The clinical features of tuberculous meningitis correlate well with the pathologic processes that occurr in the CNS: (1) hypersensitivity reaction to mycobacterial antigen which causes CSF changes; (2) vasculitis and vascular occlusion which lead to focal neurologic deficits; (3) thick basilar exudate which results in cranial nerve palsies and hydrocephalus; (4) cerebral edema which produces impaired consciousness, intracranial hypertension, and seizures; and (5) tuberculomas which act as space-occupying lesions (20).

In the elderly, the disease tends to be insidious in onset, although some patients may present as acute meningitis. Nonspecific symptoms of fatigue, weakness, and anorexia are often associated with headache, intermittent or persistent low-grade fever, altered mental status, or changes in behavior. Depending on which pathologic processes are present, the elderly patient may be alert, drowsy or comatose; have focal or generalized seizures; develop cranial nerve palsies or focal neurologic deficits including hemiplegia; or show cerebrate or decorticate posturing, coma, fixed and dilated pupils, and unstable blood pressure, pulse, and respiration. Paradoxically, in some older patients, nuchal rigidity and fever may be absent.

DIAGNOSTIC APPROACH

Differential Diagnosis. Fungal meningitis, *Listeria monocytogenes* meningitis (which can show a lymphocyte-predominance in the CSF), brain abscess, partially treated bacterial meningitis, and neurosyphilis are the major infections along with tuberculosis to consider in elderly patients who have the above-described clinical syndrome and who have a CSF examination as discussed below.

Lumbar Puncture. Like bacterial meningitis, examination of the CSF is essential to the diagnosis of mycobacterial meningitis. However, because a brain abscess (or other mass lesions) may be in the differential diagnosis, a brain CT scan should be done before a lumbar puncture. If the CT scan is negative (i.e., no mass effect), then examination of the CSF should be expedited quickly. The typical CSF findings in tuberculous meningitis are the following: (1) total white blood cell count of 100–500/mm^3 with a predominance of lymphocytes or mononuclear cells (less than 60 or 70% PMNs); (2) protein concentration of 100–500 mg/dl (higher with CSF block); (3) glucose less than 40 mg/dl or less than 40% of simultaneously measured blood glucose; and (4) positive smear for acid-fast bacilli (AFB) (which is positive in 20–40% of cases but increases up to

90% with centrifugation of 10–20 ml CSF and examining the pellet). The CSF culture for *M. tuberculosis* is positive up to 90% of cases (20) but requires incubation for at least 6 weeks. Because the initial CSF findings may be nondiagnostic, and a routine AFB smear is likely to be negative, repeat lumbar punctures with diligent and careful examination of the CSF are important in order to make a diagnosis of tuberculous meningitis. An enzyme-linked immunosorbent assay (ELISA) for mycobacterial antigen appears promising (specificity 95%; sensitivity 81%) as a diagnostic test for tuberculous meningitis (21). However, experience is limited using this test.

Other Tests. Evidence for pulmonary tuberculosis should be sought on chest x-ray. Elderly patients may have the usual or atypical sites of pulmonary tuberculosis, for example, lower lobes or bilateral involvement (20). A miliary pattern, hilar adenopathy, or no abnormalities may be seen on chest x-ray in elderly patients with tuberculous meningitis. A tuberculin skin test with intermediate strength (5 tuberculin units) purified protein derivative (PPD) should be placed and read at 48 hours. The skin test may be positive in 40 to 80% of cases (17,18).

TREATMENT

In all suspected cases of tuberculous meningitis, antituberculous chemotherapy should be initiated immediately since the AFB smear may be negative and culture data require up to 6 weeks for confirmation. The treatment of choice is isoniazid 300 mg a day taken orally and oral rifampin 600 mg a day. Pyridoxine 50 mg a day should be added to prevent the peripheral neuropathy associated with prolonged or high-dose administration of isoniazid. This daily regimen may be continued for 9 months. However, more recently, a twice-weekly regimen of these drugs has proven to be equally efficacious for extrapulmonary tuberculosis, including meningitis (22). Isoniazid and rifampin are administered daily in the above dose, for 1 month. This regimen is then followed by isoniazid, 900 mg, and rifampin, 600 mg, taken twice weekly for 8 months (22).

In order to minimize or prevent cerebral edema, hydrocephalus, or irreversible neurologic deficits, or blocks, corticosteroids have been recommended for tuberculous meningitis complicated by (*1*) altered consciousness; (*2*) focal neurologic abnormalities; (*3*) elevated CSF pressure above 300 mm water; and (*4*) CSF block (23). Prednisone in a dose of 60 mg a day is given for 1 to 2 weeks and then gradually tapered over the next 4 weeks (23).

Complications such as seizures and hydrocephalus require active treatment, that is, anticonvulsants and shunting procedures, respectively. Unfortunately, despite early therapy such complications as focal neurologic deficits (hemiplegia, paraplegia), cranial nerve palsies, visual and auditory deficits, and loss of cognitive function is common in these patients.

PREVENTION
Prevention of tuberculous meningitis can only be achieved by preventing tuberculosis in general and actively treating other sites of tuberculous infections (see Chapter 11 on tuberculosis for discussion on chemoprophylaxis).

Brain Abscess

GENERAL CONSIDERATIONS
The elderly do not appear to have an unusually high predisposition to develop brain abscesses. However, many of the predisposing factors or associated conditions for brain abscess do occur in the elderly. Since this infection is potentially curable, it is important to consider it in the differential diagnosis of CNS infections. Although the overall mortality for brain abscess had been nearly 40% (24), recent death rates due to this infection have been reported to be closer to 5 to 10% (25). This improvement appears to be due primarily to earlier recognition and diagnosis of brain abscesses from the use of CT scanning of the brain and possibly from improved understanding of the microbiology and advances in antimicrobial therapy.

ETIOLOGY
The pathogens that cause brain abscesses are diverse and often polymicrobial depending on the predisposing site of infection or the associated clinical conditions. As a general rule, streptococci and anaerobic bacteria dominate as the causes of brain abscess (25,26). These organisms are associated with brain abscesses secondary to sinusitis, dental sepsis, and pleuropulmonary infections, and they invade the brain directly or via bacteremia. *Staphylococcus aureus* can be isolated from abscesses associated with osteomyelitis, cranial trauma, postoperative infection, endocarditis, and pneumonia (25). Ear and mastoid infections can result in brain abscesses due to *Bacteroides fragilis* and aerobic gram-negative bacilli. In immunocompromised elderly patients, aerobic gram-negative bacilli, fungi (*Cryptococcus neoformans, Aspergillus* sp., *Candida* sp.) and

such unusual pathogens as *Nocardia* sp. and *Toxoplasma gondii* can be the cause of brain abscess (25).

CLINICAL MANIFESTATIONS

The clinical manifestations vary depending on the rapidity with which the infection develops; the degree of associated cerebral edema; the area of brain involvement; the number of abscesses present; the presence of a mass effect; and the occurrence of a secondary meningitis or ventriculitis (27). Symptoms may be present for 1 or 2 weeks or may develop slowly over several months. Fever is present in half the patients, and altered consciousness or impaired cognitive function may be present as well. Nausea, vomiting, and headache are common symptoms, and focal neurologic deficits may be apparent.

Clinical findings of extra-CNS infection such as sinusitis, otitis media or mastoiditis, dental abscess, pleuropulmonary infection, endocarditis, intraabdominal abscess, or osteomyelitis may be present.

DIAGNOSTIC APPROACH

Differential Diagnosis.   Such CNS infections as bacterial meningitis, tuberculous or fungal meningitis, and subdural empyema may be confused with brain abscess. Certainly in the elderly such noninfectious problems as stroke, brain tumor (primary or metastatic), and subdural hematoma must be excluded.

Computed Tomography.   A noncontrast brain CT scan should be done immediately to make the diagnosis of a brain abscess. If this result is negative or equivocal and the diagnosis is still suspected, the CT scan should be repeated with contrast dye. In some instances, particularly early in the abscess formation (i.e., "cerebritis" stage), a CT scan even with contrast may be unremarkable. In such circumstances, a radionuclide brain scan may be abnormal (25). An arteriogram should be used only if the CT scan fails to differentiate a brain abscess from other mass lesions (e.g., tumor or arteriovenous malformation). A lumbar puncture should be avoided if a mass lesion is found on CT scan because of the risk of herniation. An electroencephalogram may show focal findings, but this abnormality is nonspecific.

Other Studies.   Blood cultures should be obtained. Evaluation for other sites of infections should be initiated based on clinical findings. At operation, the abscess fluid should be immediately Gram stained and sent for aerobic, anaerobic, and fungal cultures.

TREATMENT

Once the diagnosis is made clinically, the treatment of choice is an operation. Before taking the patient for the operation, intravenous antibiotics should be initiated in order to (1) treat the associated cerebritis and (2) minimize contamination of normal brain tissue during the operation. Preoperative antibiotics rarely diminish the yield of the culture of abscess fluid. Selection of antibiotics may be guided by the associated infection or predisposing factors. However, frequently this is not practical. Under these circumstances, such as when there are no clues to a potential etiologic pathogen(s), intravenous antibiotics with the following regimen is recommended: penicillin G, 20–30 million units a day in six divided doses and metronidazole 2 g a day in four divided doses. If staphylococci are suspected, nafcillin or oxacillin 12–16 g a day in six divided doses should be added; if aerobic gram-negative bacilli are suspected, ceftazidime 6 g a day in three divided doses should be added. In patients allergic to penicillin, chloramphenicol 6 g a day in four divided doses with or without vancomycin 1.5–2.0 g a day in two to four divided doses can be used. Some investigators have suggested combining metronidazole with a third-generation cephalosporin as a regimen for empiric therapy (25). After the operation, the antibiotic regimen should be appropriately changed depending on results of the initial Gram stain and subsequent culture of the abscess fluid. Antibiotics should be continued for 4 to 8 weeks.

Under defined circumstances, some brain abscesses may be managed medically alone without an operation (27). The conditions that may permit nonsurgical intervention for brain abscess include (1) excessive risk for operation; (2) presence of multiple small abscesses; (3) abscesses located in deep or dominant location; (4) presence of meningitis or ependymitis; (5) presence of single small (less than 4 cm in diameter) abscess; and (6) presence of hydrocephalus that requires a CSF shunt that might become infected during the abscess operation (25). Medical therapy alone generally requires antibiotic administration for 8 weeks or longer (27). However, neurosurgical consultation throughout the course of illness is mandatory in all cases.

PREVENTION

Brain abscess can only be prevented by prompt recognition and treatment of those conditions that may lead to this infection.

Neurosyphilis

GENERAL CONSIDERATIONS

With the exception of the infrequent case of acute meningitis associated with secondary syphilis, neurosyphilis is a late form of syphilis. Depending on the type of neurosyphilis, the clinical manifestations may appear from months to 20 to 25 years after the primary exposure (28). Thus, neurosyphilis can potentially occur in middle- to old-aged persons. In one study the mean age of patients with neurosyphilis was 65 years (29). Approximately 10% of untreated cases of syphilis develop neurosyphilis (30).

ETIOLOGY
Treponema pallidum, a spirochete, is the etiologic pathogen of syphilis.

CLINICAL MANIFESTATIONS
The clinical features of neurosyphilis appear to have changed during the modern antibiotic era. Whereas tabes dorsalis and paresis were the dominant types of neurosyphilis in the 1930s and 1940s, meningovascular syphilis as well as seizures and neuroophthalmic involvement are the more common forms and findings of neurosyphilis in modern times (28,29). Meningovascular syphilis presents as a stroke or at times as a encephalomalacia with focal neurologic signs. Neuroophthalmic abnormalities include optic atrophy that results in vision loss, disorders of eye movement, and pupillary dysfunction (Argyll Robertson pupil).

Paresis is a form of dementia that results from syphilis. Patients develop insidious onset of deficits in memory, judgment, orientation, and cognitive function as well as behavior and personality changes. Tabes dorsalis is spinal syphilis characterized by lightning pains, ataxia, absence of stretch reflexes, pupil abnormalities, bladder dysfunction, and impotence (28).

Of note, 30 to 40% of cases of neurosyphilis may have no neurologic findings.

DIAGNOSTIC APPROACH
Differential Diagnosis.   Depending on the form of neurosyphilis, the differential diagnosis includes stroke, brain abscess, tuberculous meningitis, fungal meningitis, and the various causes of dementia.

Serology and Lumbar Puncture.   Neurosyphilis is diagnosed by one of the following criteria: (*1*) a positive serum fluorescent treponemal antibody absorption (FTA-ABS) or microhemagglutination assay for *T. pallidum* (MHA-TP) with neurologic or ophthalmologic findings consistent with neurosyphilis; (*2*) a positive serum FTA-ABS or MHA-TP with CSF abnormalities (elevated while cells and/or protein) not attributable to other causes; or (*3*) a positive serum FTA-ABS or MHA-TP with positive CSF VDRL (Veneral Disease Research Laboratory: a nontreponemal serologic test). Serum VDRL is insensitive and fails to diagnose 25% of late syphilis cases; therefore the FTA-ABS or MHA-TP should be used as the definitive test. A negative serum FTA-ABS or MHA-TP virtually excludes late syphilis including neurosyphilis. The FTA-ABS is not used for the CSF because of its lack of specificity; the CSF VDRL is specific but not sensitive (31). The activity of neurosyphilis is determined by the CSF cell count and/or protein.

Because many elderly patients have asymptomatic neurosyphilis, several questions arise: Should all asymptomatic elderly patients with a positive serology undergo a lumbar puncture to exclude or make the diagnosis of neurosyphilis and to determine its activity? Does the expense, discomfort, yield of diagnosis, and small risk warrant a lumbar puncture? (31). Some helpful guidelines follow:

1. In elderly patients with positive serology and neurologic features consistent with neurosyphilis, a lumbar puncture is mandatory.
2. In elderly patients with a positive serology and no clinical evidence of neurosyphilis, a lumbar puncture is recommended if the date of the primary infection is *less than 30 years ago or is unknown.* If the interval is over 30 years, a lumbar puncture is unnecessary. It is unusual for elderly persons to develop neurosyphilis after 30 years from the primary infection (33).

TREATMENT

Therapy should be based on whether the elderly patient has symptomatic disease or asymptomatic neurosyphilis. In patients with neurologic manifestations, treatment should be with intravenous penicillin G, 12–24 million units a day in six divided doses for 10 days followed by benzathine penicillin G 2.4 million units intramuscularly once a week for 3 weeks. In elderly asymptomatic patients, benzathine penicillin 2.4 million units intramuscularly once a week for 3 weeks is administered.

In patients with clinical neurologic findings or in asymptomatic neurosyphilis patients in whom CSF findings show activity, a repeat CSF examination should be performed every 6 months until the CSF parameters are normal. If after 3 years the patient does not improve or stabilize, or the CSF changes do not normalize, the patient should be treated again. A quantitated serum nontreponemal test (VDRL) should be checked every 3 months in the first year and every 6 months thereafter until the titer falls or becomes negative.

Patients allergic to penicillin can be given oral tetracycline or erythromycin, 2 g a day for 30 days. However, this regimen has not been proven to be efficacious for neurosyphilis.

PREVENTION

Neurosyphilis can only be prevented by identifying all cases of syphilis *before* the stage of neurosyphilis and initiating effective chemotherapy.

REFERENCES

1. Karandanis D, Shulman JA: Recent survey of infectious meningitis in adults: Review of laboratory findings in bacterial, tuberculous and aseptic meningitis. *South Med J* 69:449–457, 1969.
2. Norman DC, Yoshikawa TT: Recognizing bacterial meningitis in the elderly. *Geriatr Med Today* 3:85–88, 1984.
3. Yoshikawa TT: Meningitis and encephalitis, in Yoshikawa TT, Chow AW, Guze LB (eds): *Infectious Diseases. Diagnosis and Management.* New York, John Wiley & Sons, 1980, p 45.
4. Gorse GJ, Thrupp LD, Nudleman KL, et al: Bacterial meningitis in the elderly. *Arch Intern Med* 144:1603–1607, 1984.
5. Finland M, Barnes MW: Acute bacterial meningitis at Boston City Hospital during 12 selected years, 1935–1972. *J Infect Dis* 136:400–415, 1977.
6. Berk SL: Bacterial meningitis, in Gleckman RA, Gantz NM (eds): *Infections in the Elderly.* Boston, Little Brown and Co., 1983, p 235.
7. Bolan G, Barza M: Acute bacterial meningitis in children and adults: A perspective. *Med Clin North Am* 69:231–241, 1985.
8. Newton JE, Wilczynski RJG: Meningitis in the elderly. *Lancet* 2:157–158, 1979.
9. Cherubin CE, Marr JS, Sierra MF, et al: Listeria and gram-negative bacillary meningitis in New York City, 1972–1979. *Am J Med* 71:199–209, 1981.
10. Rubin RH, Hooper DC: Central nervous system infection in the compromised host. *Med Clin North Am* 69:281–296, 1985.
11. LeFrock JL, Smith BR, Molavi A: Gram-negative bacillary meningitis. *Med Clin North Am* 69:243–256, 1985.
12. Berk SL, McCabe WR: Meningitis caused by gram-negative bacilli. *Ann Intern Med* 93:253–260, 1980.
13. Puxty JAH, Fox RA, Horan MA: The frequency of physical signs usually attributed to meningeal irritation in elderly patients. *J Am Geriatr Soc* 31:590–592, 1983.
14. Shapiro ED: Prophylaxis for bacterial meningitis. *Med Clin North Am* 60:269–280, 1985.
15. Nagami PH, Yoshikawa TT: Tuberculosis in the geriatric patient. *J Am Geriatr Soc* 31:356–363, 1983.
16. Rich AR, McCordock HA: The pathogenesis of tuberculous meningitis. *Bull Johns Hopkins Hosp* 52:5–37, 1933.
17. Kennedy DH, Fallon RJ: Tuberculous meningitis. *JAMA* 241:264–268, 1979.
18. Haas EJ, Madhavan T, Quinn EL, et al: Tuberculous meningitis in an urban general hospital. *Arch Intern Med* 137:1518–1521, 1977.

19. Klein NG, Damsker B, Hirschman SZ: Mycobacterial meningitis. Retrospective analysis from 1970 to 1983. *Am J Med* 79:29–34, 1985.
20. Molavi A, LeFrock JL: Tuberculous meningitis. *Med Clin North Am* 69:315–331, 1985.
21. Sada E, Ruiz-Palacios GM, Lopez-Vidal Y, et al: Detection of mycobacterial antigens in cerebrospinal fluid of patients with tuberculous meningitis by enzyme-linked immunosorbent assay. *Lancet* 2:651–652, 1983.
22. Dutt AK, Moers D, Stead WW: Short-course chemotherapy for extrapulmonary tuberculosis. Nine years' experience. *Ann Intern Med* 104:7–12, 1986.
23. O'Toole RD, Thornton GF, Mukherjee MK, et al: Dexamethasone in tuberculous meningitis: Relationship of cerebrospinal fluid effects to therapeutic efficacy. *Ann Intern Med* 70:39–47, 1969.
24. Yoshikawa TT, Goodman SJ: Brain abscess. *West J Med* 121:207–219, 1974.
25. Kaplan K: Brain abscess. *Med Clin North Am* 69:345–360, 1985.
26. Mathison GE, Meyer RD, George WL, et al: Brain abscess and cerebritis. *Rev Infect Dis* 6(suppl 1):5101–5106, 1984.
27. Boom WH, Tuazon CU: Successful treatment of multiple brain abscesses with antibiotics alone. *Rev Infect Dis* 7:189–199, 1985.
28. Hotson JR: Modern neurosyphilis: A partially treated chronic meningitis. *West J Med* 135:191–200, 1981.
29. Burke JM, Schaberg DR: Neurosyphilis in the antibiotic era. *Neurology* 35:1368–1371, 1985.
30. Hooshmand H, Escobar MR, Kopf SW: Neurosyphilis. A study of 241 patients. *JAMA* 219:726–729, 1972.
31. Hart G: Syphilis tests in diagnostic and therapeutic decision making. *Ann Intern Med* 104:368–376, 1986.
32. Wiesel J, Rose DN, Silver A, et al: Lumbar puncture in asymptomatic late syphilis. An analysis of the benefits and risks. *Arch Intern Med* 145:465–468, 1985.
33. Jaffe HW, Kabins SA: Examination of cerebrospinal fluid in patients with syphilis. *Rev Infect Dis* 4(suppl)5842–5847, 1982.

SUGGESTED READINGS

Gorse GJ, Thrupp LD, Nudleman KL, et al: Bacterial meningitis in the elderly. *Arch Intern Med* 144:1603–1607, 1984.
Hotson JR: Modern neurosyphilis: A partially treated chronic meningitis. *West J Med* 135:191–200, 1981.
Kaplan K: Brain abscess. *Med Clin North Am* 69:345–360, 1985.
Klein NG, Damsker B, Hirschman SZ: Mycobacterial meningitis. Retrospective analysis from 1970 to 1983. *Am J Med* 79:29–34, 1985.
Molavi A, LeFrock JL: Tuberculous meningitis. *Med Clin North Am* 69:315–331, 1985.

Norman DC, Yoshikawa TT: Recognizing bacterial meningitis in the elderly. *Geriatr Med Today* 3:85–88, 1984.

Wiesel J, Rose DN, Silver A, et al: Lumbar puncture in asymptomatic late syphilis. An analysis of the benefits and risks. *Arch Intern Med* 145:465–468, 1985.

Chapter 10

Pneumonia

BACTERIAL PNEUMONIA

General Considerations

Pneumonia and influenza are the leading infectious disease causes of mortality in the elderly. Furthermore, they rank fourth behind cardiovascular, cancer, and cerebrovascular disease as causes of death in this age group. Older individuals not only are more susceptible to most types of pneumonia but suffer more morbidity and death than do the young (1,2). Factors responsible for the increased severity of pneumonia in the older age group are listed in Table 10.1.

One approach to better understand the pathogenesis of any infectious disease is to analyze the interrelationship between the major factors that influence the host's risk to an infection. This can be simplified by the following equation (see Chapter 2 on predisposing factors to infection):

$$\text{Infection} = \frac{\text{Inoculum} \times \text{Virulence}}{\text{Host resistance}}$$

TABLE 10.1   Factors Associated with Increased Severity and Death from Pneumonia in Elderly Persons

Massive/continuous aspiration
Nosocomial pathogens (e.g., gram-negative bacilli, *Staphylococcus aureus*)
Poor response to bacteremia
Chronic lung disease
Underlying chronic diseases
Impaired host defenses

Since the elderly are highly susceptible to lung infections, examination of these factors may provide insight to the pathogenesis of pneumonia in the aged.

In most cases of bacterial pneumonia, the type and amount (inoculum) of pathogen(s) gaining access to the lower airways is determined by colonization of the oropharynx by microbes and the subsequent aspiration of these organisms into the lungs (3). Aspiration may also be iatrogenically induced during and after introduction of nasotracheal and endotracheal tubes. In some cases, pathogens may spread to the lungs hematogenously from an extrapulmonary source of infection (e.g., septic pulmonary emboli from septic phlebitis) or bacteria may be inhaled during intermittent positive pressure breathing (particularly if aerosols are contaminated) (4).

Gram-negative bacilli (GNB) are important causes of pneumonia in the elderly (see next section on etiology). Factors that influence oropharyngeal colonization by aerobic GNB include (1) level of care and severity of illness (more seriously ill patients are more likely to be colonized) (5,6); (2) prior antimicrobial therapy (presumably through alteration of normal flora); and (3) certain life styles and diseases such as chronic alcoholism and diabetes (7,8). Whether or not advanced age in itself is a risk factor for colonization with GNB is not clear. In one prospective study, there was some evidence that the "healthy" aged may be more prone to oropharyngeal colonization by pathogenic bacteria. Normal elderly patients admitted to the hospital for elective procedures were more likely to become colonized with GNB and *Staphylococcus aureus* than are their younger controls. Several of the colonized elderly patients later developed pneumonia (10). Correlations of colonization with immune function were attempted, but could not be demonstrated in this study.

Microaspiration or macroaspiration of the oropharyngeal flora is not frequently observed clinically. In fact, the classic aspiration of gastrointestinal contents is not observed (or necessary) in most cases of bacterial pneumonia. The inapparent introduction of oropharyngeal secretions into the lung while swallowing, lying supine, or during sleep compounded by ineffective coughing is the usual mechanism for aspiration. Even healthy young individuals aspirate small amounts of oral secretions (11), and the elderly are more prone to this problem because of increased use of sedating medications and the higher frequency of impaired swallowing due to the increased prevalence of cerebrovascular disease.

The other determinant of infection is the integrity of host resistance or defenses. (See Chapter 2 on predisposing factors to infection for overview on aging and host defenses.) The cough reflex, an important mechanism for protecting the lower airway, is diminished with age (12). However, data are lacking as to whether or not other pulmonary defense mechanisms including mucociliary transport, respiratory tract secretions, alveolar macrophages, and local humoral mucosal immunity are compromised with normal aging. It is clear that lifestyle (e.g., cigarette smoking and alcohol) have a negative impact on some of these systems (13,14). In one study of bacterial clearance from the lungs of young and old mice, it was shown that resident alveolar macrophages from the aged animals (studied in vitro) were less efficient in bacterial killing. However, senescent mice actually cleared pathogenic bacteria from the lung more rapidly than did younger mice (15). Viral respiratory infection, particularly influenza, is capable of altering local pulmonary defense mechanisms. This plays a role in the occurrence of secondary bacterial pneumonia, which is responsible for most mortality from influenza (16). (Also see the section on viral pneumonia.)

Etiology

COMMUNITY-ACQUIRED PNEUMONIA

The frequency of the various bacterial pneumonias in the elderly has been reviewed recently (3). Largely because of difficulties in making a precise etiologic diagnosis, the incidence of the different bacterial pneumonias in the elderly can only be crudely estimated. Moreover, certain pathogens such as *Legionella pneumophila* have variable incidence depending on geography.

It should be emphasized that a major difference between community-acquired pneumonia in the aged versus young adults is the higher frequency of diverse etiologic pathogens. The following briefly describes the most important bacterial causes of pneumonia in the elderly.

Streptococcus pneumoniae accounts for about 50% of geriatric cases of community-acquired pneumonia (3) and may be a cause of nosocomial pneumonia in elderly patients with chronic obstructive pulmonary disease, cerebrovascular disease, or malignancy (18). *Hemophilus influenzae* has been recently recognized as an important cause of pneumonia and is responsible for between 2 and 20% of cases of community-acquired pneumonia in the aged (3). *H. influenzae* may colonize the normal respiratory tract and is commonly found in the sputum of patients with chronic bronchitis (19). Its emergence as an important pulmonary pathogen in the geriatric age group may be attributable to one or more factors: employing more precise diagnostic methods, for example, transtracheal aspiration (19–21); declining immunity to this pathogen with age; or an actual increase in incidence of pneumonias caused by this bacterium. Most pulmonary infections caused by *H. influenzae* are due to nontypable strains, but if bacteremia occurs, it is usually from the encapsulated type B strain. Clinical manifestations of *H. influenzae* pneumonia in the elderly are not distinct from other community-acquired pneumonias (20).

A major difference between the young and the elderly in terms of bacterial etiology of pneumonia is the increased prevalence of gram-negative bacilli (GNB) in community-acquired pneumonia in elderly persons. Ebright and Rytel (22) in a retrospective review found that only 8% of patients between the ages of 20 and 40 years had pneumonia caused by GNB, whereas 21% of patients over age 65 had community-acquired GNB pneumonia. Moreover, the mortality for GNB pneumonia in the elderly age group was 71% compared to a death rate of 40% for GNB pneumonia in patients less than 65 years. Another finding of this study was that when the older patients were grouped according to etiologic pathogens, the prevalence of underlying disease was similar in each age group, but mortality was highest in those infected with GNB. This confirms that GNB are particularly virulent pathogens once they are established in the lower respiratory tract, especially in the very old. Additionally, this study demonstrated that the prevalence of serious underlying diseases was similarly present in all age groups with pneumonia, suggesting that age itself is a predisposing factor for GNB pneumonia. This may reflect the increased rate of oropharyngeal colonization by GNB observed in the elderly in the community compared to younger controls. However, this study must be interpreted with some caution, as the criteria for etiologic diagnosis included the results of expectorated sputum culture, which may be unreliable (see discussion in section on diagnostic approach).

The incidence of community-acquired anaerobic pneumonia in the elderly cannot be estimated, since transtracheal aspiration (TTA) is required for accurate characterization of the anaerobic pathogens. However, it can be assumed that many pneumonias in older persons are due to anaerobic bacteria, since aspiration of oropharyngeal flora is a common event in this age group. Anaerobic pulmonary infection has been recently reviewed (23).

Legionella pneumophila may be an important cause of lower respiratory infection in the aged under select circumstances (please see Chapter 24 on Legionella infection). Similarly, *Staphylococcus aureus* may cause serious pneumonia in the elderly (see Chapter 20 on staphylococcal infections). Finally, *Branhamella catarrhalis,* an aerobic gram-negative diplococcus, has recently emerged as a pulmonary pathogen that is frequently found in the sputa of elderly persons with chronic obstructive pulmonary disease and may be responsible for some pulmonary infections in these patients (24,25).

NOSOCOMIAL PNEUMONIA

Although there are no definitive studies that compare differences in bacterial etiologies of nosocomial (hospital-acquired) pneumonia versus age, in a major survey of 170,00 patients in 338 hospitals, the risk of nosocomial pneumonia in the elderly (over age 60) was 2 to 3 times that of the young (under age 40) patients. Those with chronic obstructive pulmonary disease or who received continuous ventilatory support were at greatest risk (26).

One factor that contributes to the high mortality of nosocomial pneumonia is the high incidence of bacteremia (8–12%) (27). Bacteremia is more likely to occur in elderly men with severe underlying diseases, more likely to be due to GNB, and is associated with over a 50% mortality.

Nosocomially acquired pneumonia, like community-acquired pneumonia in the elderly, may be caused by a variety of pathogens. The bacteriology of this disease has been well documented (via culture of transtracheal aspirate, blood, or empyema fluid) in a recently published study that prospectively studied 154 episodes of pneumonia in a Veterans Administration hospital during the early 1970s (28). The median age of the patients was 68 years. Aerobic GNB were recovered in 46% of patients with (in descending order) *Klebsiella* sp., *Escherichia coli, Proteus mirabilis,* and *Pseudomonas aeruginosa* being the most common isolates. *Streptococcus pneumoniae* (31%) and *S. aureus* (26%) were the most common grampositive isolates; anaerobic bacteria were isolated in 35% of cases, but were found in "pure" culture in only 6%. Virtually all patients had underlying medical diseases, and 56 of 159 patients had conditions predisposing to aspiration (e.g., coma, general anesthesia, cerebrovascular disease, general debility, and chronic pulmonary disease). In this study, *S. pneumoniae* was more likely to be isolated from patients with underlying pulmonary disease and general debility (18). Not surprisingly, *Klebsiella* sp. were found more frequently in patients who were receiving antimicrobial agents. Anaerobic bacteria were more likely to be found in patients prone to aspiration. Of note, 20 of 159 patients with nosocomial pneumonia had been exposed to aerosols via inhalation therapy. Mortality either directly due to pneumonia or contributed to by the pneumonia process was 32%; GNB accounted for the highest mortality (3). Mixed infections occurred in 54% of cases, consistent with aspiration as a major pathogenetic mechanism in nosocomial pneumonia. Other studies have yielded similar results, and Berk, Weiner et al. (29) reported that 25% (6) of 24 elderly patients with *S. pneumoniae* grown on transtracheal aspirate culture also had concomitant growth of GNB.

PNEUMONIA IN EXTENDED CARE FACILITIES

Pneumonias that occur in extended care facilities, such as nursing homes, are more likely to be associated with previous antimicrobial therapy and to be similar in etiology to nosocomial (hospital-acquired) pneumonias; GNB (particularly *Klebsiella* sp.) and *S. aureus* are reported as frequent isolates (2,30,31). Thus, pneumonia that is acquired in the nursing home is similar to nosocomially acquired pneumonia.

Clinical Manifestations

The clinical manifestation of pneumonia in the elderly may be different from that of pneumonia in younger persons (1-3,32). These differences are summarized in Table 10.2. Briefly, while the sudden onset of fever, pleurisy, and cough productive of purulent sputum characterizes bacterial pneumonia in the young adult, in older persons the symptoms of pneumonia may be insidious. Confusion or other changes in functional status (e.g., new onset falls or sudden decompensated congestive heart failure) may be the only symptoms (2). Fever may be blunted or even absent in a significant percentage of elderly patients (20–68%) (3,32), even when bacteremia is present (33). Rigors may also be diminished in the elderly (34). Cough may be minimal (3,5,36). The physical examination, which usually shows lobar or lobular consolidation in young patients with pneumonia, is often nonspecific in the elderly, particularly if underlying cardiopulmonary disease is present (e.g., congestive heart failure, emphysema) (37). One important sign, elevated respiratory rate, may be an early clue to the diagnosis of pneumonia in the aged (38).

Diagnostic Approach

DIFFERENTIAL DIAGNOSES
Other disorders that potentially could be confused with bacterial pneumonia in the aged include pulmonary embolism, congestive heart failure, tuberculosis, mycoses, and malignancy.

TABLE 10.2   Clinical Features of Pneumonia in Elderly Versus Young Adults

PARAMETER	YOUNG ADULT	ELDERLY
Time of onset	Abrupt	May be insidious
Symptoms		
Fever and rigors	Common	May be absent
Chest pain	Common	Less common
Cough	Common	Weak or absent
Sputum	Increased	May be minimal
Mental confusion	Occasional	More common
Physical findings		
Lungs	Typical for consolidation	Variable
Hypotension	Occasional	More common

LABORATORY TESTS

Radiography. The chest x-ray frequently reveals incomplete lobar consolidation in the elderly patient with pneumonia, even in cases of *S. pneumoniae* pneumonia. Diagnosis of a specific pathogen based on x-ray findings is not possible. Moreover, differentiating pneumonia on x-ray film from preexisting chronic obstructive pulmonary disease, congestive heart failure, or tumor is often difficult.

Sputum Analysis. The value of expectorated sputum culture has been questioned in recent years, and this subject has been reviewed recently (2,3,39,40). An exhaustive review of sputum analysis is beyond the scope of this chapter, but is discussed briefly. It was shown in the past that even in cases of bacteremic pneumococcal pneumonia, in approximately one-half of cases, *S. pneumoniae* could not be isolated from sputum culture (41). This reflects both the fastidious nature of this particular pathogen and the problem of overgrowth by "normal" mouth flora that contaminate any expectorated sputum specimen. The accuracy of sputum culture can be enhanced to approach the "gold" standard of transtracheal aspiration if the criteria that were established by Murray and Washington (42) and modified by Van Scoy (43) are followed. That is, sputum specimens should be cultured only after initial screening of the sample by Gram stain shows less than 10 epithelial cells and more than 25 polymorphonuclear leukocytes per low power field (lpf) ($\times$10 objective, $\times$100 magnification). These criteria increase the probability that the specimen is from the lower respiratory tract rather than saliva, which is heavily contaminated with oral microflora.

Boernor and Zwadyk (45) divided community-acquired pneumonia cases into two groups: Group A patients had Gram stains characteristic of pneumococcal pneumonia, whereas group B patients showed no apparent pathogen or mixed flora on Gram stain (patients that had another apparent pathogen were excluded). Clinically, the two groups differed in presentation only in that Group A (pneumococcus on Gram stain) patients had shorter duration of illness before presentation (4.2 days vs. 11.9 days). As expected, group A sputum culture or transtracheal aspiration culture more often yielded *S. pneumoniae,* whereas group B sputum was more likely to grow normal oral flora (mixed anaerobes grew if TTA was performed). More importantly, clinically, group A patients tended to respond rapidly with fever reduction to a single antibiotic (usually penicillin), whereas group B patients were more likely to receive broad-spectrum antibiotic coverage and tended to respond more slowly, thus requiring over 6 days to become afebrile. Furthermore, 4 of 31 patients in group B had positive sputum cytologies, which reflected the presence of postobstructive anaerobic pneumonia in this group. Mortality was higher in group B patients as well. Thus, in community-acquired bacterial pneumonia, a carefully processed sputum Gram stain has value in directing therapy and predicting outcome.

An attempt to obtain sputum should be made on all elderly patients with suspected pneumonia. A sputum Gram stain should be performed and analyzed by the criteria of Murray and Washington (42). Additionally, a smear for acid-fast bacilli (AFB) should be performed as well (see Chapter 11 on tuberculosis). In cases of suspected legionellosis, a sputum Direct Fluorescent Antibody (DFA) should be done (see Chapter 24 on Legionella infection). Sputum should routinely be sent for directed aerobic bacterial, fungal, and mycobacterial culture.

Transtracheal Aspiration. Although open lung biopsy and percutaneous needle aspiration of the lung are the most accurate methods of determining the etiology of pneumonia, transtracheal aspiration (TTA) of lung secretion is a more convenient and less invasive procedure. In the hands of experienced physicians, TTA is relatively safe and has good diagnostic accuracy for the microbiology of pneumonia (providing colonization of the upper airways with normal flora has not occurred). Unfortunately, for a variety of reasons—including unfamiliarity with the procedure and fear of complications despite the fact that it is a relatively safe procedure (3)—housestaff and postgraduate physicians are reluctant to perform this test. Berk et al. (47) have performed TTAs on many severely ill elderly patients with pneumonia and have reported only one minor complication (self-limited subcutaneous emphysema). Contraindications to performing TTA include (*1*) arterial $PO_2 < 60$ (on supplemental oxygen), (*2*) bullous emphysema, (*3*) distorted anatomic landmarks, (*4*) uncooperative patient, and (*5*) abnormalities of hemostasis.

We believe a TTA is not indicated for most cases of pneumonia and should be strongly considered in an elderly patient under the following circumstances: (*1*) immunocompromised status, (*2*) patient not responding to initial antimicrobial therapy, and (*3*) patient who relapses after an initial clinical response to antibiotics (i.e., superinfection). TTA aspirates should be examined routinely by Gram stain, AFB smear, fungal wet mount, and DFA (in suspected Legionella cases), as well as routinely cultured for aerobes, anaerobes, mycobacteria, and fungi.

Bronchoscopy. Cultures obtained by usual bronchoscopic methods will be contaminated by oral flora as the bronchoscope is pushed through the mouth. Recently, quantitative bacteriology done on samples obtained from a specially protected catheter attached to a bronchoscope gave reliable results if cultures yielded $\geqslant 10^3$ bacteria/ml fluid (48). The accuracy of this technique is enhanced if the presence of antibody-coated bacteria is determined (49). These tests hold future promise and may become the "gold standard" for determining the etiology of pneumonia.

Other Diagnostic Tests. All elderly patients with presumptive pneumonia should have a skin test for tuberculosis performed. A skin test for coccidioidomycosis is indicated in endemic areas. Additionally, two sets of blood cultures should *always* be obtained before initiating antimicrobial therapy.

As part of the overall management of elderly patients with pneumonia, other recommended laboratory examinations include (*1*) arterial blood gas analysis; (*2*) electrocardiograph; (*3*) complete blood count; (*4*) coagulation studies (with severe sepsis); (*5*) serum electrolytes, blood urea nitrogen, serum creatinine, and liver function tests; and (*6*) urinalysis. Depending on the clinical situation, additional tests may be indicated.

Treatment

Initial empiric antimicrobial therapy for pneumonia generally is predicated on the clinical setting, as this provides the best clue to the most likely etiologic pathogens. In most cases, initial therapy should be with parenteral antibiotics.

COMMUNITY-ACQUIRED PNEUMONIA

Most elderly patients who are diagnosed as having pneumonia should be hospitalized. As part of the initial evaluation, the clinician should determine: (*1*) the underlying diseases (e.g., chronic bronchitis is likely to be associated with *H. influenzae* and *S. pneumoniae*); (*2*) the functional status of the patient (e.g., recent cerebrovascular accident that results in altered consciousness or swallowing function would imply aspiration and therefore suggest mixed anaerobic and aerobic flora); and (*3*) whether there has been recent use of antibiotics (predisposes to oropharyngeal colonization with GNB). As in younger persons, a travel history and history of exposure to tuberculosis should also be elicited. Routine laboratory and microbiologic studies should then be obtained as described in the section on diagnostic approach.

Recommendations for empiric antimicrobial therapy of community-acquired pneumonia in the elderly is outlined in Table 10.3. After culture data become available, the antimicrobial agents should be appropriately changed (if indicated). A TTA should be considered in patients who do not respond to the initial antimicrobial therapy, regardless of whether the pneumonia is acquired in the community or in an institution. Antimicrobial regimens should be adjusted according to the TTA results. Furthermore, in immunosuppressed patients who do not respond to initial antimicrobial therapy, such invasive procedures as bronchoscopy

TABLE 10.3 Recommendations for Empiric Antimicrobial Therapy of the Aged for Pneumonia Acquired in the Community or in an Extended Care Facility

PATIENT CHARACTERISTICS	DRUG(S)[a]	ALTERNATIVE DRUG(S)[a]
Clinically stable Gram stain demonstrates predominant organism	Treat according to Gram stain results	—
Good sputum is not available or no predominant organism is demonstrated	Cefuroxime (or cefoxitin)	Third-generation[b] cephalosporin; or trimethoprim-sulfamethoxazole; or clindamycin plus aminoglycoside[d]
Toxic, septic, clinically unstable, immunosuppressed or recently on antibiotics[c]	First- or second-generation cephalosporin plus aminoglycoside;[d] or third-generation cephalosporin with or without an aminoglycoside[d]	Penicillin G (or ampicillin) plus nafcillin (or oxacillin) plus aminoglycoside[d]

[a]Doses for these antibiotics are described in Chapter 5 on antimicrobial therapy: special considerations.
[b]Cefoperazone, ceftriaxone, ceftizoxime, or ceftazidime.
[c]Gram strain results are only confirmatory in these cases, regardless if good sputum demonstrates a predominant organism on the smear. Erythromycin should be added if *Legionella* suspected.
[d]Tobramycin, gentamicin, amikacin, or netilmicin.

with transtracheal biopsy, lung aspiration (needle), or open lung biopsy should be considered until a definitive diagnosis is made. Supportive therapy which includes fluids, oxygen, suction, and so on should be provided in all cases, and any complications should be vigorously treated. Although the duration of antibiotic therapy varies depending on the etiology and severity of the pneumonia as well as on the clinical response of the patient, most patients should be treated for a minimum of 2 weeks.

PNEUMONIA IN THE EXTENDED CARE FACILITY
This section is not intended as a discussion of the ethical, psychosocial, or the economic aspects of treating pneumonia in the nursing home. Once the decision is made to "treat" the nursing home resident who has pneumonia, then a decision on whether or not to hospitalize the patient becomes necessary (see Chapter 7 on infections in the nursing home population). All patients should be hospitalized if they are hemodynamically unstable, septic, or in acute respiratory distress. The patient may be

managed in the nursing home if (*1*) 24-hour monitoring of patient status is available; (*2*) supportive therapy exists (i.e., oxygen, parenteral fluids, etc.); (*3*) laboratory tests (e.g., x-ray, hematology, arterial blood gases, cultures, etc.) are available in a timely fashion; and (*4*) an interested, capable physician is willing to attend the patient (31).

As in community-acquired pneumonia, the clinician should determine the relevant clinical history and obtain the appropriate laboratory and microbiologic tests (careful attention should be made to obtain results of sputum AFB smear as well as to send the sputum for culture of mycobacteria).

Empiric antibiotic therapy is outlined as per Table 10.3, and drugs should be adjusted when culture data become available. Supportive treatment should be provided as outlined for community-acquired pneumonia.

PNEUMONIA IN THE ACUTE HOSPITAL
In the acute hospital, the evaluation and studies are the same as for the nursing home patient. Supportive care and the treatment of complications of pneumonia should be provided. Many of these patients may be severely compromised and may require continuous ventilatory support. Empiric antibiotic therapy is outlined in Table 10.4.

TABLE 10.4 Empiric Antimicrobial Therapy for Pneumonia Acquired in an Acute Hospital

PATIENT CHARACTERISTICS	DRUG(S)[a]	ALTERNATIVE DRUG(S)[a]
Clinically stable[c]	Third-generation cephalosporin; or cefuroxime (or cefoxitin) plus piperacillin (or mezlocillin)	Clindamycin plus trimethoprim-sulfamethoxazole (or aminoglycoside[b])
Toxic, septic, clinically unstable, immunosuppressed or on recent antibiotics[c]	First- or second-generation cephalosporin plus aminoglycoside;[b] or penicillin G (or ampicillin) plus nafcillin (or oxacillin) plus aminoglycoside[b]	Third-generation cephalosporin[d] with or without aminoglycoside;[b] or vancomycin plus clindamycin plus aminoglycoside[b]

[a]Doses for these antibiotics are described in Chapter 5 on antimicrobial therapy: special considerations.
[b]Tobramycin, gentamicin, amikacin, or netilmicin.
[c]Regardless of Gram stain results.
[d]Ceftazidime recommended because of risk of *Pseudomonas aeruginosa.*

Prevention

The prevention of pneumonias due to *S. pneumoniae* (pneumococcal vaccine) is discussed in Chapter 6 on prevention of infections. One potential mechanism for reducing the incidence of bacterial pneumonia would be to reduce the frequency of influenza (through vaccination), thus reducing postinfluenza bacterial pneumonia. Another mechanism for reduction of pneumonia involves eliminating or reducing risk of aspiration (e.g., avoiding or carefully monitoring drugs that depress the central nervous system) and decreasing the risk of oropharyngeal colonization by GNB and other pathogens (e.g., avoiding unnecessary antibiotic therapy).

VIRAL PNEUMONIA

General Considerations

Presumably all of the important respiratory viruses are capable of infecting elderly persons. However, only a few of these viruses have a significant impact in the older population. Influenza A and B are an enormous public health problem that account for significant morbidity and mortality in the elderly. Respiratory syncytial virus (RSV) and parainfluenza virus, which are major causes of lower respiratory tract infections in young children, occur relatively infrequently in adults. However, they have been associated with outbreaks in geriatric acute hospitals and in long-term care facilities (50,51); therefore, a brief discussion of these viral illnesses is provided.

The epidemiology and significance of influenza is covered in detail in Chapter 6 on prevention of infections. Much of the excess mortality observed during periods of influenza activity in the community is due to bacterial pneumonia that complicates influenza cases. Although not completely understood, the pathogenesis of secondary bacterial pneumonia is thought to be due to viral induced deleterious effects on host immune function (16). Some of these effects, which have been shown in both human and animal studies, include impairment of neutrophil chemotaxis and killing; suppression of macrophage and T-cell function; and perhaps more importantly, reduction of mucociliary clearance by damaging respiratory tract mucosal cells (16). Mortality resulting from infection with either RSV or parainfluenza virus in the adult appears to be largely secondary to the development of viral bronchopneumonia. In one outbreak of RSV reported in a nursing home, 40% of residents were affected, and in over one-half of cases, pneumonia was present with a 20% mortality (52). Similarly, in a report compiled by the Communicable Disease Surveillance Centre in Britain (CDSC), only 2.0% of reported cases of parainfluenza infections occurred in elderly persons, but over 50% of these had viral pneumonia or other lower respiratory tract infection (51). Also the CDSC reported five outbreaks of parainfluenza virus in the elderly that occurred in various geriatric acute and chronic health centers. The pathogenesis and effect of RSV and parainfluenza viruses on host defenses is beyond the scope of this book. These aspects are extensively reviewed in standard textbooks (53,54).

Etiology

The influenza virus is discussed in detail in Chapter 6 on prevention of infections.

RSV is an RNA virus of the paramyxovirus family that grows well in several human cell culture lines (53). It is the major pathogen recovered from infants with pneumonia and bronchiolitis. Essentially, all persons have experienced infection with this virus at an early age, but immunity is not complete and reinfection is common. Outbreaks occur on a yearly basis, usually occurring in the winter or spring. The virus is spread easily via respiratory secretions; spread from contaminated hands or fomites is possible and may play a major role in nosocomial or institutional outbreaks (53).

Parainfluenza viruses include serotypes 1, 2, 3 and are also RNA viruses of the paramyxovirus family. These viruses (like RSV) require various cell culture lines for growth (54). In contrast to influenza, these viruses are antigenically stable, and the epidemic behavior as well as age and sex distribution of severe cases is dependent on the serotype. All these serotypes are capable of infecting the elderly (51). Respiratory droplet spread from person to person, as in RSV and influenza virus, is thought to be the major mechanism of transmission.

Clinical Manifestations

After a short incubation period of 18 hours to 3 days, most patients with uncomplicated influenza experience the abrupt onset of constitutional symptoms (55,56). These initial complaints include fever (often high), chills, headache, and myalgia. Ocular symptoms such as photophobia or pain with eye movement are helpful diagnostic clues to the presence of influenza. Generally the systemic symptoms abate in 2 to 3 days and respiratory complaints dominate the clinical picture. These usually include a dry cough, which may be accompanied by chest discomfort;; this phase of the illness along with lassitude and malaise typically persists 1 to 2 weeks. It should be emphasized that even in "uncomplicated" influenza, elderly patients with chronic underlying diseases, especially chronic bronchitis, may have exacerbation of their underlying problems that lead to morbidity or mortality (e.g., decompensated congestive heart failure).

This is primarily because of pulmonary function abnormalities that can be demonstrated by using sensitive testing methods even though "uncomplicated" influenza cases may not have clinically detectable pneumonia. Thus, involvement of the lower respiratory tract is common even in "uncomplicated" cases (57).

Although nonpulmonary complications of influenza infection occur and include myositis, myocarditis, Guillain Barré, and Reyes' syndrome, they are not particularly relevant to the elderly population. Pulmonary complications in the elderly include viral pneumonia, which tends to be fulminant in patients with cardiovascular disease. As alluded to above, secondary bacterial pneumonia is the most important pulmonary complication of influenza, especially in the elderly, and is usually caused by *S. pneumoniae, S. aureus,* or *H. influenzae.* Typically, secondary bacterial pneumonia occurs in the elderly person with chronic cardiopulmonary disease. Most patients who develop secondary bacterial infection initially appear to improve after acquiring the viral infection with resolution of fever. They usually relapse with fever, cough, and purulent sputum production, which is suggestive of bacterial pneumonia. However, in the elderly, the manifestations of bacterial pneumonia may be atypical (see Table 10.2). At this time, a chest x-ray film will reveal an infiltrate.

Both RSV and parainfluenza viruses are capable of causing an influenza-like illness in elderly persons (50,51). However, nosocomial and extended care facility outbreaks of these viruses have been particularly severe with symptoms and signs of lower respiratory tract infection being most often present. In the case of RSV pneumonia, a high mortality has been observed (52,58).

Diagnostic Approach

During periods in which influenza virus is confirmed to be present in the community by the local or state health department or by the Centers for Disease Control (CDC), the diagnosis can be made clinically. Detection of virus in respiratory secretions can easily be accomplished in viral diagnostic laboratories that are equipped for cell culture. Cultures are usually positive within 3 to 7 days. (Swabs must be placed in special viral transport medium and sent as soon as possible to the laboratory for inoculation into cell cultures.) A rapid direct immunofluorescence test for influenza A antigen has been developed (59). Serologic diagnosis that uses complement fixation titer tests requires acute and convalescent serum specimens and is, therefore, of value only for epidemiologic purposes. The diagnosis of RSV or parainfluenza infection, like influenza, is best made by isolating the virus in cell culture. However, rapid diagnostic

122 PNEUMONIA

tests that detect viral antigen in respiratory secretions are available for RSV (53,54).

Treatment

Amantadine hydrochloride is the only antiviral agent approved for the prophylaxis and therapy of influenza A (Amantadine has no effect on influenza B). Its value (and dose) in the prophylaxis of influenza A is discussed in Chapter 6 on prevention of infections. Rimantadine, a newer antiviral agent with activity against influenza A, may have less side effects than amantadine (e.g., insomnia, difficulty with concentration, irritability), but it is not yet approved for influenza A therapy (60).

There is no effective antiviral agent for parainfluenza virus, but recently aerosolized ribavirin has been shown to be effective in treating infants with underlying cardiopulmonary disease who had become infected with RSV (61). Whether or not this agent is effective in adults with severe RSV infection needs to be determined.

Prevention

The prevention of influenza is discussed in detail in Chapter 6 on prevention of infections. Vaccines are currently being developed and tested for RSV and parainfluenza. Nosocomial spread of RSV can be limited through careful handwashing by health care personnel and through isolation of index cases.

REFERENCES

1. Marrie TJ, Haldane EV, Faukner RS, et al: Community-acquired pneumonia requiring hospitalization. Is it different in the elderly? *J Am Geriatr Soc* 33:671-680, 1985.
2. Bentley DW: Bacterial pneumonia in the elderly: Clinical features, diagnosis, etiology, and treatment. *Gerontology* 30:297-307, 1984.
3. Verghese A, Berk SL: Bacterial pneumonia in the elderly. *Medicine* 62:271-285, 1983.
4. Lerner AM: The gram-negative bacillary pneumonias, in Weinstein L, Fields BN (eds): *Seminars in Infectious Diseases. Pneumonias.* New York, Thieme-Stratten, Inc., 1983, vol 5, p 159.
5. Johanson WG, Pierce AK, Sanford JP: Changing pharyngeal bacterial flora of hospitalized patients. Emergence of gram-negative bacilli. *N Engl J Med* 281:1137-1140, 1969.
6. Valenti WM, Trudell RG, Bentley DW: Factors predisposing to oropharyngeal colonization with gram-negative bacilli in the aged. *N Engl J Med* 298:1108-1111, 1978.

7. Mackowiak PA, Martin RM, Jones SR, et al: Pharyngeal colonization by gram-negative bacilli in aspiration-prone persons. *Arch Intern Med* 138: 1224–1227, 1978.

8. Fuxench-López Z, Ramirez-Ronda CH: Pharyngeal flora in ambulatory alcoholic patients: Prevalence of gram-negative bacilli. *Arch Intern Med* 138:1815–1816, 1978.

9. Laforce FM, Hopkins J, Trow R, et al: Human oral defenses against gram-negative rods. *Am Rev Respir Dis* 114:929–935, 1976.

10. Phair JP, Kauffman CA, Bjornson A: Investigation of host defense mechanisms in the aged as determinants of nosocomial colonization and pneumonia. *J Reticuloendothel Soc* 23:397–405, 1978.

11. Huxley EJ, Viroslav J, Gray WR, et al: Pharyngeal aspiration in normal adults and patients with depressed consciousness. *Am J Med* 64:564–566, 1978.

12. Pontoppidan H, Beecher HK: Progressive loss of protective reflexes in the airway with the advance of age. *JAMA* 174:2209–2213, 1960.

13. Newhouse M, Sanchis J, Bienenstock J: Lung defense mechanisms. Part 1. *N Engl J Med* 295:990–998, 1976.

14. Newhouse M, Sanchis J, Bienenstock J: Lung defense mechanisms. Part 2. *N Engl J Med* 295:1045–1052, 1976.

15. Esposito AL, Pennington JE: Effects of aging on antibacterial mechanisms in experimental pneumonia. *Am Rev Respir Dis* 128:662–667, 1983.

16. Couch RB: The effects of influenza on host defenses. *J Infect Dis* 144:284–291, 1981.

17. Gardner ID: The effect of aging on susceptibility to infection. *Rev Infect Dis* 2:801–809, 1980.

18. Berk SL, Gallemore GM, Smith JK: Nosocomial pneumococcal pneumonia in the elderly. *J Am Geriatr Soc* 29:319–321, 1981.

19. Hirschmann JV, Everett ED: Hemophilus influenzae infections in adults: Report of nine cases and review of the literature. *Medicine* 58:80–94, 1979.

20. Everett ED, Rahm AE, Adaniya R, et al: Haemophilus influenzae pneumonia in adults. *JAMA* 238:319–321, 1977.

21. Berk SL, Holtsclaw SA, Wiener SL, et al: Nontypeable Haemophilus influenzae in the elderly. *Arch Intern Med* 142:537–539, 1982.

22. Ebright JR, Rytel MW: Bacterial pneumonia in the elderly. *J Am Geriatr Soc* 28:220–223, 1980.

23. Finegold SM, George WL, Mulligan ME: Anaerobic infections. Part I. *Disease-a-Month* 31(10):1–77, 1985.

24. Louie MH, Gabay EL, Mathisen GE, et al: Branhamella catarrhalis pneumonia. *West J Med* 138:47–49, 1983.

25. Nicotra B, Rivera M, Lumen JI, et al: Branhamella catarrhalis as a lower respiratory tract pathogen in patients with chronic lung disease. *Arch Intern Med* 146:890–893, 1986.

26. Haley RW, Hooton TM, Culver DH, et al: Nosocomial infections in U.S. hospitals, 1975–1976. Estimated frequency by selected characteristics of patients. *Am J Med* 70:946–959, 1981.

27. Bryan CS, Reynolds KL: Bacteremic nosocomial pneumonia. Analysis of

172 episodes from a single metropolitan area. *Am Rev Respir Dis* 129:668–671, 1984.

28. Bartlett JG, O'Keefe P, Tally FP, et al: Bacteriology of hospital-acquired pneumonia. *Arch Intern Med* 146:868–871, 1986.

29. Berk SL, Wiener SL, Eisner LB, et al: Mixed Streptococcus pneumoniae and gram-negative bacillary pneumonia in the elderly. *South Med J* 74:144–146, 1981.

30. Garb JL, Brown RB, Garb JR, et al: Differences in etiology of pneumonias in nursing home and community patients. *JAMA* 240:2169–2172, 1978.

31. Castle S: Pneumonia in the elderly nursing home patient. *Geriatr Med Today* 5:70–79, 1986.

32. Berk SL: Bacterial pneumonia in the elderly: The observations of Sir William Osler in retrospect. *J Am Geriatr Soc* 32:683–685, 1984.

33. Finkelstein MS, Petkun WM, Freedman ML, et al: Pneumococcal bacteremia in adults. Age dependent differences in presentation and in outcome. *J Am Geriatr Soc* 31:19–27, 1983.

34. Esposito AL: Community acquired bacteremic pneumococcal pneumonia. Effect of age on manifestations and outcome. *Arch Intern Med* 144:945–948, 1984.

35. Dhar S, Shastri SR, Lenora RA: Aging and the respiratory system. *Med Clin North Am* 60(6):1121–1139, 1976.

36. Horton JM, Pankey GA: Pneumonia in the elderly. *Postgrad Med* 71:114–122, 1982.

37. Murphy TF, Fine BC: Bacteremic pneumococcal pneumonia in the elderly. *Am J Med Sci* 288:114–118, 1984.

38. McFadden JP, Price R, Eastwood HD, et al: Raised respiratory rate in elderly patients: A valuable physical sign. *Br Med J* 284:626–627, 1982.

39. Rozas CJ, Goldman AL: Responses to bacterial pneumonia. *Geriatrics* 37:61–66, 1982.

40. Stulbarg MS: Problems in diagnosing pneumonia. *West J Med* 140:594–601, 1984.

41. Barrett-Connor E: The nonvalue of sputum culture in the diagnosis of pneumococcal pneumonia. *Am Rev Respir Dis* 103:845–848, 1971.

42. Murray PR, Washington JA: Microscopic and bacteriologic analysis of expectorated sputum. *Mayo Clin Proc* 50:339–344, 1975.

43. Van Scoy RE: Bacterial sputum cultures. A clinician's viewpoint. *Mayo Clin Proc* 52:39–41, 1977.

44. Heineman HS, Chawla JK, Lofton WM: Misinformation from sputum cultures without microscopic examination. *J Clin Microbiol* 6:518–527, 1977.

45. Boerner DF, Zwadyk P: The value of sputum Gram's stain in community acquired pneumonia. *JAMA* 247:642–645, 1982.

46. Davidson M, Tempest B, Palmer DL: Bacteriologic diagnosis of acute pneumonia. Comparison of sputum, transtracheal aspirates, and lung aspirates. *JAMA* 235:158–163, 1976.

47. Berk SL, Holtsclaw SA, Kahn A, et al: Transtracheal aspiration in the severely ill elderly patient with bacterial pneumonia. *J Am Geriatr Soc* 29:228–231, 1981.

48. Pollock HM, Hawkins EL, Bonner JR, et al: Diagnosis of bacterial pulmonary infections with quantitative protected catheter cultures obtained during bronchoscopy. *J Clin Microbiol* 17:255–259, 1983.
49. Winterbauer RH, Hutchison JF, Reinhardt GN, et al: The use of quantitative cultures and antibody coating of bacteria to diagnose bacterial pneumonia by fiberoptic bronchoscopy. *Am Rev Respir Dis* 128:98–103, 1983.
50. Public Health Laboratory Service Communicable Disease Surveillance Centre: Respiratory syncytial virus infection in the elderly 1976–1982. *Br Med J* 287:1618–1619, 1983.
51. Public Health Laboratory Service Communicable Disease Surveillance Centre: Parainfluenza infections in the elderly 1976–1982. *Br Med J* 287: 1619, 1983.
52. Sorvillo FJ, Huie SF, Strassburg MA, et al: An outbreak of respiratory syncytial virus pneumonia in a nursing home for the elderly. *J Infect* 9:252–256, 1984.
53. Hall CB: Respiratory syncytial virus, in Mandell GL, Douglas RG, Bennett JE (eds): *Principles and Practice of Infectious Diseases.* New York, John Wiley & Sons, 1985, p 877–888.
54. Hendley JO: Parainfluenza virus, in Mandall GL, Douglas RG, Bennett JE (eds): *Principles and Practice of Infectious Diseases.* New York, John Wiley & Sons, 1985, p 868–871.
55. Seneca H: Influenza: Epidemiology, etiology, immunization and management. *J Am Geriatr Soc* 28:241–250, 1980.
56. Weitekamp MR, Aber RC: Nonbacterial and unusual pneumonias in the elderly. *Geriatrics* 39:87–100, 1984.
57. Douglas RG, Betts RF: Influenza virus, in Mandell GL, Douglas RG, Bennett JE (eds): *Principles and Practice of Infectious Diseases.* New York, John Wiley & Sons, 1985, p 846–866.
58. Morales F, Calder MA, Inglis JM, et al: A study of respiratory infections in the elderly to assess the role of respiratory syncytial virus. *J Infect* 7:236–247, 1983.
59. Centers for Disease Control: Update: Influenza activity—United States—and the role of rapid virus typing in improving amantadine use. *MMWR* 35:46–47, January 24, 1986.
60. Hayden FG, Douglas RG: Antiviral agents, in Mandell GL, Douglas RG, Bennett JE (eds): *Principles and Practice of Infectious Diseases.* New York, John Wiley & Sons, 1985, p 270–286.
61. Hall CB, McBride JT, Gala CL, et al: Ribavirin treatment of respiratory syncytial viral infection in infants with underlying cardiopulmonary disease. *JAMA* 254:3047–3051, 1985.

SUGGESTED READINGS

Bentley DW: Bacterial pneumonia in the elderly: Clinical features, diagnosis, etiology, and treatment. *Gerontology* 30:297–307, 1984.
Castle S: Pnemonia in the elderly nursing home population. *Geriatr Med Today* 5:70–79, 1986.

Finkelstein MS, Petkun WM, Freedman ML, et al: Pneumococcal bacteremia in adults. Age dependent differences in presentation and in outcome. *J Am Geriatr Soc* 31:19–27, 1983.

Garb JL, Brown RB, Garb JR, et al: Differences in etiology of pneumonias in nursing home and community patients. *JAMA* 240:2169–2172, 1978.

Marrie TJ, Haldane EV, Faukner RS, et al: Community-acquired pneumonia requiring hospitalization. Is it different in the elderly? *J Am Geriatr Soc* 33:671–680, 1985.

Public Health Laboratory Service Communicable Disease Surveillance Centre: Respiratory syncytial virus infection in the elderly 1976–1982. *Br Med J* 287:1618–1619, 1983.

Seneca H: Influenza: Epidemiology, etiology, immunization and management. *J Am Geriatr Soc* 28:241–250, 1980.

Sorvillo FJ, Huie SF, Strassburg MA, et al: An outbreak of respiratory syncytial virus pneumonia in a nursing home for the elderly. *J Infect* 9:252–256, 1984.

Centers for Disease Control: Update: Influenza activity—United States—and the role of rapid virus typing in improving amantadine use. *MMWR* 35:46–47, January 24, 1986.

Verghese A, Berk SL: Bacterial pneumonia in the elderly. *Medicine* 62:271–285, 1983.

Chapter 11

Tuberculosis

GENERAL CONSIDERATIONS

The overall incidence of tuberculosis is declining in industrialized nations (1,2). However, the rate of this decline is not paralleled in the aging population. Consequently, the frequency of new cases of tuberculosis is disproportionately higher (and usually highest) in the elderly (3). Studies that report on patients with active tuberculosis confirm that persons 55 years and older make up over 50% of all cases (4,5) and furthermore indicate that persons 60 years and older comprise 25 to 50% of all cases of tuberculosis (6–8). Unfortunately, the higher incidence of this disease in the elderly is also followed by a significantly higher death rate due to tuberculosis in this age group (4,9). Not surprisingly then, clinically undiagnosed tuberculosis (subsequently diagnosed at autopsy) occurs more frequently in the aged (10–12).

The current elderly population comprises many individuals who were infected with tuberculosis in the early 1900s. These aged persons usually have tuberculin skin test positivity and are at risk for active tuberculosis by reactivation of dormant infection. Thus, reactivation tuberculosis is the major, but not sole, pathogenetic mechanism for most cases of tuberculosis in the elderly. Tubercle bacilli in these older infected persons may die off over the years resulting in gradual waning of the skin test reactivity (and hence the cell-mediated immunity). If these individuals are able to mount a booster skin test response (a second tuberculin skin test that gives a significant positive response), they will likely be protected from reinfection due to exposure to an index case. Furthermore, they should also maintain tuberculin sensitivity and cellular immunity against possible active disease (13). The booster effect is explained in detail at the end of this chapter. If there is no booster response (and hence diminished immune resistance), these elderly persons would be at risk to acquire new infection (13). This has been verified by studies of tuberculosis in nursing home patients based on tuberculin skin test reactivity (14,15). Indeed, outbreaks of active tuberculosis in nursing homes have been documented in susceptible (skin-test negative) hosts (16).

ETIOLOGY

Human tuberculosis is caused almost exclusively by *Mycobacterium tuberculosis*. In countries outside the United States, a few cases of tuberculosis may be a result of infection by *M. bovis*. Infections caused by mycobacteria other than *M. tuberculosis* and *M. bovis* are called nontuberculous mycobacteriosis (formerly atypical mycobacteriosis or atypical tuberculosis). Although nontuberculous mycobacteriosis does occur in the elderly, its frequency is much less than tuberculosis, and thus the discussion in this chapter is limited to tuberculosis.

   M. tuberculosis are aerobic, thin bacilli. They stain variably with Gram stain; therefore, this method is unreliable for demonstrating the organism. The lipid and wax constituents of this organism's cell wall are remarkable for their acid-fast properties. *M. tuberculosis* grows slowly (replicates every 16–20 hours) on artificial media; hence, cultures are held for at least 6 weeks before a final interpretation is made (as either positive or negative).

CLINICAL MANIFESTATIONS

General Features

Tuberculosis should be considered as a diagnostic possibility in any elderly patient who has a subacute (weeks to months) change in well being, health status, or functional status. Clinical manifestations can be quite varied and nonspecific including: fever of unknown origin; weight loss; unexplained gastrointestinal symptoms (anorexia, nausea); change in cognitive function or personality; or progressive weakness.

Pulmonary Tuberculosis

REACTIVATION PULMONARY INFECTION
This most common form of pulmonary tuberculosis in the elderly may present with progressive cough with or without sputum production. Hemoptysis, dizziness, fever, night sweats, weight loss, and fatigue may also be present. However, there may be a paucity of respiratory symptoms, which may delay both the patient and physician from considering pulmonary tuberculosis as a cause of the patient's change in health status

(9); this may be disastrous both for the patient and for susceptible contacts.

PRIMARY PULMONARY INFECTION
The clinical manifestations in primary infection are similar to those of reactivation disease. Many of these patients are those who reside in nursing homes, and they may have lower lobe involvement with tuberculosis (14–16).

Miliary and Extrapulmonary Tuberculosis

MILIARY OR DISSEMINATED TUBERCULOSIS
Patients over 60-years old comprise the largest group of people who contract miliary tuberculosis (10,17,18). Features of miliary disease in adults range from those with insidious onset of malaise, weakness, weight loss, and fever to those with severe illness, acute respiratory failure, toxicity, and fever. Depending on which organ system is involved, there may be tachycardia, tachypnea, lymphadenopathy, hepatomegaly, or splenomegaly. In elderly patients, atypical forms of miliary tuberculosis may occur (19). These patients may have progressive cachexia and weight loss with or without fever, and the chest x-ray film may not show a characteristic miliary pattern.

TUBERCULOUS MENINGITIS
Please refer to Chapter 9 on central nervous system infections for discussion of tuberculous meningitis.

SKELETAL (BONE AND JOINT) TUBERCULOSIS
Skeletal tuberculosis is reported more frequently in older patients (20,21). The weight-bearing bone and joints are most frequently involved, such as the vertebrae, hips, and knees (19,21). The clinical features are not unique in the elderly, and pain with or without an inflammatory response at the site of involvement is the most common finding. Fever or other systemic complaints may be absent. Not infrequently, the complaints may be erroneously attributed to other age-related skeletal diseases, for example, osteoarthritis, gout, or osteoporosis, which delays or confuses the diagnosis.

GENITOURINARY TUBERCULOSIS
Tuberculosis that involves the genitourinary tract may be the most common site of infection for extrapulmonary tuberculosis (22). Again, as with other forms of tuberculosis, the elderly are disproportionately more affected with genitourinary *M. tuberculosis* infection (23). Although there

are no clinical studies of this infection in the elderly alone, it appears that
the aged experience similar clinical manifestations as the general population. The majority of patients complain of inflammatory or irritative
symptoms of the genitourinary tract, that is, dysuria, frequency, hematuria, and urgency (24,25). Some patients experience flank pains, fever,
weight loss, or symptoms related to tuberculous involvement of another
site (e.g., epididymitis, orchitis). Physical findings are generally unreveal-
ing, and 20% of these patients may be totally asymptomatic (25).

OTHER SITES OF TUBERCULOSIS
Although virtually any organ may be involved with tuberculosis, this infection has been reported to occur in the elderly in the following organs
or organ sites: cervical lymph nodes (26), pleura as bronchopleural fistula
(27), liver as hepatitis (28) or abscesses/nodules (29), gallbladder, and
common bile duct (29), small and large intestine (30,31), pericardium (32),
middle ear (33), and carpal tunnel (34).

DIAGNOSTIC APPROACH

Differential Diagnosis

It is beyond the scope of this chapter to list the differential diagnosis for
tuberculous involvement of all the aforementioned organ sites. Nevertheless, it should be stated that the nonspecific symptoms that frequently ac-
company many forms of tuberculosis as they occur in the elderly are
similarly encountered in such diseases as fungal infections, malignancy,
bacterial infections, and chronic anemia.

Laboratory Tests

All patients suspected of tuberculosis, regardless of the site of involvement, should have the following tests performed: chest x-ray, PPD intermediate skin test with dermal control antigens, complete blood count,
urinalysis, renal function tests, and liver function tests.

SPECIFIC SITES OF INFECTION
   Lungs and Pleura.   Sputum examination for acid-fast bacilli and culture for *M. tuberculosis* is mandatory for suspected pleuropulmonary disease. Three early morning sputum collections are generally sufficient for
most cases of suspected tuberculosis. Elderly patients who cannot produce an expectorated sputum may require induced sputa or, in some
cases, sputa obtained by fiberoptic bronchoscopy (9). Pleural effusion

should be drained by thoracentesis; if the elderly patient is cooperative and clinically stable, a pleural biopsy specimen for culture and histology is diagnostically helpful.

Cerebrospinal Fluid. See Chapter 9 on central nervous system infections.

Genitourinary. Urinalysis invariably shows pyuria with or without hematuria or proteinuria. Three morning urine specimens for *M. tuberculosis* culture should be obtained. An intravenous pyelogram with a voiding cystourethrogram is essential to observe for typical abnormalities of genitourinary tuberculosis (24,25). Further invasive diagnostic procedures is indicated depending on the severity of disease.

Bone and Joint. Plain x-ray films of the bones and joints are helpful; radionuclide bone scanning should also be done. Joint fluid should be aspirated, analyzed, and sent for mycobacteria studies. Synovial biopsy specimens from accessible sites (knees) may be helpful in yielding a diagnosis.

Miliary or Disseminated. In patients without miliary changes on the chest x-ray film, percutaneous needle biopsy of the liver should be done. The presence of caseating or noncaseating granuloma (with or without acid-fast bacilli) strongly suggest the diagnosis. In some patients, especially those with hematologic changes, a bone marrow biopsy is positive on histologic examination (9). In patients with miliary changes on the chest x-ray film, sputum should be collected for smear and culture. If acid-fast bacilli smears are negative, bronchoscopy with transbronchial biopsy should be performed.

SPECIFIC TESTS

Tuberculin Skin Test. The tuberculin skin test is the procedure of choice for testing the presence of past or recent tuberculous infection. Although a positive test does not indicate the activity of tuberculous disease, it does show that the host is capable of maintaining a cellular immune response to this infection (35). In proven cases of active tuberculosis, the tuberculin skin test may be negative in up to 28% of cases (36). This appears to be related to serious protein deficiencies that cause impaired lymphocyte function (36,37).

With advancing age, the frequency of false-negative tuberculin skin test results with active disease increases (38–41). However, if these elderly patients with active disease are able to respond to tuberculin antigen at all, the degree of skin reactivity does not decrease with age (41). In some individuals with a history of infection, the tuberculin skin reactivity may wane. However, if a repeat skin test is applied at some time after 1 week from the initial test, a "booster effect" may be observed. That is, the initial tuberculin skin test reactivity is less than 10 mm of induration, and the repeat skin test results in an increase of skin reactivity of at least 6 mm with the total size of induration being 10 mm or more. This booster effect is more frequently seen with advancing age (42). Thus, for routine screening purposes for tuberculosis (e.g., in nursing homes), a two-step skin test program should be used. This avoids (1) missing cases of patients with a past history of tuberculosis and (2) misinterpreting repeat skin tests that become positive (from a previous negative test) as a true conversion (recent infection). Nontuberculous mycobacteria infection may also cause a booster effect.

The skin test should be done using the Mantoux method with Tween-80 stabilized purified protein derivative (PPD) that contains 5 tuberculin units (intermediate strength) (43). The test is performed by injecting 0.1 ml of PPD intracutaneously on either the volar or dorsal forearm (creating a wheal). A 26- or 27-gauge needle is recommended. The test is read after 48 hours. A positive test is 10 mm or more of induration; 5–9 mm induration is a borderline or doubtful reaction; and 0–4 mm is a negative test.

Chest X-Rays.   Chest x-rays should be done on every geriatric patient in whom active tuberculosis is being considered and in all elderly patients who have a positive tuberculin skin test result. It is no longer recommended for purposes of surveillance screening to detect tuberculosis (44). Furthermore, patients with positive skin tests in whom chemoprophylaxis may be considered, repeat chest x-rays are not needed if the initial roentgenogram was negative (44).

Serologic Tests.   Serologic tests for purposes of diagnosis of tuberculosis appear promising. Currently, an enzyme-linked immunosorbent assay (ELISA) and a latex particle agglutination test have been tested and have shown a high sensitivity and specificity (45,46).

TREATMENT

Pulmonary Tuberculosis

Most elderly patients with active tuberculosis secondary to reactivation most likely have an organism that is susceptible to isoniazid (INH) and rifampin (RIF), since the *M. tuberculosis* would have been acquired before the introduction of these drugs. INH and RIF are highly mycobactericidal and have been shown to be efficacious in treating clinical tuberculosis. In order for antituberculous drugs to be considered acceptable for clinical use, they must be effective with a relapse rate lower than 5%, and they must have a low risk of side effects. The current recommended treatment for active pulmonary tuberculosis is INH 300 mg and RIF 600 mg taken orally once a day (a combination capsule containing 150 mg of INH and 300 mg of RIF is available; it adds convenience and improves drug compliance in the elderly). These drugs are taken for 9 months. An alternative and equally acceptable regimen (which might again improve drug compliance) is to administer daily INH and RIF for 1 month, followed by INH 900 mg with RIF 600 mg taken twice weekly for 8 months (47). The latter regimen has been efficacious and safe in patients 60 years and older (48). The pharmacokinetics of INH and RIF in the elderly differ only slightly from younger adults; thus, the dose administered to the elderly patient requires no modification (49–51). However, elderly patients, while receiving INH, should also take pyridoxine 50 mg a day to minimize the dose-related neurotoxicity of this drug.

Some experts in the field of tuberculosis recommend two additional drugs, pyrazinamide (PZA), 30 mg/kg a day plus streptomycin, 500–1,000 mg a day (or PZA plus ethambutol, 15–25 mg/kg a day) to the daily INH–RIF regimen during the initial 2 months of therapy (47). However, for the elderly, we would recommend these additional drugs only if (*1*) the patient had been on antituberculous drugs previously; (*2*) the patient was from an area or country with significant drug-resistant tuberculosis (e.g., Southeast Asia or Latin America); (*3*) the patient appears to have acquired the disease from a person with drug-resistant *M. tuberculosis;* or (*4*) the patient lives in an area where INH resistance is common (5% or more) (52).

Recently, several studies have shown the efficacy and safety of a 6-month drug regimen (47,53). The regimen includes four drugs, INH, RIF, PZA, and streptomycin (or INH, RIF, PZA plus ethambutol) taken daily for 2 months, followed by INH and RIF only, either daily or twice weekly for 4 months. However, a regimen of INH and RIF only for 6 months, or any drug regimen (2–4 drugs) for less than 6 months is not recommended at this time (47,54).

Elderly patients who receive INH alone (see later section on prophylactic chemotherapy) or in combination with RIF should have routine liver function tests (serum transaminase levels) at 1, 3, 6, and 9 months (55). If symptoms of liver toxicity (anorexia, nausea, vomiting, jaundice, etc.) develop (with a concurrent rise in transaminase levels), or if the transaminase levels increase to five times normal, the medications should be stopped. When the liver function tests normalize, then INH *only* should be instituted at a lower dose (e.g., 50–100 mg a day) and gradually increased while monitoring liver function tests. If no adverse effect develops with INH, then RIF can be added, again at a low dose (e.g., 200 mg a day) and gradually increased with careful monitoring for hepatotoxicity. If the elderly patient develops hepatotoxicity with the second rechallenge of INH, the drug should be stopped and RIF given as stated above. In cases of INH hepatotoxicity without RIF side effects, the patient should be treated with a two-drug regimen of RIF and ethambutol (or RIF plus streptomycin) for a minimum of 12 months. Similarly, if RIF is responsible for the hepatotoxicity, INH plus ethambutol (or INH plus streptomycin) can then be substituted for a 12-month-treatment period. The addition of PZA depends on whether this drug also causes abnormalities in liver function tests.

Table 11.1 summarizes adverse effects of the major antituberculous drugs.

Extrapulmonary Tuberculosis

Extrapulmonary tuberculosis is effectively and safely treated with the same 9-month INH–RIF regimen prescribed for pulmonary tuberculosis (52,56).

TABLE 11.1 Adverse Effects of Major Antituberculous Drugs

DRUG	ADVERSE EFFECTS	COMMENT
Isoniazid	Peripheral neuritis, hyperexcitability, hepatitis, rash, drug fever	Give pyridoxine, monitor liver function tests
Rifampin	Hepatitis; drug fever; rarely, thrombocytopenia; orange color to urine	Monitor liver function tests
Ethambutol	Reversible optic neuritis (rare at 15 mg/kg dose)	Monitor color vision, and visual acuity
Streptomycin	Eighth nerve damage especially vestibular; rarely renal failure	Do baseline and follow-up tests on hearing and vestibular functions, reduce dose if renal impairment is present
Pyrazinamide	Hyperuricemia, occasionally hepatitis, flushing, skin rash	Monitor serum uric acid levels in patients with gout or on diuretics

TABLE 11.2 Indications for Chemoprophylaxis for Tuberculosis

Elderly contacts of newly discovered case(s) of tuberculosis.
  Contacts with positive tuberculin skin test: give isoniazid (INH) for 12 months.
  Contacts with negative skin test: repeat skin test in 1 week with control dermal antigen to exclude booster effect and cutaneous anergy. Then, if negative, hold chemotherapy, repeat skin test in 3 months. Prescribe INH only if skin test converts to positive at 3 months.
Elderly who convert their skin test.
Elderly with positive skin test and who have
  Chest x-ray abnormalities consistent with tuberculosis (excluding calcified granuloma as the sole abnormality)
  Hematologic or reticuloendothelial malignancy
  Been receiving immunosuppressive therapy
  Silicosis
  Nutritional deficiency, gastrectomy, and intestinal bypass
  Poorly controlled diabetes mellitus
  Chronic renal failure

Chemoprophylaxis for Tuberculosis

Table 11.2 summarizes the clinical circumstances in which chemo-prophylaxis for tuberculosis is recommended (55). Standard chemo-prophylaxis is with INH, 300 mg a day, for 12 months. However, INH taken regularly for 6 or 9 months may still provide significant (but less than 12-month prophylaxis) protection against active tuberculosis (57). INH chemoprophylaxis is also recommended for nursing home patients who are at risk to develop active tuberculosis (58).

Because the risk for INH-associated hepatitis has a direct age relationship, controversy exists as to whether or not elderly patients without chest x-ray abnormalities but with a positive tuberculin skin test should receive INH chemoprophylaxis. It is our practice to recommend INH chemo-prophylaxis under the circumstances given in Table 11.2 unless there are compelling reasons not to give it, that is, active liver disease, poor compliance, inability to take oral medications, or history of allergy to INH. If INH is administered, monitoring for *both* clinical symptoms and laboratory evidence of hepatotoxicity is recommended as discussed previously (55,59). Some clinicians do not recommend routine monitoring for liver function tests (52), because mild transaminase abnormalities do occur commonly and usually return to normal despite continuation of INH. However, because clinical symptoms are so unreliable in the elderly, it is best to monitor liver function tests as well as clinical manifestations.

If elderly patients are unable to tolerate INH administration (because of hepatotoxicity, allergic reaction, drug fever, etc.), it is best to discontinue further consideration of chemoprophylaxis. But, if chemoprophylaxis appears absolutely necessary, the combination of RIF and ethambutol might be an alternative regimen (60).

REFERENCES

1. Centers for Disease Control: Tuberculosis—United States, 1984. *MMWR* 34:86–87, 1985.
2. Horne NW: Problem of tuberculosis in decline. *Br Med J* 288:1249–1251, 1984.
3. Powell KE, Farer LS: The rising age of the tuberculosis patient: A sign of success and failure. *J Infect Dis* 142:946–948, 1980.
4. MacKay AD, Cole RB: The problems of tuberculosis in the elderly. *Q J Med* 53:497–510, Autumn 1984.
5. Medical Research Council Tuberculosis and Chest Diseases Unit: Treatment of pulmonary tuberculosis in patients notified in England and Wales in 1978–9: Chemotherapy and hospital admissions. *Thorax* 40:113–120, 1985.
6. Page MI, Lunn JS: Experience with tuberculosis in a public teaching hospital. *Am J Med* 77:667–670, 1984.
7. DeBuitleir M, Fitzgerald MN: The changing profile of tuberculosis in a general teaching hospital: A five-year review of 121 cases. *Irish Med J* 75: 390–399, 1982.
8. Dutt AK, Jones L, Stead WW: Short-course chemotherapy for tuberculosis with largely twice-weekly isoniazid-rifampin. *Chest* 75:441–447, 1979.
9. Nagami PH, Yoshikawa TT: Tuberculosis in the geriatric patient. *J Am Geriatr Soc* 31:356–363, 1983.
10. Bobrowitz ID: Active tuberculosis undiagnosed until autopsy. *Am J Med* 48:72:650–658, 1982.
11. Rudd A: Tuberculosis in a geriatric unit. *J Am Geriatr Soc* 33:566–569, 1985.
12. Davis CE, Jr, Carpenter JL, McAllister CK, et al: Tuberculosis. Cause of death in antibiotic era. *Chest* 88:726–729, 1985.
13. Stead WW, Lofgren JP: Does the risk of tuberculosis increase in old age? *J Infect Dis* 147:951–955, 1983.
14. Narain JP, Lofgren JP, Warren E, et al: Epidemic tuberculosis in a nursing home. A retrospective cohort study. *J Am Geriatr Soc* 33:258–263, 1985.
15. Stead WW, Lofgren JP, Warren E, et al: Tuberculosis as an endemic and nosocomial infection among the elderly in nursing homes. *N Engl J Med* 312:1483–1487, 1985.
16. Stead WW: Tuberculosis among elderly persons: An outbreak in a nursing home. *Ann Intern Med* 94:606–610, 1981.
17. Edlin GP: Active tuberculosis unrecognized until autopsy. *Lancet* 1:650–652, 1978.
18. Proudfoot AT, Aktar AJ, Douglas AC, et al: Miliary tuberculosis in adults. *Br Med J* 1:273–276, 1969.
19. Nagami P, Yoshikawa TT: Aging and tuberculosis. *Gerontology* 30:308–315, 1984.

20. Kelly PJ, Karlson AG: Musculoskeletal tuberculosis. *Mayo Clin Proc* 44:73–80, 1967.
21. Davies PDO, Humphries MJ, Byfield SP, et al: Bone and joint tuberculosis. A survey of notifications in England and Wales. *J Bone Joint Surg* 66-B:326–330, 1984.
22. Weir MR, Thornton GF: Extrapulmonary tuberculosis. Experience of a community hospital and review of the literature. *Am J Med* 79:467–478, 1985.
23. Wong SH, Lau WY, Poon GP, et al: Treatment of urinary tuberculosis. *J Urol* 131:297–301, 1984.
24. Christiansen WF: Genitourinary tuberculosis: Review of 102 cases. *Medicine* 53:377–390, 1974.
25. Simon HB, Weinstein AJ, Pasternak MS, et al: Genitourinary tuberculosis. Clinical features in a general hospital population. *Am J Med* 63:410–420, 1977.
26. Lai KK, Stottmeier KD, Sherman IH, et al: Mycobacterial cervical lymphadenopathy. Relation of etiologic agents to age. *JAMA* 251:1286–1288, 1984.
27. Donath J, Kahn FA: Tuberculous and posttuberculous bronchopleural fistula. Ten year clinical experience. *Chest* 86:697–703, 1984.
28. Essop AR, Posen JA, Hodkinson JH, et al: Tuberculous hepatitis: A clinical review of 96 cases. *Q J Med* 53:465–477, Autumn 1984.
29. Alvarez SZ, Carpio R: Hepatobiliary tuberculosis. *Dig Dis Sci* 28:193–200, 1983.
30. Schulze K, Warner HA, Murray D: Intestinal tuberculosis. Experiences at a Canadian teaching hospital. *Am J Med* 63:735–745, 1977.
31. Sherman S, Rohwedder JJ, Ravikrishnan KP, et al: Tuberculous enteritis and peritonitis. Report of 36 general hospital cases. *Arch Intern Med* 140:506–508, 1980.
32. Rooney JJ, Crocco JA, Lyons HA: Tuberculous pericarditis. *Ann Intern Med* 72:73–78, 1970.
33. Case Records of the Massachusetts General Hospital: Case 5-1976. *N Engl J Med* 294:267–274, 1976.
34. Klofkorn RW, Steigerwald JC: Carpal tunnel syndrome as the initial manifestation of tuberculosis. *Am J Med* 60:583–586, 1976.
35. Chaparas SD: Immunity in tuberculosis. Bull World Health Organization 60:447–462, 1982.
36. Rooney JJ, Crocco JA, Kramer S, et al: Further observations on tuberculin reactions in active tuberculosis. *Am J Med* 60:517–522, 1976.
37. Chandra RK, Baker M, Kumar V: Body composition, albumin levels, and delayed cutaneous cell-mediated immunity. *Nutr Res* 5:679–684, 1985.
38. Woodruff CE, Chapman PT: Tuberculin sensitivity in elderly patients. *Am Rev Respir Dis* 104:261–263, 1971.
39. Johnston RN, Ritchie RT, Murray IHF: Declining tuberculin sensitivity with advancing age. *Br Med J* 2:720–724, 1963.
40. Nash DR, Douglas JE: Anergy in active pulmonary tuberculosis. A comparison between positive and negative reactors and an evaluation of 5 TU and 250 TU skin test doses. *Chest* 77:32–37, 1980.

41. Battershill JH: Cutaneous testing in the elderly patient with tuberculosis. *Chest* 77:188–189, 1980.
42. Thompson NJ, Glassroth JL, Snider DE Jr, et al: The booster phenomenon in serial tuberculin testing. *Am Rev Respir Dis* 119:587–597, 1979.
43. Committee on Diagnostic Skin Testing of the American Thoracic Society. The tuberculin skin test. *Am Rev Respir Dis* 104:769–775, 1971.
44. Lordi GM, Reichman LB: Tuberculosis. When not to order roentgenograms. *JAMA* 253:1780–1781, 1985.
45. Daniel TM, Debanne SAM, van der Kuyp F: Enzyme-linked immunosorbent assay using *Mycobacterium tuberculosis* antigen 5 and PPD for serodiagnosis of tuberculosis. *Chest* 88:388–392, 1985.
46. Krambovitis E, McIllmurray MB, Lock PE, et al: Rapid diagnosis of tuberculous meningitis by latex particle agglutination. *Lancet* 2:1229–1231, 1984.
47. Committee on Chemotherapy of Tuberculosis: Standard therapy for tuberculosis 1985. *Chest* 87(suppl):117S–124S, 1985.
48. Dutt AK, Jones L, Stead WW: Short-course chemotherapy for tuberculosis with largely twice-weekly isoniazid-rifampin. *Chest* 75:441–447, 1979.
49. Advenier C, Saint-Aubin A, Gobert C, et al: Pharmacokinetics of isoniazid in the elderly. *Br J Clin Pharmacol* 10:167–168, 1980.
50. Kergueris MF, Bourin M, Larousse C: Pharmacokinetics of isoniazid: Influence of age. *Eur J Clin Pharmacol* 30:335–340, 1986.
51. Advenier C, Gobert C, Houin G, et al: Pharmacokinetic studies of rifampicin in the elderly. *Ther Drug Monit* 5:61–65, 1983.
52. Dutt AK, Stead WW: Tuberculosis, in Kass EH, Platt R (eds): *Current Therapy in Infectious Disease.* Toronto, B.C. Decker, Inc., 1986, vol 2, p 319.
53. British Thoracic Society: A controlled trial of 6 months' chemotherapy in pulmonary tuberculosis. Final report: results during the 36 months after the end of chemotherapy and beyond. *Br J Dis Chest* 78:330–336, 1984.
54. Snider DE Jr, Long MA, Cross FS, et al: Six-month isoniazid-rifampin therapy for pulmonary tuberculosis. Report for a United States Public Health Service Cooperative Trial. *Am Rev Respir Dis* 129:573–579, 1984.
55. Committee on Isoniazid Preventive Treatment: Preventive treatment of tuberculosis. *Chest* 87(suppl):1285–1325, 1985.
56. Dutt AS, Moers D, Stead WW: Short-course chemotherapy for extrapulmonary tuberculosis. Nine years' experience. *Ann Intern Med* 104:7–12, 1986.
57. International Union Against Tuberculosis Committee on Prophylaxis. Efficacy of various durations of isoniazid preventive therapy for tuberculosis: five years of follow-up in the IUAT trial. *Bull World Health Organization* 60:555–564, 1982.
58. Cooper JK: Decision analysis for tuberculosis preventive treatment in nursing homes. *J Am Geriatr Soc* 34:814–817, 1986.
59. Byrd RB, Horn BR, Solomon DA, et al: Toxic effects of isoniazid in tuberculous chemoprophylaxis. Role of biochemical monitoring in 1,000 patients. *JAMA* 241:1239–1241, 1979.
60. Livengood JR, Sigler TG, Foster LR, et al: Isoniazid-resistant tuberculosis. A community outbreak and report of a rifampin prophylaxis failure. *JAMA* 253:2847–2849, 1985.

SUGGESTED READINGS

Battershill JH: Cutaneous testing in the elderly patient with tuberculosis. *Chest* 77:188–189, 1980.

Committee on Chemotherapy of Tuberculosis: Standard therapy for tuberculosis 1985. *Chest* 87(suppl):117S–124S, 1985.

Committee on Isoniazid Preventive Treatment: Preventive treatment of tuberculosis. *Chest* 87(suppl):1285–1325, 1985.

Dutt AS, Moers D, Stead WW: Short-course chemotherapy for extrapulmonary tuberculosis. Nine years' experience. *Ann Intern Med* 104:7–12, 1986.

Nagami PH, Yoshikawa TT: Tuberculosis in the geriatric patient. *J Am Geriatr Soc* 31:356–363, 1983.

Stead WW, Lofgren JP: Does the risk of tuberculosis increase in old age? *J Infect Dis* 147:951–955, 1983.

Stead WW, Lofgren JP, Warren E, et al: Tuberculosis as an endemic and nosocomial infection among the elderly in nursing homes. *N Engl J Med* 312:1483–1487, 1985.

Thompson NJ, Glassroth JL, Snider DE Jr, et al: The booster phenomenon in serial tuberculin testing. *Am Rev Respir Dis* 119:587–597, 1979.

Weir MR, Thornton GF: Extrapulmonary tuberculosis. Experience of a community hospital and review of the literature. *Am J Med* 79:467–478, 1985.

Chapter 12

Infective Endocarditis

GENERAL CONSIDERATIONS

Epidemiology

Infective endocarditis refers to infection of the endocardial surface of the heart. Since the beginning of the antibiotic era, the mean age of patients diagnosed as having natural valve infective endocarditis (henceforth referred to as *IE*) has increased, particularly if drug addicts with IE are excluded (1) (Fig. 12.1). In fact, several studies indicate that over 50% of the patients with IE are age 60 years or older (3–6). Some factors that contribute to this demographic change include: (*1*) decline in rheumatic fever in industrialized nations and hence a reduction in rheumatic valvular disease; (*2*) increased longevity of people with congenital or rheumatic heart disease; (*3*) rise in age-related degenerative valvular disease as a predisposition to IE; and (*4*) emergence of nosocomial endocarditis as a result of newer therapeutic modalities (pacemakers, intravenous catheters, dialysis shunts, etc.) (2,7).

Similarly, prosthetic valve endocarditis (hereafter referred to as *PVE*) occurs with increasing frequency in the elderly age groups and parallels the increasing number of older persons that receive prosthetic heart valves (1,8,9).

The mortality of elderly patients with IE ranges from 40 to 70% (10–13), far surpassing that of the younger population with IE. For PVE, the overall mortality may approach 50% (14).

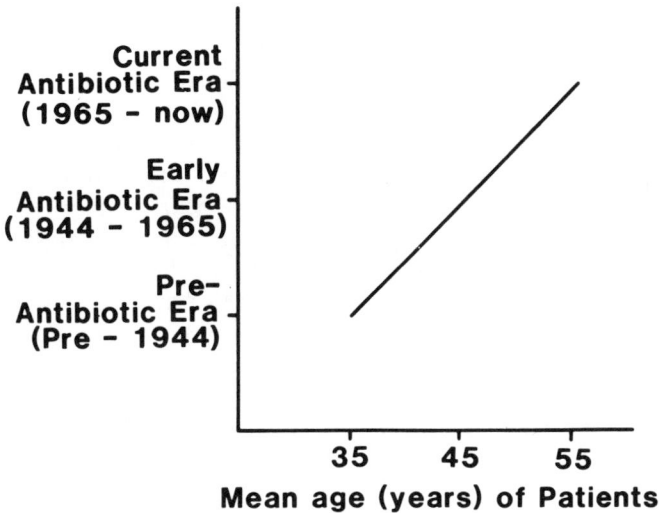

Figure 12.1. Mean age of patients with infective endocarditis who were reported in the literature during different study periods.

Pathogenesis

It is beyond the scope of this book to discuss in detail the pathogenesis of IE (or PVE). (The reader may find a full description in most standard references on infectious disease or infective endocarditis.) Nevertheless, an understanding of the presumed pathogenetic mechanisms of IE in humans (most data come from experimental animal models of IE) is important in order to better understand the natural history and clinical aspects of this infection. For IE to develop, the endocardial surface must first be altered (usually secondary to cardiac defects or therapeutic devices that create turbulent blood flow), which then permits the deposition of platelets and fibrin and subsequent formation of nonbacterial thrombotic endocarditis (1,2). If bacteremia (or fungemia) occurs, microorganisms can reach the valve and adhere to the nonbacterial thrombotic lesion, replicate, and eventually form a vegetation. Thus, factors that influence or modulate the development of IE include the degree of blood flow turbulence related to the valve lesion or dysfunction and the ability of the organism to adhere to the nonthrombotic lesion. Also, immunologic responses of the host to the etiologic pathogen are important (15).

Etiology

Aerobic gram-positive coccal bacteria account for the majority of cases of IE and PVE, regardless of age (2,16,17). In the elderly, infection on natural valves is dominated by streptococci, particularly viridans streptococci as is the case in younger patients with IE (3,13,18). However, in the elderly, other streptococci are more likely to be isolated as a cause of IE (13). For example, *S. bovis* is the most common cause of IE in patients over 55 years in some studies (16). More importantly, *S. bovis* bacteremia and endocarditis is associated with colorectal disease, primarily colorectal carcinoma (19–22), and this association occurs primarily in the elderly. Enterococcal (primarily *S. faecalis*) endocarditis is largely a disease of elderly patients (23,24). *S. faecalis* is a frequent cause of urinary tract infection in the elderly (see Chapter 14 on urinary tract infection); it may be a cause of biliary sepsis in the aged, and it is part of the normal gastrointestinal microflora. Other streptococci that are reported as a cause of IE in the elderly include group B, C, and G streptococci (25–27). Whether this represents an actual change in pathogens or is due to better laboratory methods of streptococcal identification is unclear. Finally, *Staphylococcus aureus* may be responsible for 20 to 30% of IE in the geriatric age group (2,28,29). Moreover, the older population (60 years and older) may account for over 50% of all cases of *S. aureus* endocarditis (7) with a mortality of 88% (7). They are more likely to have *S. aureus* endocarditis that is undiagnosed clinically as well as acquire the infection in the hospital (7).

In elderly patients with PVE, the etiologic pathogens are the same as for younger patients. *Staphylococcus epidermidis* is the single most frequently isolated pathogen, followed by *S. aureus*. Various species of streptococci, gram-negative bacilli, and occasionally fungi (*Candida* and *Aspergillus*) are less common isolates (13,30–32).

CLINICAL MANIFESTATIONS

The classic manifestations of IE (fever, changing or new murmurs, embolic manifestations, splenomegaly, mucocutaneous findings, and constitutional symptoms) may be seen in elderly patients. However, a significant number of older patients with IE have atypical and/or nonspecific symptoms and signs (10–13,17,33). The diagnosis may not be suspected clinically in as many as 60% of elderly patients with proven IE (33). Symptoms in this older age group may be vague and nondescript, for example, weakness, malaise, easy fatigueability, anorexia, or unexplained weight loss. Fever may be absent in as many as one-third of elderly patients with IE (4), although other studies report an absence of fever in 9 to 17% of geriatric cases (17,34). Alternatively, IE was the cause of *fever of unknown origin* (FUO) in 8% of 111 patients aged 65 years and older who had prolonged and perplexing fevers (35). A heart murmur due to congenital heart disease, degenerative or atherosclerotic valvular disease, rheumatic fever, syphilis, idiopathic hypertrophic subaortic stenosis, or mitral valve prolapse is generally found in most cases of IE in the elderly. However, as many as 37% of elderly IE cases may not have any underlying heart disease, and 32% may not demonstrate a heart murmur on clinical examination (33). In one recent study of 119 cases of *S. aureus* endocarditis, 65 patients with a median age of 65 did not have their infection diagnosed clinically (7). Of those undiagnosed cases, 56% of the patients failed to demonstrate a heart murmur.

Neurologic symptoms and signs are commonly seen in elderly patients either as a presenting manifestation or as a later complication of IE. More importantly, the presence of a neurologic abnormality in older patients with IE dramatically increases the mortality to 75% (13). Typical neurologic manifestations found in this age group with IE include confusion, delirium, coma, depression or paranoia, aphasia, and hemiplegia. Pathologic changes in the brain that may result from IE include embolic infarcts, subarachnoid blood, mycotic aneurysm, intracerebral bleeding, and brain abscess.

Other important manifestations of IE in the aged include unexplained heart failure or arrhythymias, renal abnormalities (hematuria, pyuria, proteinuria, oliguria, azotemia), and musculoskeletal complaints (arthralgia, low back pain, myalgia).

The clinical findings of PVE in the elderly are similar to those of natural valve endocarditis. Additionally, depending on the type of prosthetic valve, there may be changes in valve opening and closing sounds as well as in new systolic and/or diastolic murmurs.

DIAGNOSTIC APPROACH

Differential Diagnosis

The differential diagnosis of IE includes any infectious process that can cause bacteremia. Additionally, cerebrovascular accidents and collagen vascular disease may be considered in the elderly patient who develops the manifestations of IE.

Laboratory Tests

The diagnosis of IE is *definite* if there is histologic and/or microbiologic evidence of valve infection. (The valve would have to be biopsied or surgically removed.) The diagnosis of IE is *probable* when one of the following conditions exists: (*1*) persistently positive blood cultures are found in a patient with a new regurgitant murmur or in a patient with a predisposing heart lesion and peripheral manifestations of IE; or (*2*) if blood cultures are negative or only intermittently positive, the patient must have fever, new regurgitant murmurs, and peripheral manifestations of IE (34).

BLOOD CULTURES

Blood cultures are the single most important laboratory test for the diagnosis of IE. Bacteremia in IE is usually continuous and low grade (less than 100 organisms/ml blood) (36). In IE patients with documented bacteremia, the first two sets of blood cultures are positive in over 90% of cases (2,5,37). Therefore, three sets of blood cultures (two bottles, one for aerobic organisms and one for anaerobic bacteria per venipuncture) drawn from different venipuncture sites at different times during the first 24 hours are recommended. This method documents the presence of continuous bacteremia and facilitates the interpretation of a positive blood culture as true bacteremia versus skin contamination. In patients who have received antibiotics in the preceeding 2 weeks, additional blood cultures may be necessary to demonstrate bacteremia. If a patient is acutely ill and the clinical diagnosis of IE is rather obvious, empiric antimicrobial therapy within hours of the clinical diagnosis may be appropriate. Under these circumstances, the three sets of blood cultures should be obtained at intervals of every 15 minutes from different venous sites.

OTHER TESTS

Echocardiography should be used as an adjunctive tool for the diagnosis and follow-up of IE cases. The sensitivities of M-mode and two-dimensional echocardiography for detecting valve vegetation range from 40 to 50% and 43 to 79%, respectively (38,39). Therefore, the absence of a vegetation on echocardiography does not exclude the diagnosis of IE. Conversely, false-positive studies are extremely rare (2). However, there have been no studies on the diagnostic accuracy of echocardiography in elderly patients with IE.

Anemia, leukocytosis, renal abnormalities, autoantibodies, and circulating immune complexes are commonly associated with IE. Therefore, a complete blood count, serum creatinine, urinalysis, rheumatoid factor, and serum complement should be obtained. Serial electrocardiograms and chest x-rays should be part of the diagnostic evaluation and management of IE.

A careful gastrointestinal evaluation, particularly the colon for carcinoma, is essential in all elderly patients who have *S. bovis* isolated from the blood. With enterococcal bacteremia, a urine culture as well as an evaluation of the biliary tract should be part of the diagnostic management.

TREATMENT

Antimicrobial Therapy

SPECIFIC PATHOGENS

Viridans Streptococci.   Most of these organisms are sensitive to penicillin G (minimal inhibitory concentration [MIC] equal to or less than 0.2 µg/ml). If the minimal bactericidal concentration (MBC) of the streptococci is also low, then the treatment of choice for the elderly patient with IE is intravenous aqueous penicillin G 10–20 million units a day in four to six divided doses. Patients with a serious penicillin allergy (e.g., anaphylaxis, urticaria, angioedema) should be treated with vancomycin 1.5–2.0 g a day in two to four divided doses. A small but significant percentage of strains of viridans streptococci are resistant to penicillin G (MIC > 0.2 µg/ml), show evidence of "tolerance" (inhibited but not killed by penicillin G; MBC to MIC ratio exceeds 10:1), or are nutritionally dependent (also showing tolerance). These organisms should be treated with the same regimen as for enterococcal endocarditis.

Streptococcus bovis.   These organisms may be treated with the same regimen prescribed for penicillin-sensitive viridans streptococci.

Enterococci.   The enterococci are relatively resistant to penicillin G and also demonstrate tolerance. Therefore, the treatment of choice for elderly persons with enterococcal endocarditis is a combination of intravenous aqueous penicillin G 20–30 million units a day *or* ampicillin 12 g a day, both given in six divided doses, *plus* intramuscular streptomycin 1 g in two divided doses (40). In elderly patients with significant renal impairment, the dose of penicillin and streptomycin may have to be reduced, and careful monitoring of eighth nerve function should be implemented. In some strains of enterococci, there may be resistance to streptomycin (MIC > 2,000 µg/ml). With these streptomycin-resistant strains, the patient should receive gentamicin 3 mg/kg a day in three divided doses (or dose adjusted for level of renal function) (40). Penicillin-allergic patients should receive vancomycin 1.5–2.0 g a day in two to four divided doses *plus* streptomycin or gentamicin.

Staphylococcus aureus.   Most strains of *S. aureus* are resistant to penicillin G; therefore, they should be treated with other beta-lactam drugs. For the elderly with *S. aureus* endocarditis, treatment should be with intravenous nafcillin or oxacillin, 12 g a day in six divided doses

(41). High-dose cefazolin, 6–8 g a day in three to four divided doses, is also effective. The value of adding an aminoglycoside to these beta-lactam antibiotics is controversial (2); however, tolerant strains of *S. aureus* should be treated with the addition of an aminoglycoside or rifampin. Patients allergic to penicillin or who have IE caused by methicillin-resistant (and therefore, also resistant to oxacillin and nafcillin) *S. aureus* should be given vancomycin 1.5–2.0 g a day.

Staphylococcus epidermidis.   This organism is frequently resistant to methicillin and cephalosporins. The treatment of choice is then vancomycin 1.5–2.0 g a day combined with rifampin 600 mg a day. If the organism is methicillin sensitive, then nafcillin or oxacillin, 12 g a day, should be administered.

Gram-Negative Bacilli.   Treatment is dependent on antibiotic susceptibility studies. Most patients require an aminoglycoside plus either an antipseudomonas penicillin (piperacillin, mezlocillin, or azlocillin) or a third-generation cephalosporin (e.g., ceftazidime). Of course, in the elderly, drug toxicity is a major concern with administration of an aminoglycoside (see Chapter 5 for details on aminoglycoside usage).

EMPIRIC TREATMENT
Empiric antibiotic treatment (before blood culture data return) should be started in an elderly person suspected of IE if any of the following conditions are present: (*1*) shock due to sepsis; (*2*) significant congestive heart failure; (*3*) new regurgitant murmurs; (*4*) embolization to a major organ (e.g., brain, lung, kidneys); or (*5*) the patient is extremely toxic.

Natural Valve IE.   Since the primary organisms to be considered are viridans streptococci, *S. bovis,* enterococci, and *S. aureus,* the elderly patient should be treated with aqueous penicillin G, 10–20 million units a day, nafcillin or oxacillin, 12 g a day, and streptomycin 1 g a day until culture data become available. Penicillin-allergic patients should receive vancomycin, 1.5–2.0 g a day plus streptomycin 1 g a day.

Prosthetic Valve Endocarditis.   Vancomycin 1.5–2.0 g a day, and gentamicin, 5 mg/kg a day (three divided doses) are the drugs of choice until culture data become available.

Culture-Negative Endocarditis.   If after initiating empiric therapy, the blood cultures return negative and IE or PVE is still considered as a primary diagnosis, the above regimen should be continued.

DURATION OF TREATMENT

All elderly patients with endocarditis should be treated with antibiotics for a minimum of 4 weeks. Under select circumstances, 6 weeks (or longer) of treatment may be indicated. These cicumstances include (*1*) all prosthetic valve endocarditis treated medically alone; (*2*) any natural aortic valve endocarditis except if the etiology is a penicillin-sensitive streptococci; (*3*) all gram-negative bacillary endocarditis; (*4*) all culture-negative endocarditis; and (*5*) all cases of endocarditis associated with major complications (e.g., heart failure, embolization).

Surgery

For natural valve IE, surgery is indicated for the following complications: (*1*) progressive congestive heart failure (especially aortic valve); (*2*) microbiologic failure on adequate doses of antibiotics; (*3*) fungal endocarditis; (*4*) myocardial abscess; and (*5*) repeated embolization on therapy (42). With PVE, surgical replacement of the infected valve is indicated if the following conditions are present: (*1*) hemodynamic instability; (*2*) new regurgitant murmur; (*3*) myocardial abscess; (*4*) repeated episodes of major embolization; and (*5*) the etiology is an organism that is not highly susceptible to the available antibiotics (1).

Supportive Care

Supportive care and special attention to potential complications of IE is equally important in managing these elderly patients. In all cases, proper oxygenation is required. Observation for and vigorous treatment of heart failure, arrhythmias, and aspiration should be done. Prevention of thrombophlebitis and decubitus ulcers with correction of anemia, poor nutritional status, and fluid and electrolyte disorders is essential in the elderly as these patients are least likely to tolerate these complications.

Follow-Up Management

After appropriate antimicrobial therapy is begun, the elderly patient's clinical status should be closely monitored; the important parameters are fever, mental status, functional level, appetite, status of murmur and cardiac hemodynamics, and evidence for any new clinical symptoms or signs. Additionally, complete blood count, renal function test and urinalysis, blood cultures, and serum bactericidal concentration (SBC) should be obtained weekly. The clinical utility of the SBC has been debated by some investigators (43); however, we do recommend this test. A SBC titer of 1:8 or higher has been shown to be associated with improved results in some clinical and in many animal studies of IE. If aminoglycosides are administered, drug levels as well as renal and eighth nerve function should be closely monitored. (Preventive management for IE is discussed in Chapter 6.)

REFERENCES

1. Cantrell M, Yoshikawa TT: Aging and infective endocarditis. *J Am Geriatr Soc* 31:216–222, 1983.
2. Scheld WM, Sande MA: Endocarditis and intravascular infections, in Mandell GL, Douglas RG, Jr, Bennett JE (eds): *Principles and Practice of Infectious Diseases,* ed 2. New York, John Wiley & Sons, 1985, p 504.
3. Garvey GJ, Neu HC: Infective endocarditis—an evolving disease: A review of endocarditis at the Columbian-Presbyterian Medical Center. *Medicine* 57:105–127, 1978.
4. Lowes JA, Williams G, Tabaqchali S, et al: 10 years of infective endocarditis at St. Bartholomew's Hospital: Analysis of clinical features and treatment in relation to prognosis and mortality. *Lancet* 1:133–136, 1980.
5. Weinstein L, Rubin RH: Infective endocarditis—1973. *Prog Cardiovasc Dis* 16:239–274, 1973.
6. Venezio FR, Westenfelder GO, Cook FV, et al: Infective endocarditis in a community hospital. *Arch Intern Med* 142:789–792, 1982.
7. Espersen F, Frimodt-Moller N: *Staplylococcus aureus* endocarditis: A review of 119 cases. *Arch Intern Med* 146:1118–1121, 1986.
8. Karchmer AW, Dismukes WE, Buckley MJ, et al: Late prosthetic valve endocarditis: Clinical features influencing therapy. *Am J Med* 64:199–206, 1978.
9. Jamieson WRE, Thompson DM, Munro HI: Cardiac valve replacement in the elderly. *Can Med Assoc J* 123:628–632, 1980.
10. Glecker WJ: Diagnostic aspects of subacute bacterial endocarditis in the elderly. *Arch Intern Med* 102:761–765, 1958.
11. Cummings V, Furman S, Dunst M, et al: Subacute bacterial endocarditis in the older age group. *JAMA* 172:137–141, 1960.
12. Applefeld MM, Hornick RB: Infective endocarditis in patients over 60. *Am Heart J* 88:90–94, 1974.
13. Robbins N, DeMaria A, Miller MH: Infective endocarditis in the elderly. *South Med J* 73:1335–1338, 1980.
14. Watanakunakorn C: Prosthetic valve infective endocarditis. *Prog Cardiovasc Dis* 22:181–192, 1979.
15. Sande MA, Korzeniowski DM, Scheld WM: Factors influencing the pathogenesis and prevention of infective endocarditis. *Scand J Infect Dis* 31(suppl):48–54, 1984.
16. Cantrell M, Yoshikawa TT: Infective endocarditis in the aging patient. *Gerontology* 30:316–326, 1984.
17. Ries K: Endocarditis in the elderly, in Kaye D (ed): *Infective Endocarditis.* Baltimore, University Park Press, 1976, p 143.

18. Parker MT, Ball LC: Streptococci and aerococci associated with systemic infections in man. *J Med Microbiol* 9:275–302, 1976.
19. Dunham WR, Simpson JH, Feest TG, et al: *Streptococcus bovis* endocarditis and colorectal disease. *Lancet* 1:421–422, 1980.
20. Klein RS, Recco RA, Catalan MT, et al: Association of *Streptococcus bovis* with carcinoma of the colon. *N Engl J Med* 297:800–802, 1982.
21. Murray HW, Roberts RB: *Streptococcus bovis* bacteremia and underlying gastrointestinal disease. *Arch Intern Med* 138:1097–1099, 1978.
22. Silver SC: *Streptococcus bovis* endocarditis and its association with colonic carcinoma. *Dis Colon Rectum* 27:613–614, 1984.
23. Moellering RC, Watson RK, Kunz LJ: Endocarditis due to group D streptococci: Comparison of disease caused by *Streptococcus bovis* with that produced by the enterococci. *Am J Med* 57:239–250, 1974.
24. Mandell GL, Kaye D, Levison ME, et al: Enterococcal endocarditis: An analysis of 38 patients observed at the New York Hospital-Cornell Medical Center. *Arch Intern Med* 125:258–264, 1970.
25. Gallagher PG, Watanakunakorn C: Group B streptococcal endocarditis: Report of seven cases and review of the literature, 1962–1985. *Rev Infect Dis* 8:175–188, 1986.
26. Stein DS, Panwalker AP: Group C streptococcal endocarditis: Case report and review of the literature. *Infection* 13:282–285, 1985.
27. Vartian C, Lerner PI, Shlaes DM, et al: Infections due to Lancefield group G streptococci. *Medicine* 64:75–88, 1985.
28. Watanakunakorn C, Tan JC, Phair JP: Some salient features of *Staphylococcus aureus* endocarditis. *Am J Med* 54:473–481, 1973.
29. Watanakunakorn C, Tan JC: Diagnostic difficulties of staphylococcal endocarditis in geriatric patients. *Geriatrics* 28:168–173, 1973.
30. Wilson WR, Danielson GK, Guiliane ER, et al: Prosthetic valve endocarditis. *Mayo Clin Proc* 57:155–161, 1982.
31. Wilson WR, Jaumin PM, Danielson GK, et al: Prosthetic valve endocarditis. *Ann Intern Med* 82:751–756, 1975.
32. Rubenstein E, Noriega ER, Simberkoff M, et al: Fungal endocarditis: Analysis of 24 cases and review of the literature. *Medicine* 54:331–344, 1974.
33. Thell R, Martin FH, Edwards JE: Bacterial endocarditis in subjects 60 years of age and older. *Circulation* 51:174–182, 1975.
34. Von Reyn K, Levy BS, Arbert RD, et al: Infective endocarditis. I. An analysis based on strict case definitions. *Ann Intern Med* 94:505–518, 1981.
35. Esposito AL, Gleckman RA: Fever of unknown origin in the elderly. *J Am Geriatr Soc* 26:498–505, 1978.
36. Werner AS, Cobbs CG, Kaye D, et al: Studies on bacteremia of bacterial endocarditis. *JAMA* 202:127–131, 1967.
37. Washington JA, II: Blood cultures: Principles and techniques. *Mayo Clin Proc* 50:91–98, 1975.
38. Gilbert BW, Haney RS, Crawford F, et al: Two-dimensional echocardiographic assessment of vegetative endocarditis. *Circulation* 55:346–353, 1977.
39. Mintz GS, Kotler MN: Clinical value and limitations of echocardiography:

Its use in the study of patients with infective endocarditis. *Arch Intern Med* 140:1022–1027, 1980.

40. Scheld WM, Mandell GL: Enigmatic enterococcal endocarditis. *Ann Intern Med* 100:904–906, 1984.
41. Thompson RL: Staphylococcal endocarditis. *Mayo Clin Proc* 57:106–114, 1982.
42. Weinstein L: Life-threatening complications of infective endocarditis and their management. *Arch Intern Med* 146:953–957, 1986.
43. Coleman DL, Horwitz RI, Andriole VT: Association between serum inhibitory and bactericidal concentration and therapeutic outcome in bacterial endocarditis. *Am J Med* 73:260–268, 1982.

SUGGESTED READINGS

Cantrell M, Yoshikawa TT: Aging and infective endocarditis. *J Am Geriatr Soc* 31:216–222, 1983.

Klein RS, Recco RA, Catalan MT, et al: Association of *Streptococcus bovis* with carcinoma of the colon. *N Engl J Med* 297:800–802, 1982.

Ries K: Endocarditis in the elderly, in Kaye D (ed): *Infective Endocarditis.* Baltimore, University Park Press, 1976, p 143.

Robbins N, DeMaria A, Miller MH: Infective endocarditis in the elderly. *South Med J* 73:1335–1338, 1980.

Scheld WM, Sande MA: Endocarditis and intravascular infections, in Mandell GL, Douglas RG, Jr, Bennett JE (eds): *Principles and Practice of Infectious Diseases,* ed 2. New York, John Wiley & Sons, 1985, p 504.

Thell R, Martin FH, Edwards JE: Bacterial endocarditis in subjects 60 years of age and older. *Circulation* 51:174–182, 1975.

Watanakunakorn C: Prosthetic valve infective endocarditis. *Prog Cardiovasc Dis* 22:181–192, 1979.

Chapter 13

Intraabdominal Infection

Intraabdominal infections in the elderly often present difficult diagnostic and therapeutic problems. This chapter focuses on those infections of particular relevance to the aged, which include biliary sepsis, diverticulitis, appendicitis, and intraabdominal abscess. Clearly, geriatric patients with intraabdominal infection have both higher morbidity and mortality than do similarly affected younger patients. Elderly patients are more likely to have atypical presentation, delays in definitive surgery, complicating chronic diseases, and postoperative complications (e.g., pneumonia) (1) as well as factors that contribute to the higher morbidity and mortality usually observed for intraabdominal infections in this population (2–5).

However, recently two studies of acute abdominal disease in the elderly (6) and emergency abdominal procedures in patients above 70 (7) reported more encouraging outcomes. In the former study, Fenyö looked at two large groups of elderly patients with acute abdominal disease (series I studied patients between 1960 and 1968, and series II looked at patients between 1977 and 1978) (6). Biliary sepsis accounted for most cases of acute abdomens in both groups. Significant reductions in mortality were observed for biliary sepsis (6 to 2%), acute appendicitis (12 to 9%), and diverticulitis (12 to 3%) between series I and series II patients. Overall mortality was not dramatically lower between the two series (although reduced by 2.7%) because a substantial portion of patients in series II had malignant diseases.

Similarly, in the latter study, Reiss and Deutsch evaluated 200 consecutive emergency abdominal surgeries in patients over age 70, and, again, biliary sepsis accounted for the most cases (7). If patients with malignancy are excluded, mortality was low (biliary sepsis, 3%; appendicitis, 0%); these authors recommended *early* surgery in elderly patients with 'acute' abdomens (7). Nevertheless, when patients with intraabdominal infections are stratified according to parameters that measure severity of illness (e.g., the recently developed acute physiology score (APS), which gives numerical weight to multiple physiologic and laboratory test values), *advanced age,* as well as presence of chronic diseases, malnutrition, and poor APS correlate with increased mortality (8,9). The highest mortality rates are in patients greater than age 70 with dramatic increases with each successive decade (7).

BILIARY SEPSIS

General Considerations

The incidence of gallstones increases with age, and autopsy studies indicate that fully 30% of individuals over age 70 have cholelithiasis (10). Thus, it is not surprising that inflammatory disease of the biliary tract also increases with advanced age and that biliary tract disease is the most common cause for both emergency and elective abdominal surgery in the elderly (6,7). Furthermore, morbidity and mortality for biliary sepsis are highest in the elderly largely due to complications of infection and coexisting cardiopulmonary disease (3).

Etiology

Bile is normally sterile. However, the risk of bacterial colonization of the bile with intestinal microflora is increased in the presence of inflammatory disease of the biliary tract, obstruction (e.g., from stones), previous biliary surgery, and particularly if there is an anastomosis between the bile ducts and the bowel (11–13). Moreover, with increasing age, the risk of bacterial infection of the bile similarly increases. Approximately 70% of patients over the age of 70 years compared to 35% of patients under the age of 70 have positive bile cultures at the time of cholecystectomy (11,12). The presence of bacteria in the bile contributes to inflammatory biliary disease as well as to such septic complications as wound infection and bacteremia (12–14), especially in those patients who require emergency surgery (15).

Typically, aerobic bacteria are the main isolates from bile with (in descending order) *Escherichia coli, Klebsiella* sp., and *Streptococcus faecalis* (enterococcus) as the most common isolates (see Table 13.1) (13,14). Although there are no studies directly comparing the microbiology of bile of young and old patients who underwent biliary surgery, the micro-

TABLE 13.1 Microorganisms Commonly Isolated
From Intraabdominal Infections in Descending Order of Frequency

| TYPE OF INFECTION | MICROORGANISMS | |
	FACULTATIVE ANAEROBES OR AEROBES	STRICT ANAEROBES
Intraabdominal abscess (including diverticular and appendiceal abscess, or gangrenous or perforated appendices)	*Escherichia coli* *Streptococcus* sp. (including enterococcus) *Proteus* sp. *Klebsiella* sp.	*Bacteroides* sp. *Bacteroides fragilis* *Peptococcus* sp. *Peptostreptococcus* sp. *Fusobacterium* sp. *Eubacterium* sp. *Clostridium* sp.
Biliary sepsis	*Escherichia coli* *Klebsiella* sp. *Streptococcus faecalis* (enterococcus) *Enterobacter* sp.	*Bacteroides fragilis*[a] *Clostridium* sp.
Early appendicitis (no perforation or gangrene)	*Escherichia coli*	

SOURCE: Adapted from references 3, 50, and 61.
[a]Anaerobes are more likely to be isolated in elderly patients with biliary carcinoma or prior biliary tract surgery.

organisms isolated from elderly patients are similar to those from younger patients (16). However, anaerobic bacteria including *Bacteroides fragilis* and *Clostridium* sp. appear to be more likely to be isolated in elderly patients with complicated, severe biliary tract disease (e.g., obstructions due to carcinoma or associated with previous biliary surgery) (17,18).

Clinical Manifestations

ACUTE CHOLECYSTITIS
The clinical features of acute cholecystitis are shown in Table 13.2, which summarizes the results of two recent studies (16,19). Classic symptoms and findings of right upper quadrant pain, nausea and vomiting, right upper quadrant tenderness, fever, and leukocytosis may not be present in elderly patients with cholecystitis. Morrow et al. (Table 13.2), in their series of geriatric patients who underwent emergency cholecystectomy for acute cholecystitis, reported that abdominal tenderness and focal peritoneal signs were not present in a substantial number of cases (16). Furthermore, fever may be absent in over 30% of these patients (Table 13.2).

TABLE 13.2   Clinical Features of Elderly
Patients Undergoing Emergency Cholecystectomy

	STUDY (REFERENCE)			
	MORROW ET AL. (16)		HUBER ET AL. (19)	
PARAMETER	(N)	(%)	(N)	(%)
Total patients	39	100	43	100
Fever	24	62	30	70
Abdominal pain	38	97	42	97
Abdominal tenderness	29	74	—	—
Peritonitis	16	41	—	—
Jaundice	11	28	10	23
Mass	7	18	—	—
Disorientation	5	13	—	—
Hypotension	2	5	—	—
WBC >10,000/mm^3	24	62		
Increased bilirubin or alkaline phosphatase	21	54	—	—
Increased serum glutamic pyruvic transaminase (SGPT) or serum glutamic oxalacetic transaminase (SGOT)	23	60	—	—
Pathology showing only simple acute cholecystitis (e.g., no empyema, gangrene, or perforation)	17	44	—	—
Complications (e.g., wound infection)	17	44	14	33
Mortality	4	10[a]	6	14[a]

[a]Mortality for acute cholecystitis for the population as a whole has been reported to be 3.5% (28).

ACALCULOUS CHOLECYSTITIS

Although it appears that in most cases acute cholecystitis is caused by obstruction of the cystic duct by a stone, the pathogenesis is not completely understood (20). However, a small percentage (approximately 2.3–6%) (20,21) of cases of acute cholecystitis have acalculous cholecystitis. Furthermore, acalculous cholecystitis is often complicated by gangrene of the gallbladder (22,23). This disease usually occurs in elderly, debilitated, or critically ill patients, and diagnosis is often difficult because clinical signs can be obscured by systemic disease. Mortality is high, ranging from 9 to 67% (22–24).

ACUTE SUPPURATIVE CHOLANGITIS
Acute suppurative cholangitis results from concurrent biliary obstruction (usually calculous, stricture, or neoplasm) and infection. Although it is potentially life threatening, acute cholangitis has a wide spectrum of severity (25,26), the most severe of which is acute suppurative cholangitis (ASC). Clinically, ASC is a pentad of symptoms that include fever (and chills), jaundice, and right upper quadrant pain (Charcot's triad) with hypotension and central nervous system depression. ASC is defined pathologically by obstruction and pyogenic infection of the biliary tract (27). Fortunately, ASC occurs in only a small percentage (15%) of cholangitis cases (25). Yet this disease, which has an associated mortality of 17 to 30% (27) rarely occurs before the seventh decade of life, which makes it a geriatric disease.

Though classically patients with ASC present as described above, in many elderly patients the complete pentad of clinical features may not be present (25,26). Generally, in cases of ASC, findings are more severe than in nonsuppurative cholangitis (25). But fever may be low grade, jaundice may be mild, or the symptoms and signs of sepsis may obscure the biliary tract features (2). Bacteria are usually present in the bile, and blood cultures are frequently positive (see the section on etiology). It should be noted that anaerobes are more frequently present in ASC than in cases of simple acute cholecystitis.

Diagnostic Approach

DIFFERENTIAL DIAGNOSIS
The differential diagnosis of biliary tract disease in the elderly include gallbladder malignancy, liver abscess, hepatitis, primary or secondary carcinoma of the liver, pancreatic disease, acute appendicitis, and intraabdominal abscess.

LABORATORY TESTS
Rapid diagnosis is essential to reduce the high morbidity and mortality associated with biliary sepsis. Fortunately, diagnosis has been facilitated with the widespread availability of ultrasonography and sensitive and specific radionuclide scanning techniques, which can be used even if jaundice is present. When intravenous cholescintigraphy demonstrates nonvisualization of the gallbladder, but shows prompt visualization of the common bile duct, then the diagnosis of acute cholecystitis is strongly supported (30). Moreover, in the presence of a compatible syndrome, the demonstration of gallstones on abdominal ultrasonography also supports the diagnosis.

Similarly, in cases of suspected ASC, the absence of radioactivity in the biliary and gastrointestinal tract when intravenous cholescintigraphy is performed or the presence of a dilated common duct with ultrasonography support the diagnosis of biliary obstruction (27). Although endoscopic retrograde cholangiopancreatography (ERCP) and percutaneous transhepatic cholangiography are useful diagnostic tools in cholangitis, they have the potential of increasing biliary tract pressure and may exacerbate ASC.

Treatment

Significantly, acute cholecystitis in the elderly is associated with high morbidity and mortality compared to the population as a whole (28) (see Table 13.2). This is caused in part by the presence of advanced pathology of the gallbladder that is found at operation in elderly patients even when the clinical presentation is relatively benign. In the series reported by Morrow et al., 21% of patients had empyema, 10% had perforation, and 8% had gangrene of the gallbladder (16). Fry et al. reviewed 18 cases of gangrenous cholecystitis (taken from a series of 310 patients who underwent cholecystectomy) and found the mean age of patients to be 69-years old with a mortality of 22% (29). Since elective cholecystectomy in the elderly (usually because of chronic cholecystitis or symptomatic cholelithiasis) is associated with a much lower morbidity and mortality (16,19) than emergency cholecystectomy, an elective procedure is much more desirable. Moreover, because of the high incidence of suppurative gallbladder disease in elderly patients, an early operation is preferred, as medical therapy alone is associated with a high failure rate (16). Early operation also reduces the length of hospital stay. Norrby et al. reported on acute cholecystitis in patients *less than 75-years old* and showed that early operation resulted in 6.4 fewer hospital days compared to delayed operation (30). Although this study did not include patients over 75 years of age, it does point out another benefit of early surgical intervention.

Thus, the management of acute cholecystitis in the elderly includes: (*1*) rapid confirmation of the diagnosis by ultrasonography or radionuclide scanning; (*2*) stabilization of hemodynamic and cardiopulmonary status; (*3*) initiation of empiric antimicrobial therapy; and (*4*) performance of cholecystectomy (with intraoperative bile Gram stain and culture). In cases of ASC, a similar approach is warranted and the definitive surgical procedure is decompression of the biliary duct.

The role of the antimicrobial therapy in biliary sepsis has been thoroughly reviewed recently and is summarized in Table 13.3 (2,14). Prophylactic antibiotics are recommended for elderly patients who undergo elective cholecystectomy because of the higher incidence of bacterial colonization of the bile. Prophylactic antimicrobial agents clearly reduce

TABLE 13.3 Antimicrobial Therapy for
Elective Cholecystectomy and for Biliary Sepsis

CLINICAL CONDITION	REGIMEN[a]
Elective cholecystectomy	A first- or second-generation cephalosporin given in a single preoperative dose (e.g., cefazolin or cefuroxime). A third-generation cephalosporin (e.g., cefoperazone or ceftriaxone) is also effective
Acute cholecystitis	
Clinically stable	Ampicillin plus any second generation (or third-generation) cephalosporin; OR cefoperazone (or ceftriaxone) plus mezlocillin (or piperacillin)
Clinically unstable	Ampicillin and clindamycin (or metronidazole) plus an aminoglycoside;[b] OR ampicillin and cefoxitin; OR mezlocillin (or piperacillin) PLUS an aminoglycoside[b]
Acute suppurative cholangitis	Same as for clinically unstable acute cholecystitis

[a]Other regimens may equally be effective. Only a few are shown here. Please refer to Chapter 5 on antimicrobial therapy: special considerations for specific doses for each antibiotic.
[b]Gentamicin, tobramycin, amikacin, or netilmicin.

wound infection associated with biliary tract surgical procedures (31).

Prevention

The prevention of gallstones and the issue of whether or not asymptomatic cholelithiasis merits treatment is beyond the scope of this chapter. However, in view of the high morbidity and mortality observed with biliary sepsis, a strong argument can be made for elective cholecystectomy in elderly persons with mildly symptomatic cholelithiasis and in elderly diabetic patients with gallstones even though asymptomatic.

DIVERTICULITIS

General Considerations

Diverticuli are rare before the age of 40, but thereafter the prevalence of diverticulosis increases with age. Between the fifth and ninth decades, the prevalence of diverticuli in the population increases from 5 to 50% (32). The incidence of diverticulitis, the most common complication of diverticulosis, increases with time such that between 10 to 25% of persons with diverticulosis develop diverticulitis during their lifetime (32–34). The pathophysiology of diverticulitis is not well understood, but it is thought to result from diverticular inspissation of fecal matter, which leads to obstruction of the orifice and mucosal abrasion of the diverticulum with eventual perforation (35). Thus, diverticulitis is not an intraluminal infection, but it is a pericolitis, that results from micro- or macroperforation of a diverticulum.

Morbidity and mortality for acute diverticulitis vary considerably depending on the severity of the disease (e.g., whether or not macroperforation with resulting intraabdominal abscess or sepsis is present), occurrence of recurrent attacks (recurrence occurs in one-third of cases [36]), and the presence of concomitant diseases.

Etiology

Pericolitis, intraabdominal abscess, or peritonitis caused by perforation of a diverticulum involve the normal colonic microflora (aerobic and anaerobic enteric bacteria) (see section on intraabdominal abscess and Table 13.1). If sepsis occurs, bacteremia may be polymicrobial.

Clinical Manifestations

The clinical manifestation of diverticulitis varies depending on the severity of disease. Microperforation of the colon may be subclinical or may be characterized by left lower quadrant abdominal pain and altered bowel habits (35). On physical examination, left lower quadrant tenderness and an abdominal mass may be appreciated. However, some elderly patients may express more nonspecific signs of infection as well as features of their underlying disease(s) that may overshadow the abdominal findings (3). Moreover, in elderly women, the presence of a pelvic mass may lead the clinician to make the erroneous diagnosis of a gynecologic disorder (37).

Generalized abdominal guarding or rigidity, adynamic ileus, or signs of sepsis suggest macroperforation with large intraabdominal abscess and/or peritonitis.

Diagnostic Approach

DIFFERENTIAL DIAGNOSIS
The differential diagnosis of diverticulitis includes ischemic bowel disease, carcinoma of the colon, inflammatory bowel disease, renal colic, urinary tract infection, pelvic disease, and fecal impaction.

LABORATORY TESTS

The diagnosis of diverticulitis is essentially made clinically. However, upright abdominal radiographs should be obtained to look for intraperitoneal free air, ileus, obstruction, or mass effect. Barium enema studies and endoscopy should be avoided if possible. If contrast-medium studies are done, they should be performed using water-soluble agents such as Hypaque. Ultrasonography, computed tomography, and gallium scan are useful for identifying mass lesions and localizing abscesses. (See the section on intraabdominal abscess.)

Treatment

Larson et al. studied 132 patients with acute diverticulitis (38). Ninety-nine of these patients were initially treated medically and 33 were treated surgically. Over a period of 9.2 years, 73% of the medical patients and 79% of the surgical patients were either symptom free, had mild symptoms, or had died of unrelated causes (see Table 13.4). Since outcomes were similar in either treatment group, it can be inferred that medical therapy should be the initial treatment modality for uncomplicated acute diverticulitis. Surgery is indicated for recurrent disease, large abscess, generalized peritonitis, fistula formation, bowel obstruction, or suspected coexisting carcinoma. Immunocompromised patients who develop acute diverticulitis also merit early surgery (39). The surgical management of diverticulitis has been reviewed recently (40).

One approach to the medical treatment of uncomplicated diverticulitis is to treat mild illness on an outpatient basis with a high-fiber diet. The role of antibiotics for mild cases has not been established. More severely ill patients (e.g., fever, leukocytosis) should be hospitalized, placed on nasogastric suction and intravenous fluids, and treated with broad-spectrum antibiotics that are active against colonic bacteria (see the section on intraabdominal abscess).

TABLE 13.4 Long-Term Follow-Up of Medical Versus Surgical Management of Acute Diverticulitis

	MANAGED MEDICALLY INITIALLY	MANAGED SURGICALLY INITIALLY
	N (%)	N (%)
Total patients	99 (100)	33 (100)
Number of patients with favorable outcomes[a]	72 (73)	26 (79)

SOURCE: Adapted from reference 38.
[a]No severe recurrences or hospitalizations related to colonic problems.

TABLE 13.5 Frequency of Perforation and Mortality of Appendicitis in Elderly Versus Younger Patients (or Population as a Whole)

STUDY (AUTHOR, YEAR, REFERENCE NO.)	NUMBER OF ELDERLY PERSONS	% PERFORATION		% MORTALITY	
		OLD	YOUNG	OLD	YOUNG
Wood, 1934 (44)	43	65	—	28	—
Wollf et al., 1985 (45)	88	58	24	4.5	0.7
Peltokallio et al., 1970 (42)	300	32	6	2.0	0
Albano et al., 1975 (46)	93	38	—	20.0	0
Freund et al., 1984 (47)	77	38	7	1.3	—
Burns et al., 1985 (48)	96	65	—	3	0

SOURCE: Adapted from reference 43.

APPENDICITIS

General Considerations

Although older persons constitute only 5% of all cases of appendicitis (41,42), virtually all deaths occur in the older age group (43). The mortality for acute appendicitis in the elderly ranges from 1.3% to 28% (see Table 13.5) compared to a negligible mortality for this disease in younger persons (43–48). A higher mortality is observed for patients over the age of 30 (49).

The most striking feature of acute appendicitis in the aged, which accounts, in part, for the higher observed morbidity (25–61%) (47) and mortality, is a high perforation rate. Numerous studies have reported higher frequencies of advanced disease in the appendix of the elderly patients with acute appendicitis compared to their younger counterparts. This finding has been consistent, occurring through the preantibiotic era to the present. The reasons for the high incidence of gangrenous or perforated appendixes found at surgery in the elderly with acute appendicitis are multifactorial. Table 13.5 lists perforation rates for appendicitis described in a few selected studies, and Table 13.6 summarizes the factors that contribute to the high morbidity and mortality of appendicitis in the elderly.

Etiology

There are no studies that directly compare the bacteriology of appendicitis in old versus young patients; nevertheless, it is assumed to be

TABLE 13.6   Factors that Contribute to Morbidity
and Mortality of Appendicitis in the Elderly

Prolonged diagnostic delay
  Failure of patients to seek medical evaluation
  Failure of physicians to consider or make a clinical diagnosis (e.g., other
    diseases causing abdominal pain in this group are more common)
  Atypical clinical presentation
  Excessive laboratory tests, radiographic studies, and medical consultation
  Reluctance to operate on elderly patients
Increased frequency of gangrene or perforation of appendix
  Prolonged diagnostic delay
  Anatomic changes of the appendix with age that lead to increased susceptibility
    to obstruction with vascular occlusion
  Narrowing of appendiceal lumen
  Loss of lymphoid tissue
  Thinning of mucosa
  Fatty infiltration plus fibrosis of appendiceal wall
  Sclerosis of arterial and venous vessels
Concomitant chronic diseases (e.g., arteriosclerotic heart diseases, malnutrition)
Postoperative complications
  Septic (e.g., wound infection, sepsis or peritonitis due to gangrene or
    perforation of appendix)
  Nonseptic

---

similar. Intraoperative cultures in cases of simple inflammation of appendix (i.e., no gangrene or perforation) yield predominantly aerobic organisms (usually *E. coli*) (50). In advanced cases where gangrene or perforation are present (as in elderly patients), mixed aerobic and anaerobic flora are present with *B. fragilis* as the dominant anaerobic isolate (50,51). Thus, in most cases of appendicitis in the elderly, empiric antimicrobial therapy should be directed against aerobic and anaerobic bacteria (see the section on treatment).

Clinical Manifestations and Diagnostic Approach

Despite advances in laboratory tests and procedures, the early diagnosis of appendicitis is made clinically (52). Classically, appendicitis presents with anorexia and periumbilical pain that localizes to the right lower quadrant within 12 hours. Focal peritoneal signs are invariably present. However, older patients tend to have more atypical presentations than do younger patients. For example, "typical" appendicitis occurred in only 22% of elderly appendicitis cases in a study reported by Albano et al. (46) and in 25% of cases of elderly appendicitis in a study published by Burns et al. (48). However, the majority of elderly appendicitis patients do present with complaints of abdominal pain. The frequency of nausea, vomiting, fever, anorexia, and leukocytosis vary considerably in various series and do not appear to differ from younger patients with acute appendicitis (43). Localization of symptoms and signs to the right lower quadrant eventually occurs in over 80% of patients (41,48), but may not be as impressive and may be significantly delayed compared to the rapid localization observed in younger patients (53). Radiographic tests such as a plain upright abdominal x-ray should be performed, which occasionally will reveal an obstructing fecalith, a localized ileus, or free air. A barium enema demonstrating an extrinsic pericecal mass may be of diagnostic value, but is hazardous because of potential barium leak; the risk of the procedure should be considered carefully before being performed (43).

Misdiagnosis occurs most often in elderly patients (particularly at the extreme of old age). It ranges between 5 and 48% as reported by Freund et al., who published their own series and compared their low diagnostic error rate with past series (47). Their low (5%) diagnostic error rate was attributed to an aggressive surgical approach that minimized the delay from hospitalization to definitive surgery. Moreover, the mortality in this series was only 1.3%. As a general recommendation, appendicitis should be considered in any elderly patient with complaints of unexplained abdominal pain or acute signs of infection (including acute confusional state) in whom prior appendectomy has not been performed. The differential diagnosis of appendicitis in the aged is similar to that described for diverticulitis (see the section on diverticulitis).

Treatment

Prompt diagnosis and surgical intervention is the mainstay of therapy for acute appendicitis. Avoidance of unnecessary radiologic studies, laboratory tests, and consultations (unless it is clinically indicated because findings suggest other diagnoses) cannot be overemphasized, as this will delay definitive operation, thus increasing the likelihood of morbidity and mortality (Table 13.6).

As mentioned above, because of the likelihood of advanced disease of the appendix by the time a clinical diagnosis is made, empiric antimicrobial therapy of acute appendicitis in the elderly should be begun (after blood cultures are obtained). Furthermore, the antimicrobial regimen should include an antibiotic with activity against enteric aerobic (particularly gram-negative bacilli) and anaerobic (especially *B. fragilis*) flora. Traditionally, these regimens have included such anti-anaerobic drugs as clindamycin (1,200–2,400 mg a day), chloramphenicol (4–6 g a day), or metronidazole (1.5–2.0 g a day), plus an anti-gram-negative bacilli drug such as an aminoglycoside. In recent years, monotherapy with newer penicillins or certain second- or third-generation cephalosporins have been used with success in treating intraabdominal infections, and this approach is attractive in managing elderly patients with intraabdominal infection because of the problem of aminoglycoside toxicity (see the section on intraabdominal abscess). However, monotherapy of acute gangrenous or perforated appendicitis with certain third-generation cephalosporins has been disappointing and compares poorly with traditional regimens in both efficacy and cost (when antibiotic failure costs are considered) (54–57). Thus, monotherapy for the elderly should be used only when the risk of nephrotoxicity due to an aminoglycoside outweighs the risk of death from septic complications of appendicitis. The duration of therapy and any adjustments in particular antibiotics is dependent on what is found at the operation, the results of intraoperative and blood cultures, and the clinical course.

Prevention

In the case of acute appendicitis, prevention is not possible. However, the severity of this disease can be reduced in the elderly population with early diagnosis and prompt surgical intervention.

INTRAABDOMINAL ABSCESS

General Considerations

With the exception of pyogenic liver abscess, which is discussed separately in this section, data are not available in the elderly on the relative frequency of various primary infection sites that result in intraabdominal abscesses (IAA). However, it is a reasonable assumption that most IAA in elderly patients result from diverticulitis, appendicitis, perforating ulcer or colonic tumors, and abdominal operations (3,58). Hepatic pyogenic abscesses that result from biliary sepsis occur less frequently.

Mortality from IAA is dependent on multiple factors, but age in and of itself is an important risk factor (see introduction to chapter) (59). It is clear that early diagnosis and therapy is imperative to diminish the mortality and morbidity for IAA. Nonetheless, despite early diagnosis and aggressive therapy, in a recent series of IAA reported by Saini et al., IAA still had a mortality of 12% and morbidity of 20%. Encouragingly, this mortality is an improvement over the 28% mortality for IAA observed in the same hospital in an earlier period before advances in diagnostic imaging techniques facilitated early diagnosis of IAA (60).

Etiology

The microbiology of intraabdominal abscess not surprisingly reflects the colonic microflora, which usually consists of mixed aerobic and anaerobic flora (see Table 13.1) (61,62).

Clinical Manifestations

Clinical manifestations of IAA in the elderly varies considerably depending on the severity and anatomy of the infection. However, it is important to remember that nonspecific symptoms and signs may be present including "failure to thrive," altered mental status, or fever of unknown origin (63).

Diagnostic Approach

In suspected cases of IAA, plain films of the abdomen (upright position) should be obtained to find free air, extraluminal air/fluid levels, soft tissue densities, and bowel displacement (resulting from inflammatory mass) (64). An upright chest x-ray may show elevation or obliteration of the right hemidiaphragm, which is suggestive of a subphrenic abscess (64). Water-soluble dye contrast films may be helpful in distinguishing intraluminal gas from extraluminal gas when plain films are positive. Leaks or mass distortion of bowel may also be demonstrated. Furthermore, water-soluble contrast studies through stomas or sinus tracts may show an abscess cavity. These studies should be performed before ordering the more costly ultrasonography or computed tomography (CT) scans. In addition, the accuracy of CT and ultrasonography are enhanced when directed by clinical and plain film findings. CT scanning of the abdomen in suspected cases of IAA has high sensitivity and specificity (>85%) with an added advantage that directed percutaneous drainage may be facilitated (65,66). CT has been shown to be particularly helpful in patients with sepsis and multiple organ failure postlaparotomy (66). However, ultrasonography, though less sensitive and specific than CT, has the advantages of being less costly and more rapid than CT, and it can be portable (67). Imaging with radionuclide scanning may be helpful, though less so than CT or ultrasonography. Scanning with Indium-111-labeled leukocytes is superior to scanning with gallium-67 citrate, because gallium is excreted in the normal gastrointestinal tract (67). Laparotomy with surgical exploration may be indicated in difficult cases in which radiographic tests either cannot be performed or are not diagnostically helpful.

Treatment

The primary modes of therapy are surgical drainage and antibiotics (68). Percutaneous catheter drainage directed by CT (or ultrasonography) has been used successfully, with one series employing CT and percutaneous catheter drainage to drain satisfactorily 86% of 71 abscesses (69). This procedure has some therapeutic advantage in elderly patients who are generally severely ill or who cannot tolerate general anesthesia. However, open drainage is necessary in cases of IAA when the abscesses contain thick necrotic debris and multiple loculations (64).

Empiric antimicrobial therapy for IAA in severely ill, compromised elderly patients should include an aminoglycoside directed at aerobic gram-negative bacilli plus either clindamycin (1,200–2,400 mg a day), chloramphenicol (4–6 g a day) or metronidazole* (1.5–2.0 g a day) to cover anaerobes (68). The role of enterococci in intraabdominal infection is controversial (68,70). However, enterococcal bacteremia in one reported surgical series was associated with a mortality of 54% (71). Fortunately, enterococcal bacteremia from IAA is unusual (70), and antimicrobial regimens without additional coverage of the enterococcus (e.g., adding ampicillin [8–12 g a day]) have been used successfully to treat IAA (70). Nonetheless, ampicillin should be added to a regimen containing an aminoglycoside if enterococcal bacteremia is proven or the organism is repeatedly isolated from a wound infection or abscess.

Recently, certain newer penicillins (e.g., piperacillin, mezlocillin [12–18 g a day]) and third-generation cephalosporins have been used alone (monotherapy) with success in treating *community-acquired* intraabdominal infections (72–75). Monotherapy for IAA in the aged is recommended only if the risk of nephrotoxicity due to an aminoglycoside outweighs the risk of death from sepsis, or if the suspicion of IAA is low in a relatively stable elderly patient.

Prevention

The role of antimicrobial prophylaxis in elderly persons who undergo elective cholecystectomy has been discussed in the section on biliary sepsis. Antimicrobial prophylaxis to prevent wound infection and IAA in patients who undergo elective colorectal surgery is firmly established. Various short-course or single-dose regimens used alone or combined with whole gut irrigation have been used successfully in these cases (76–78) (also, see Chapter 6 on prevention of infections). Finally, tetracycline lavage was found to reduce significantly postoperative IAA (in combination with systemic antimicrobial agents) in patients who undergo a wide variety of elective and emergency intraabdominal operations (79). This procedure merits further study before it can be widely recommended.

---

*If metronidazole is used in combination with an aminoglycoside to treat severely ill patients, some clinicians would recommend adding penicillin G for improved coverage against gram-positive anaerobes.

PYOGENIC LIVER ABSCESS

General Consideration

In recent years, the epidemiology and pathophysiology of pyogenic liver abscess has changed dramatically (80). Though the incidence of this disease has remained constant, in the past this disease occurred predominantly in younger patients with intraabdominal infection (usually appendicitis), which was complicated by septic portal vein thrombosis (pyelephlebitis) with resultant hepatic abscesses. Currently, most cases of pyogenic liver abscess occur in elderly individuals, usually as a complication of biliary infection and less commonly diverticulitis or appendicitis. Despite advances in diagnosis and therapy, the mortality in one recent series was 57% with the mean age of nonsurvivors being 77 years (81). In another recent study, McDonald et al. reported an overall mortality of 25% in 55 patients with pyogenic abscesses, which increased to 41% in the 22 patients with multiple abscesses. Of note, biliary disease and underlying malignancy were present in 45% and 32%, respectively, in the multiple-abscess group (82). Thus, pyogenic liver abscess is a life-threatening disease with a high mortality, particularly in the older age group and in cases complicated by multiple abscesses or malignancy. Failure to make an early diagnosis further contributes to this high mortality.

Etiology

The bacteriology of liver abscesses reflects the bacteriology of biliary and colonic infection (see Table 13.1). Facultative anaerobic or aerobic gram-negative bacilli, anaerobes (particularly *B. fragilis*), and a variety of streptococci are usually present as a mixed infection; therefore, multiple isolates may be recovered from the abscess (82). Blood cultures are positive in nearly 50% of cases, particularly if abscesses are multiple, and these cultures may be polymicrobial (82,83).

Clinical Manifestations

Even in nonelderly patients, the diagnosis of pyogenic liver abscess may be difficult. Most patients, however, have fever, chills, nonspecific gastrointestinal symptoms, and tender hepatomegaly. Table 13.7 summarizes the clinical features of three selected series of pyogenic liver abscess (82–84). It should be noted that a substantial number of patients do not have symptoms and signs localizing to the right upper quadrant. Some have a fever of unknown origin. In elderly patients, the presence of these clinical signs in the presence of suspected intraabdominal infection (especially

TABLE 13.7   Clinical Features of Pyogenic Liver Abscess

	PERCENT POSITIVE		
SYMPTOMS AND SIGNS	SERIES 1[a]	SERIES 2[b]	SERIES 3[c]
Fever[d]	87	93	87
Chills	61	44	53
Chest or abdominal pain	77	16	45
Anorexia	39	97	—
Nausea and vomiting	53	24	—
Weight loss	52	76	51
Right upper quadrant tenderness	77	65	53
Hepatomegaly	69	52	60
Jaundice	43	26	22

[a]Lazarchick et al., 1973 (83); 75 patients with 52% over age 60.
[b]Miedema et al., 1984 (84); 106 patients, mean age equaled 60.
[c]McDonald et al., 1984 (82); 55 patients, median age equaled 53.
[d]Either by history or noted on admission.

biliary sepsis) should lead to the consideration of pyogenic liver abscess (3).

Diagnostic Approach

DIFFERENTIAL DIAGNOSIS
The other diagnostic considerations include biliary tract disease, primary or secondary liver malignancy, hepatitis, cirrhosis, amebic liver abscess, subphrenic abscess, and acute pyelonephritis.

LABORATORY TESTS
A chest x-ray film that reveals right basal atelectasis, elevated right hemi-diaphragm, or pleural effusion is diagnostically helpful and should be performed first. In a series of patients reported by McDonald et al., 41% had abnormal chest films (82). Computed tomography (CT), radionuclide scanning, and ultrasonography are all useful techniques for diagnosing the presence of focal defects in the liver, with CT being the most sensitive for detecting small abscesses (82).

Treatment

Surgical drainage along with empiric broad-spectrum antimicrobial therapy directed against facultative anaerobic or aerobic bacteria and anaerobic flora (after blood cultures are obtained) is the treatment of choice (see the treatment section on intraabdominal abscess for specific antibiotic regimens). Antibiotic therapy should be adjusted according to the results of cultures of pus or blood. Percutaneous catheter drainage of abscesses, directed by CT or ultrasound, especially in cases of solitary abscesses, is replacing operative drainage as the drainage method of choice (82,85).

Prevention

Pyogenic liver abscess can only be prevented by promptly and appropriately treating the primary sites of infection.

REFERENCES

1. Martin LF, Asher EF, Casey JM, et al: Postoperative pneumonia. Determinants of mortality. *Arch Surg* 119:379–383, 1984.
2. Norman DC, Yoshikawa TT: Intraabdominal infections in the elderly. *J Am Geriatr Soc* 31:677–684, 1983.
3. Norman DC, Yoshikawa TT: Intraabdominal infection: Diagnosis and treatment in the elderly patient. *Gerontology* 30:327–338, 1984.
4. Vartian CV, Septimus EJ: Intraabdominal infections in the elderly: Diagnosis and management. *Geriatrics* 41:51–56, 1986.
5. Glew RH: Abdominal infections, in Gleckman RA, Gantz NM (eds): *Infections in the Elderly*. Boston, Little, Brown and Co, 1983, p 177.
6. Fenyö G: Acute abdominal disease in the elderly. Experience from two series in Stockholm. *Am J Surg* 143:751–754, 1982.
7. Reiss R, Deutsch AA: Emergency abdominal procedures in patients above 70. *J Gerontol* 40:154–158, 1985.
8. Dellinger EP, Wertz MJ, Meakins JL, et al: Surgical infection stratification system for intra-abdominal infection. Multicenter Trial. *Arch Surg* 120:21–29, 1985.
9. Skau T, Nyström P, Carlsson C: Severity of illness in intra-abdominal infection. *Arch Surg* 120:152–158, 1985.
10. Amberg JR, Zboralski FF: Gallstones after 70. Requiescat in pace. *Geriatrics* 20:539–542, 1965.
11. Mason RG: Bacteriology and antibiotic selection in biliary tract surgery. *Arch Surg* 97:533–537, 1968.
12. Chetlin SM, Elliott DW: Biliary bacteremia. *Arch Surg* 102:303–307, 1971.
13. Keighley MRB, Drysdale RB, Quoraishi AH, et al: Antibiotic treatment of biliary sepsis. *Surg Clin North Am* 55:1379–1390, 1975.
14. Keighley MRB, Rogers W: Preventing infection in biliary surgery. *Infect Surg* 2:711–719, 1983.
15. Willis RG, Lawson WC, Hoare EM, et al: Are bile bacteria relevant to septic complications following biliary surgery? *Br J Surg* 71:845–849, 1984.
16. Morrow DJ, Thompson J, Wilson SE: Acute cholecystitis in the elderly. A surgical emergency. *Arch Surg* 113:1149–1152, 1978.
17. Shimada K, Inamatsu T, Yamashiro M: Anaerobic bacteria in biliary disease in elderly patients. *J Infect Dis* 135:850–854, 1977.

18. Bourgault AM, England DM, Rosenblatt JE, et al: Clinical characteristics of anaerobic bactibilia. *Arch Intern Med* 139:1346-1349, 1979.
19. Huber DF, Martin EW, Cooperman M: Cholecystectomy in elderly patient. *Am J Surg* 146:719-722, 1983.
20. Matolo NM, LaMorte WW, Wolfe BM: Acute and chronic cholecystitis. *Surg Clin North Am* 61:875-883, 1981.
21. Holt S, Diaz MC, Eckhauser ML, et al: Acute acalculous cholecystitis. *IM (Internal Medicine for the Specialist)* 7:128-145, 1986.
22. Orlando R, Gleason E, Drezner AD: Acute acalculous cholecystitis in the critically ill patient. *Am J Surg* 145:472-476, 1983.
23. Fox MS, Wilk PJ, Weissman HS, et al: Acute acalculous cholecystitis. *Surg Gynecol Obstet* 159:13-16, 1984.
24. Glenn F, Becker CG: Acute acalculous cholecystitis. An increasing entity. *Ann Surg* 195:131-136, 1982.
25. Boey JH, Way LW: Acute cholangitis. *Ann Surg* 191:264-270, 1980.
26. Thompson JE, Tompkins RK, Longmire WP: Factors in management of acute cholangitis. *Ann Surg* 195:137-145, 1982.
27. Chock E, Wolfe BM, Matolo NM: Acute suppurative cholangitis. *Surg Clin North Am* 61:885-892, 1981.
28. Arnold DJ, Zollinger RW, Bartlett RM, et al: 28,621 cholecystectomies in Ohio. Results of a survey in Ohio hospitals by the Gallbladder Survey Committee, Ohio Chapter, American College of Surgeons. *Am J Surg* 119: 714-717, 1970.
29. Fry DE, Cox RA, Harbrecht PJ: Gangrene of the gallbladder: A complication of acute cholecystitis. *South Med J* 74:666-668, 1981.
30. Norrby S, Merlin P, Holmin T, et al: Early or delayed cholecystectomy in acute cholecystitis? A clinical trial. *Br J Surg* 70:163-165, 1983.
31. Harnoss BM, Hirner A, Krüselmann M, et al: Antibiotic infection prophylaxis in gallbladder surgery: A prospective randomized study. *Chemotherapy* 31:76-82, 1985.
32. Parks TG: Natural history of diverticular disease of the colon. *Clin Gastroenterol* 4:53-69, 1975.
33. Boles RS, Jordan SM: The clinical significance of diverticulosis. *Gastroenterology* 35:579-582, 1958.
34. Horner JL: Natural history of diverticulosis of the colon. *Am J Dig Dis* 3:343-350, 1958.
35. Cello JP: Diverticular disease of the colon. *West J Med* 134:515-523, 1981.
36. Almy TP, Howell DA: Diverticular disease of the colon. *N Engl J Med* 302:324-331, 1980.
37. Walker JD, Gray IA, Polk HC: Diverticulitis in women: An unappreciated clinical presentation. *Ann Surg* 185:402-405, 1977.
38. Larson DM, Masters SS, Spiro HM: Medical and surgical therapy in diverticular disease. A comparative study. *Gastroenterology* 71:734-737, 1976.
39. Perkins JD, Shield CF, Chang FC, et al: Acute diverticulitis. Comparison of treatment in immunocompromised and nonimmunocompromised patients. *Am J Surg* 148:745-748, 1984.
40. Killingback M: Management of perforative diverticulitis. *Surg Clin North Am* 63:97-115, 1983.

41. Owens BJ, Hamit HF: Appendicitis in the elderly. *Ann Surg* 187:392–396, 1978.
42. Peltokallio P, Jauhiainen K: Acute appendicitis in the aged patient. Study of 300 cases after the age of 60. *Arch Surg* 100:140–143, 1970.
43. Norman DC, Yoshikawa TT: Acute appendicitis in the elderly, in Meakins JL, McClaren J (eds): *Surgical Care of the Elderly.* Chicago, Year Book Medical Publications, in press.
44. Wood CB: Acute appendicitis in the aged. A study of 43 cases occurring after the age of sixty. *Am J Surg* 26:321–325, 1934.
45. Wolff WI, Hindman R: Acute appendicitis in the aged. *Surg Gynecol Obstet* 94:239–247, 1952.
46. Albano WA, Zielinski CM, Organ CH: Is appendicitis in the aged really different? *Geriatrics* 30:81–88, 1975.
47. Freund H, Rubinstein E: Appendicitis in the aged. Is it really different? *Am Surg* 50:573–576, 1984.
48. Burns PR, Cochran JL, Russell WL et al: Appendicitis in mature patients. *Ann Surg* 201:695–704, 1985.
49. Smithy WB, Wexner SD, Dailey TH: The diagnosis and treatment of acute appendicitis in the aged. *Dis Colon Rectum* 29:170–173, 1986.
50. Lau WY, Tech-Chan CH, Fan ST, et al: The bacteriology of septic complication of patients with appendicitis. *Ann Surg* 200:576–581, 1984.
51. Arnbjörnsson E: Appendicitis in the elderly: Part II—Special considerations in diagnosis and management. *Geriatr Med Today* 5:62–68, 1986.
52. Buchman TG, Zuidema GD: Reasons for delay of the diagnosis of acute appendicitis. *Surg Gynecol Obstet* 158:260–266, 1984.
53. Arnbjörnsson E: Recognizing appendicitis in the elderly. *Geriatr Med Today* 3:72–79, 1984.
54. Lau WY, Fan ST, Chu KW, et al: Randomized, prospective double-blind trial of new beta-lactams in the treatment of appendicitis. *Antimicrob Agents Chemother* 28:639–642, 1985.
55. Berne TV, Yellin AW, Appleman MD, et al. Antibiotic management of surgically treated gangrenous or perforated appendicitis. Comparison of gentamicin and clindamycin versus cefamandole versus cefoperazone. *Am J Surg* 144:8–13, 1982.
56. Heseltine PNR, Yellin AE, Appleman MD, et al: Perforated and gangrenous appendicitis: An analysis of antibiotic failures. *J Infect Dis* 148:322–329, 1983.
57. Gill MA, Chenella FC, Heseltine PNR, et al: Cost analysis of antibiotics in the management of perforated or gangrenous appendicitis. *Am J Surg* 151:200–203, 1986.
58. Altmeier WA, Culbertson WR, Fullen WD, et al: Intra-abdominal abscesses. *Am J Surg* 125:70–79, 1973.
59. Fry DE, Garrison RN, Heitsch RC, et al: Determinants of death in patients with intraabdominal abscess. *Surgery* 88:517–523, 1980.
60. Saini S, Kellum JM, O'Leary MP, et al: Improved localization and survival in patients with intraabdominal abscesses. *Am J Surg* 145:136–142, 1983.
61. Lorber B, Swenson RM: The bacteriology of intra-abdominal infections. *Surg Clin North Am* 55:1349–1354, 1975.

62. Nichols RL: Intraabdominal infections: An overview. *Rev Infect Dis* 7:(S)709–(S)715, 1985.
63. Esposito AL, Gleckman RA: Fever of unknown origin in the elderly. *J Am Geriatr Soc* 26:498–505, 1978.
64. Herman CM: Detection and management of intraabdominal abscess. *Infect Surg* 2:737–755, 1983.
65. Dobrin PB, Gully PH, Greenlee MB, et al: Radiologic diagnosis of intra-abdominal abscess. Do multiple tests help? *Arch Surg* 121:41–46, 1986.
66. Hoogewood HM, Rubli E, Terrier F, et al: The role of computerized tomography in fever, septicemia, and multiple system organ failure after laparotomy. *Surg Gynecol Obstet* 162:539–543, 1986.
67. Joseph AEA: Imaging of abdominal abscesses. *Br Med J* 291:1446–1447, 1985.
68. Nichols RL: Management of intraabdominal sepsis. *Am J Med* 80(Suppl B):204–209, 1986.
69. Gerzof SG, Robbins AH, Johnson WC, et al: Percutaneous catheter drainage of abdominal abscesses. A five year experience. *N Engl J Med* 305:653–657, 1981.
70. Dougherty SH: Role of enterococcus in intraabdominal sepsis. *Am J Surg* 148:308–312, 1984.
71. Garrison RN, Fry DE, Berberich S, et al: Enterococcal bacteremia. Clinical implications and determinants of death. *Ann Surg* 196:43–47, 1982.
72. Stone HH, Strom PR, Fabian TC, et al: Third-generation cephalosporins for polymicrobial surgical sepsis. *Arch Surg* 118:193–200, 1983.
73. Yoshikawa TT, Norman DC: Antimicrobial therapy of surgical infection in the elderly. *Infect Surg* 3:805–812, 1984.
74. Dunn DL, Simmons RL: Empiric therapy of peritonitis and intraabdominal infection. *Infect Surg* 2:466–483, 1983.
75. Najem AZ, Kaminiski ZC, Spillert CR: Comparative study of parenteral piperacillin and cefoxitin in the treatment of surgical infections of the abdomen. *Surg Gynecol Obstet* 157:423–425, 1983.
76. Mitchell NJ, Evans DS, Pollock D: Single dose metronidazole with and without cefuroxime in elective colorectal surgery. *Br J Surg* 70:668–669, 1983.
77. Gottrup F, Diederich P, Sørensen K, et al: Prophylaxis with whole gut irrigation and antimicrobials in colorectal surgery. A prospective, randomized double-blind clinical trial. *Am J Surg* 149:317–322, 1985.
78. McColloch PG, Blamey SL, Finlay IG, et al: A prospective comparison of gentamicin and metronidazole and moxalactam in the prevention of septic complications associated with elective operations of the colon and rectum. *Surg Gynecol Obstet* 162:521–524, 1986.
79. Silverman SH, Ambrose NS, Youngs DJ, et al: The effects of peritoneal lavage with tetracycline solution on post operative infection. *Dis Colon Rectum* 29:165–169, 1986.
80. Rubin RH, Swartz MN, Malt R: Hepatic abscess: Changes in clinical, bacteriologic and therapeutic aspects. *Am J Med* 57:601–610, 1974.
81. Sandford NL, Bradbear RA, Powell LW: Pyogenic liver abscess: A neglected diagnosis. *Aust NZ J Med* 14:597–621, 1984.

82. McDonald MI, Corey GR, Gallis HA, et al: Single and multiple pyogenic liver abscess. Natural history, diagnosis and treatment with emphasis on percutaneous drainage. *Medicine* 63:291–302, 1984.
83. Lazarchick J, de Souza e Silva NA, Nichols DR: Pyogenic liver abscess. *Mayo Clin Proc* 48:349–355, 1973.
84. Meidema BW, Dineen P: The diagnosis and treatment of pyogenic liver abscess. *Ann Surg* 200:328–335, 1984.
85. Bertel CK, van Heerden JA, Sheedy PF II: Treatment of pyogenic hepatic abscess. *Arch Surg* 121:554–558, 1986.

SUGGESTED READINGS

Arnbjörnsson E: Appendicitis in the elderly: Part II—Special considerations in diagnosis and management. *Geriatr Med Today* 5:62–68, 1986.
Huber DF, Martin EW, Cooperman M: Cholecystectomy in elderly patient. *Am J Surg* 146:719–722, 1983.
Killingback M: Management of perforative diverticulitis. *Surg Clin North Am* 63:97–115, 1983.
Larson DM, Masters SS, Spiro HM: Medical and surgical therapy in diverticular disease. A comparative study. *Gastroenterology* 71:734–737, 1976.
Morrow DJ, Thompson J, Wilson SE: Acute cholecystitis in the elderly. A surgical emergency. *Arch Surg* 113:1149–1152, 1978.
Nichols RL: Intraabdominal infections: An overview. *Rev Infect Dis* 7:(S)709–(S)715, 1985.
Norman DC, Yoshikawa TT: Intraabdominal infection: Diagnosis and treatment in the elderly patient. *Gerontology* 30:327–338, 1984.
Reiss R, Deutsch AA: Emergency abdominal procedures in patients above 70. *J Gerontol* 40:154–158, 1985.
Smithy WB, Wexner SD, Dailey TH: The diagnosis and treatment of acute appendicitis in the aged. *Dis Colon Rectum* 29:170–173, 1986.

Chapter 14

Genitourinary Tract Infection

This chapter focuses on urinary tract infection and prostatitis.

URINARY TRACT INFECTION

General Considerations

Although pneumonia is the leading infectious disease that causes death in the elderly, bacteriuria or urinary tract infection (UTI) is a more frequent infection. *Bacteriuria,* as it is used in this chapter, refers to the presence of significant numbers of bacteria in the urine without reference to symptoms. Symptomatic bacteriuria or bacteriuria causing clinical manifestations is referred to as *UTI.* The prevalence of bacteriuria in the geriatric population varies considerably and depend on several factors. These factors include sex, functional level, nature of underlying diseases, functional or anatomic status of genitourinary tract, and the presence of an indwelling bladder catheter (1). In an acute hospital setting, the prevalence of bacteriuria for both elderly men and women is approximately 30%, whereas in nursing homes or extended care facilities, the prevalence of bacteriuria for old men and old women is 15 to 20% and 25 to 50%, respectively. In a community setting in which the elderly are ambulatory and usually more functional, the prevalence of bacteriuria is approximately 5 to 10% in men and 15 to 30% in women (1). These epidemiologic data are in contrast to the prevalence of bacteriuria in younger adults. Bacteriuria or UTI in young adults is a disease primarily of sexually active women, with a prevalence of 5%; women outnumber men by a ratio of 30:1 (1).

In elderly patients, UTI is the most common cause of bacteremia or sepsis (2–5). Bacteremia is more likely to complicate UTI in the elderly than in younger adults (6). Moreover, urosepsis, particularly gram-negative (bacillary) sepsis, has a significantly higher mortality in the aged than in younger cohorts (see Chapter 18 on sepsis). Separate from sepsis-related deaths, bacteriuria is associated with higher mortality (regardless of cause of death) not only in the general population but particularly in the elderly (7–11). This same bacteriuria-mortality relationship has also been shown with nosocomial UTI that is associated with indwelling bladder catheters (12), a form of bacteriuria most common in elderly patients in nursing homes (see Chapter 7 on infections in the nursing home population). The clinical course of bacteriuria in the elderly is poorly understood, since bacteriuria, like other infections in the elderly patient, may be asymptomatic (see the section on clinical manifestations). Some limited data suggest that persistent or recurrent bacteriuria and UTI is common in the elderly (13,14). Recurrent UTI due to relapse (as opposed to reinfection, which occurs more commonly in women) is a frequent problem in elderly men (15,16).

Etiology

As stated earlier, in the general adult population, UTI is a disease primarily of healthy, ambulatory, sexually active women. In this group, *Escherichia coli* accounts for over 80% of all cases of UTI (17,18). However, UTI that is associated with recurrence, urologic abnormalities, stone formation, catheter usage, chronic antibiotic usage, severe underlying disease, or nosocomial acquisition has a decreased frequency of *E. coli* and an increased prevalence of other gram-negative bacilli (20,21).

Elderly patients with bacteriuria or UTI have uropathogens that are similar to adults with complicated UTI. That is, there is a decreased frequency of *E. coli* and an increased isolation rate of other important urinary pathogens that include *Klebsiella* sp., *Proteus* sp., *Enterobacter* sp., *Citrobacter* sp., *Serratia marcescens, Pseudomonas aeruginosa,* and coagulase-negative staphylococci (1,22). In elderly persons with a chronic indwelling bladder catheter, these gram-negative bacilli as well as enterococci (in 30–40% of patients) are the common urinary isolates (23,24).

Clinical Manifestations

The typical symptoms of UTI involving the bladder in young women are dysuria, lower abdominal pain, urgency, frequency, and nocturia. With upper genitourinary tract infection (pyelonephritis), symptomatic patients typically complain of fever, chills, or flank pain. However, in the geriatric population, particularly the very old, bacteriuria independent of the source (i.e., bladder, kidney, and prostate) is frequently present in the *absence* of genitourinary complaints (25–30). When genitourinary symptoms are present with bacteriuria, stress incontinence, urgency, or nocturia may be present. To further add confusion, many elderly persons have these same genitourinary complaints in the absence of bacteriuria (25,26). Furthermore, such vague or nonspecific complaints as confusion, lethargy, falls, anorexia, weakness, or reduced mobility (1,31) may indicate serious UTI in older persons. These clinical findings are not uncommon in nursing home patients with chronic indwelling bladder catheters in whom bacteremia (or possibly endotoxemia) occurs from bacteriuria. Therefore, any elderly patient, especially those with a bladder catheter or history of recurrent or persistent bacteriuria, who manifests a change in clinical or functional status regardless of the symptoms, should be evaluated for a UTI.

Diagnostic Approach

DIFFERENTIAL DIAGNOSIS
In elderly patients with nonspecific symptoms, the differential diagnosis would include any serious infectious disease as well as most noninfectious illness that affects the aged (e.g., heart failure, anemia, dehydration) and drug reactions. As stated above, genitourinary complaints that are consistent with UTI may be present in the elderly in the absence of bacteriuria. These symptoms may be related to bladder dysfunction due to other causes, such as diuretics, congestive heart failure, or diabetes mellitus.

LABORATORY TESTS
Urine. All patients suspected of UTI require a careful urinalysis and urine culture. Elderly patients who are functionally capable of voiding spontaneously should have urine collected by the voided midstream method. If a voided specimen cannot be obtained, the patient should be catheterized (using careful aseptic techniques). The catheter should then be removed. In patients with a chronic indwelling bladder catheter, the old catheter should be removed and a new catheter inserted. Urine for urinalysis and culture should then be obtained from this new catheter (see the section on urinary tract infection in Chapter 7 on infections in the nursing home population) (24).

Blood. Blood cultures (two sets) should be obtained. Renal function tests, complete blood count, and electrolytes are useful tests to monitor the elderly patient's state of hydration, renal function, and therapeutic response.

Other Tests. In elderly women with infrequent occurrences of UTI that involve only the bladder, further diagnostic evaluation (i.e., cystoscopy and intravenous pyelogram) is not necessary. However, if elderly women have frequent recurrent UTIs (or have UTI associated with sepsis, stones, gross hematuria, or acute urinary retention) it is valuable to have a genitourinary tract evaluation performed by a skilled urologist to exclude any identifiable and correctable anatomic or functional abnormality. Elderly men with bacteriuria or UTI not related to catheterization or instrumentation should have a thorough genitourinary tract evaluation with special attention focused on the prostate gland (hypertrophy, carcinoma, or prostatitis).

Attempts to differentiate upper (pyelonephritis) versus lower tract (cystitis) infection by clinical evaluation and simple noninvasive tests have been generally unsuccessful. Such tests as antibody-coated bacteria, beta-2-microglobulin excretion, antibodies to "O" antigens and Tamm-Horsfall protein, and urinary lactic dehydrogenase and beta-glucuronidase are flawed by problems of lack of availability, specificity, sensitivity, and cost (32). Therefore, currently we would not recommend these tests for the elderly.

Treatment

Antibiotic therapy for UTI has undergone some changes in recent times. Although the majority of patients with UTI still receive 7 to 14 days of antibiotics, select individuals can be treated with shorter courses of chemotherapy. Several studies have documented that healthy, young women (nonpregnant) with uncomplicated cystitis may be effectively treated for UTI with single-dose or short-course (for 3 days) chemotherapy (19,33–35). However, single-dose or single-day therapy in elderly men or women has an unacceptably low cure rate and high relapse rate (36,37). Certainly, short-course antibiotic regimens have no role in elderly patients with a structural abnomality of the genitourinary tract or a chronic indwelling bladder catheter (38).

In elderly patients with uncomplicated UTI (ambulatory, clinically stable, noncatheterized), treatment may begin with trimethoprim-sulfamethoxazole (TMP-SMZ), 160 mg TMP and 800 mg SMZ, twice a day until urine culture and sensitivity data become available. Other drugs that can also be used under these clinical circumstances include cefadroxil 500 mg orally once or twice a day, or oral amoxicillin 500 mg three times a day.

Elderly patients with more severe illness or who are clinically unstable should be hospitalized and empirically given a parenteral second- or third-generation cephalosporin. (See Chapter 5 on antimicrobial therapy.) Patients who are hypotensive, who have been on recent antibiotics, or who have a history of recurrent infection should also receive an aminoglycoside pending culture and sensitivity results.

Patients with chronic indwelling bladder catheters should be empirically treated with ampicillin 500–1,000 mg three or four times a day plus a third-generation cephalosporin (if clinically stable) or an aminoglycoside (if ill or unstable) until culture data become available. It should be emphasized that patients with chronic bladder catheters almost always have bacteriuria even if suppressive or prophylactic antibiotics are administered. Therefore, these patients should *only* be fully treated when they become ill or symptomatic or have a change in functional status.

All patients should be treated for 7 to 14 days, depending on the severity of disease, the clinical response of the patient, and the presence of any complications. Elderly patients who have recurrent UTI (without structural abnormalities or stones) due to relapse may be treated for 3 to 12 weeks (15,16,22,39). Some of these patients may warrant suppressive therapy (see the next section on prevention).

In noncatheterized elderly patients with chronic *asymptomatic* bacteriuria, the role of antibiotic therapy is unclear. The justification for chemotherapy would be to prevent symptomatic UTI or urosepsis, chronic pyelonephritis with renal failure, and/or unexplained excessive mortality associated with bacteriuria. Treatment would have to be balanced against the cost of drugs, possible development of resistant organisms, adverse drug effects, and the efficacy of treatment. The risk of developing symptomatic UTI or urosepsis from asymptomatic bacteriuria in the elderly is unknown. The association of bacteriuria and mortality has been previously discussed. From epidemiologic, clinical, autopsy, transplantation, and dialysis data, it appears that recurrent or chronic bacteriuria may lead to end-stage chronic pyelonephritis if there is obstruction to urine flow, bladder reflux, or underlying primary renal disease or damage (40,41). Despite these data, the risks and cost of treatment of asymptomatic bacteriuria is undefined. One recent study on short-course therapy for asymptomatic bacteriuria in the ambulatory elderly showed a cure rate of 64% (compared to 35% for untreated controls) (42). However, in other studies using short-course treatment regimens or antibiotic therapy for 2 weeks to 3 months, the therapeutic outcome was dismal with relapses occurring at very high rates (36,37). From these data, we would recommend a short-term trial of antibiotic therapy in only two types of elderly patients:

1. Elderly women who are otherwise healthy, functional, and without clinical evidence of urologic abnormalities (e.g., incontinence) may be given a short (3-day) course of an appropriate antibiotic (based on culture and sensitivity data). If there is no response or

a relapse occurs, the patient should then be evaluated urologically for abnormalities, and no further antibiotics should be given. If there is sterilization of the urine, the patient should simply be followed clinically.

2. Elderly men who have documented obstructive uropathy with asymptomatic bacteriuria but who refuse or are unable to undergo a drainage procedure (e.g., transurethral prostatic resection) should be given a 10 to 14 day trial of an appropriate antibiotic. If there is a response, with sterilization of the urine, chronic suppressive therapy would be indicated (see the next section on prevention). However, if no microbiologic response occurs, then further chemotherapy should be abandoned.

Prevention

Prevention of bacteriuria using antimicrobial therapy is termed *chemoprophylaxis. Suppressive chemotherapy* is frequently used synonymously with *chemoprophylaxis* However, suppressive therapy may be effective in preventing symptomatic disease (UTI) (by decreasing the number of organisms in the urine), but not in preventing bacteriuria. Therefore, a clear distinction should be made between chemoprophylaxis and suppressive therapy.

Chemoprophylaxis would be indicated for elderly patients who have frequent recurrent infections due to *reinfection,* but who have relatively normal genitourinary tracts and who are not chronically catheterized. Trimethoprim-sulfamethoxazole, one-half tablet (40 mg TMP and 200 mg SMZ) at bedtime is recommended.

Suppressive chemotherapy would be recommended for elderly men who have asymptomatic bacteriuria with obstructive uropathy, but who will not or cannot undergo surgery. After the patient receives antibiotics for 10 to 14 days, and if the urine becomes sterile, suppressive therapy with TMP-SMZ (1 tablet twice a day) or other antibiotics should be initiated. Patients should be monitored with periodic urine cultures. If the patient becomes bacteriuric, the suppressive therapeutic regimen should be discontinued. The patient may be retreated with an appropriate drug, and suppression attempted again, possibly with a different antibiotic. Suppressive therapy may also be indicated for chronic bacterial prostatitis that fails to be cured with antibiotics (see the next section on prostatitis).

PROSTATITIS

General Considerations

Prostatitis, inflammation of the prostate, occurs as two types, acute or chronic. Since the diagnosis of chronic bacterial prostatitis is often difficult to confirm, the exact frequency of prostatitis is not known. One source estimates the prevalence of prostatitis is as high as 35% in men over the age of 50 years (43). Although acute prostatitis may occur in elderly men, chronic bacterial prostatitis is the most important form of prostatic infection in this group. Significantly, this infection is the most common cause of relapsing urinary tract infection in men (44).

Etiology

In acute bacterial prostatitis, uropathogens are common etiologic organisms. In chronic bacterial prostatitis, aerobic gram-negative bacilli (uropathogens) are again the most common cause of infection, though *Staphylococcus saprophyticus,* enterococcus, and diphtheroids may be isolated occasionally (45,46). However, a specific etiology of chronic prostatitis may often not be found, and it is not clear whether organisms other than bacteria, for example, *Chlamydia trachomatis* or *Mycoplasma* sp., play a role in this disease (47).

Clinical Manifestations

Acute bacterial prostatitis is not difficult to diagnose. Patients are often symptomatically ill with fever, chills, and toxicity. They may complain of urinary symptoms and lower abdominal, perineal, and/or back pain. Some patients may have urinary obstruction (48). Rectal examination reveals a very tender prostate gland. (Prostatic massage or vigorous palpation should be avoided in acute bacterial prostatitis because bacteremia may be precipitated.)

Some elderly patients with chronic bacterial prostatitis may be totally asymptomatic except during exacerbations of urinary tract infection. However, most patients complain of mild low back pain, urinary urgency, frequency, nocturia, or perineal discomfort (45). The digital prostate examination frequently is completely normal.

Diagnostic Approach

DIFFERENTIAL DIAGNOSIS
Acute bacterial prostatitis may be confused with acute urinary tract infection, prostatic abscess, or granulomatous prostatitis. Chronic bacterial prostatitis may be clinically indistinguishable from nonbacterial prostatitis and prostadynia (perineal, ejaculatory, and urinary compaints with no evidence of inflammation of the prostate gland) (44).

LABORATORY TESTS

Acute Bacterial Prostatitis.   Urinalysis is abnormal with this infection; pyuria and bacteriuria are present, and urine cultures are positive. Occasionally, blood cultures show the presence of bacteria. A brisk peripheral leukocytosis is common.

Chronic Bacterial Prostatitis.   Expressed prostatic secretions should be obtained by prostatic massage. The prostatic expressate should be examined on a glass slide with a cover slip under high-power magnification. The finding of 10 to 20 white blood cells per high-power field (hpf) is suggestive of prostatitis (49). Quantitative bacteriologic localization culture is currently the standard and accepted laboratory test to diagnose bacterial prostatitis (50). Segmented urine specimens are collected and cultured quantitatively for bacteria. Elderly men who are uncircumcised should have the foreskin retracted and the glans cleansed with soap; the soap should then be removed. When the patient states he has a full bladder, he is asked to void on three occasions. The following specimens are collected: (*1*) the first 5–10 ml is collected and labeled VB_1 (voided bladder 1). This represents urethral organisms; (*2*) next, the patient voids 150–200 ml and then 5–10 ml of a midstream specimen is obtained (VB_2, voided bladder 2), which represents bladder organisms; (*3*) prostatic massage is performed, and the prostatic expressate is collected for smear (at this time, the white blood cells can be estimated in the fluid) and culture. The patient is then asked to void again, and the first 5–10 ml of urine are collected (VB_3, voided bladder 3), which represents prostatic organisms (mixed with some urethral urine; bladder urine should be sterile). Bacterial prostatitis is diagnosed if the quantity of organisms in the prostatic expressate or VB_3 specimen exceeds that of the VB_1 specimen by at least ten times (one log). Patients who might have bladder bacteriuria at the time of the study should be given 2 or 3 days of ampicillin, nitrofurantoin, or an oral cephalosporin to sterilize the urine. These agents fail to penetrate into prostatic tissue or fluid in a patient with chronic bacterial prostatitis and thus do not affect the bacterial counts in the prostatic expressate or VB_3 specimen.

Needle biopsy of the prostate gland has limited value in diagnosing bacterial prostatitis.

Treatment

ACUTE BACTERIAL PROSTATITIS

In contrast to chronic prostatitis, with acute infection, many drugs penetrate the inflamed prostate gland. Thus, most antibiotics that are used to treat urinary tract infections are effective in treating acute bacterial prostatitis. Empiric treatment may be initiated with oral TMP-SMZ or parenteral third-generation cephalosporins depending on the clinical status of the patient. An aminoglycoside may be recommended if the patient is severely ill with bacteremia. The drug regimen can be appropriately changed after culture data return.

Bedrest or hospitalization, analgesia, and hydration are also indicated.

CHRONIC BACTERIAL PROSTATITIS
Treatment of the chronic form of this infection is difficult and unsatisfactory. Because chronic bacterial prostatitis has focal and less intense inflammation than acute prostatitis, antibiotic penetration is variable and limited (51,52). Of the numerous antibiotics tested, TMP-SMZ and oral carbenicillin appear to be the most successful in curing this infection (53–56). However, long-term follow-up studies show that despite treatment for 4 to 16 weeks with these agents, the relapse rate is very high, with cure rates reaching only 30 to 40%. Despite these poor treatment results, it is recommended that all patients should be treated with TMP-SMZ, 2 tablets (160 mg TMP, 800 mg SMZ) twice a day for at least 4 weeks (assuming organism is susceptible to this agent). If relapse occurs, treatment should be restarted and continued for 3 months. Alternatively, oral carbenicillin 764 mg (one 500 mg tablet has 382 mg of carbenicillin) taken four times a day for 4 weeks may be given. Currently, some clinicians recommend oral carbenicillin as the treatment of choice for chronic bacterial prostatitis.

If patients fail on either TMP-SMZ or oral carbenicillin, low-dose antimicrobial therapy with a drug (e.g., TMP-SMZ, 1/2 tablet a day; cefadroxil 250 mg a day) to which the organism is sensitive should be provided as suppressive therapy (47). The suppressive therapeutic approach may reduce the incidence of symptomatic UTI, provided that superinfection with resistant organisms does not develop.

Prevention

Prevention of *acute* bacterial prostatitis is not feasible, since its pathogenesis and primary source of infection is not known. *Chronic* bacterial prostatitis may be prevented in a small number of patients in whom acute bacterial prostatitis is promptly treated. Otherwise, this is likewise not a preventable infection. Because its pathogenesis is poorly understood, many patients are asymptomatic, and the diagnosis is difficult to confirm.

REFERENCES

1. Yoshikawa TT: Unique aspects of urinary tract infection in the geriatric population. *Gerontology* 30:339–344, 1984.

2. Esposito AL, Gleckman RA, Cram S, et al: Community-acquired bacteremia in the elderly: Analysis of one hundred consecutive episodes. *J Am Geriatr Soc* 28:315–319, 1980.
3. Madden JW, Croker JR, Beynon GPJ: Septicemia in the elderly. *Postgrad Med J* 57:502–506, 1981.
4. Windsor ACM: Bacteremia in a geriatric unit. *Gerontology* 29:125–130, 1983.
5. Shimada K: Geriatric sepsis. Sixth International Cefoperazone Symposium. Princeton, NJ. Medica Excerpta, 1983, p 264.
6. Gleckman RA, Bradley PJ, Roth RM, et al: Bacteremic uropsepsis. A phenomenon unique to elderly women. *J Urol* 133:174–175, 1985.
7. Evans DA, Hennekins CH, Miao L, et al: Bacteriuria and subsequent mortality in women. *Lancet* 1:156–158, 1982.
8. Sourander LB, Ruikka I, Kasanen A: A health survey in the aged with a five-year follow-up. Acta Socio-medica Scand 3(suppl):5–40, 1970.
9. Dontas AS, Kasviki-Charvati P, Papanayiotou PC, et al: Bacteriuria and survival in old age. *N Engl J Med* 304:939–943, 1981.
10. Kass EH: Bacteriuria and excess mortality: What should the next steps be? *Rev Infect Dis* 7(suppl 4):S762–S766, 1985.
11. Nordenstam GR, Brandberg CA, Odén AS, et al: Bacteriuria and mortality in an elderly population. *N Engl J Med* 314:1152–1156, 1986.
12. Platt R, Polk BF, Murdock B, et al: Mortality associated with nosocomial urinary-tract infection. *N Engl J Med* 307:637–642, 1982.
13. Kasviki-Charvati P, Drolette-Kefaskis B, Papanayiotou P, et al: Turnover of bacteriuria in old age. *Age Ageing* 11:169–174, 1982.
14. Sourander LB, Kasanen A: A five-year follow-up of bacteriuria in the aged. *Gerontologica Clinica* 14:274–281, 1972.
15. Smith JW, Jones SR, Reed WP, et al: Recurrent urinary tract infections in men. Characteristics and response to therapy. *Ann Intern Med* 91:544–548, 1979.
16. Gleckman R, Crowley M, Natsios GA: Therapy of recurrent invasive urinary-tract infections of men. *N Engl J Med* 301:878–880, 1979.
17. Kumar A, Shah Y: Twice-a-day cefaclor in treatment of urinary tract infections: A prospective study. *Curr Ther Res* 35:932–936, 1984.
18. Latham RH, Wong ES, Larson A, et al: Laboratory diagnosis of urinary tract infection in ambulatory women. *JAMA* 254:3333–3336, 1985.
19. Greenberg RA, Reilly PM, Luppen KL, et al: Randomized study of single-dose, three-day and seven-day treatment of cystitis in women. *J Infect Dis* 153:277–282, 1986.
20. Brumfitt W, Hamilton-Miller JMT: A review of the problem of urinary infection management and the evaluation of a potential new antibiotic. *J Antimicrob Chemother* 13(suppl B):121–133, 1984.
21. Bryon CS, Reynolds KL: Hospital-acquired bacteremic urinary tract infection: epidemiology and outcome. *J Urol* 132:494–498, 1984.
22. Kaye D: Urinary tract infections in the elderly. *Bull NY Acad Med* 56:209–220, 1980.
23. Breitenbucher RB: Bacterial changes in the urine samples of patients with long-term indwelling catheters. *Arch Intern Med* 144:1585–1588, 1984.
24. Grahn D, Norman DC, White ML, et al: Validity of urinary catheter speci-

men for diagnosis of urinary tract infections in the elderly. *Arch Intern Med* 145:1858–1860, 1985.

25. Sourander LB: Urinary tract infection in the aged: An epidemiological study. *Annales Medicinae Internae Fenniae* 55(suppl 45):7–55, 1966.
26. Aktar AJ, Andrews GR, Caird FJ, et al: Urinary tract infection in the elderly: A population study. *Age Ageing* 1:48–54, 1972.
27. Brocklehurst JC, Dillane JB, Griffiths LL, et al: The prevalence and symptomatology of urinary infection in an aged population. *Gerontological Clinica* 10:242–253, 1968.
28. Klarsov P: Bacteriuria in elderly women. *Dan Med Bull* 23:200–204, 1976.
29. Wolfson SA, Kalmanson GM, Rubini ME, et al: Epidemiology of bacteriuria in a predominantly geriatric male population. *Am J Med Sci* 250: 168–173, 1965.
30. Heinämäki P, Haavisto M, Mattila K, et al: Urinary characteristics and infection in the very aged. *Gerontology* 30:403–407, 1984.
31. Bendall MJ: A review of urinary tract infection in the elderly. *J Antimicrob Chemother* 13(suppl B):69–78, 1984.
32. Norman DC: *In vitro* diagnostic tests for urinary tract infections. *Infect Med* 3:69–74, 1986.
33. Souney P, Polk BF: Single-dose antimicrobial therapy for urinary tract infections in women. *Rev Infect Dis* 4:29–34, 1982.
34. Pfau A, Sacks TG, Shapiro A, et al: A randomized comparison of 1-day versus 10-day antibacterial treatment of documented lower urinary tract infection. *J Urol* 132:931–933, 1984.
35. Wong ES, McKervitt M, Running K, et al: Management of recurrent urinary tract infections with patient-administered single-dose therapy. *Ann Intern Med* 102:302–307, 1985.
36. Nicole LE, Bjornson J, Harding GKM, et al: Bacteriuria in elderly institutionalized men. *N Engl J Med* 309:1420–1475, 1983.
37. Rennenberg J, Paerregaard A: Single-day treatment with trimethoprim for asymptomatic bacteriuria in the elderly patient. *J Urol* 132: 934–935, 1984
38. Lacey RW, Simpson MHC, Lord VL, et al: Comparison of single-dose trimethoprim with five-day course for the treatment of urinary tract infection in the elderly. *Age Ageing* 10:179–185, 1981.
39. Kunin CM: Duration of treatment of urinary tract infections. *Am J Med* 71:849–854, 1981.
40. Freedman LR: Natural history of urinary infections in adults. *Kidney Int* 8:S96–S100, 1975.
41. Dontas AS, Papanayiotou P, Marketos SG, et al: The effect of bacteriuria on renal functional patterns in old age. *Clin Sci* 34:73–81, 1968.
42. Kobasa W, Abrutyn E, Levison M, et al: Treatment of asymptomatic bacteriuria in elderly ambulatory women. *Clin Res* 34:675A, 1986.
43. Alyea EP: Infections and inflammation of the prostate and seminal vesicle, in Campbell MF, Harrison JH (eds): *Urology*. Philadelphia, W.B. Saunders, 1970, p 554.
44. Kreiger JN: Prostatitis syndromes: Pathophysiology, differential diagnosis and treatment. *Sex Transm Dis* 11:100–112, 1984.

45. Meares EM Jr: Prostatitis syndromes: New perspectives about old woes. *J Urol* 132:141–147, 1980.
46. Drach GW: Prostatitis: Man's hidden infection. *Urologic Clin North Am* 2:499–520, 1975.
47. Greenberg RN, Reilly PM, Luppen KL, et al: Chronic prostatitis: Comments on infectious etiologies and antimicrobial treatment. *The Prostate* 6:445–448, 1985.
48. Shortliffe LMD: Prostatitis: Still a diagnostic and therapeutic dilemma. *West J Med* 39:542–544, 1983.
49. Drach GW: Prostatitis and prostadynia. Their relationship to benign prostatic hypertrophy. *Urologic Clin North Am* 7:79–88, 1980.
50. Meares EM, Stamey TA: Bacteriologic localization patterns in bacterial prostatitis and urethritis. *Invest Urol* 5:492–518, 1968.
51. Winningham DG, Nemoy NJ, Stamey TA: Diffusion of antibiotics from plasma into prostatic fluid. *Nature* 219:139–143, 1968.
52. Barza M, Cuchural G: The penetration of antibiotics into the prostate in chronic bacterial prostatitis. *Eur J Clin Microbiol* 3:503–505, 1984.
53. Meares EM Jr: Long-term therapy of chronic bacterial prostatitis with trimethoprim-sulfamethoxazole. *Can Med Assoc J* 112:22S–25S, 1975.
54. Drach GW: Trimethoprim-sulfamethoxazole therapy of chronic bacterial prostatitis. *J Urol* 111:637–639, 1974.
55. Oliveri RA, Sachs RM, Castle PG: Clinical experience with geocillin in the treatment of bacterial prostatitis. *Curr Ther Res* 25:415–421, 1979.
56. Mobley DF: Bacterial prostatitis treatment with carbenicillin indanyl sodium. *Invest Urol* 19:31–33, 1981.

SUGGESTED READINGS

Freedman LR: Natural history of urinary infections in adults. *Kidney Int* 8: S96–S100, 1975.
Gleckman RA, Bradley PJ, Roth RM, et al: Bacteremic uropsepsis. A phenomenon unique to elderly women. *J Urol* 133:174–175, 1985.
Kaye D: Urinary tract infections in the elderly. *Bull NY Acad Med* 56:209–220, 1980.
Kreiger JN: Prostatitis syndromes: Pathophysiology, differential diagnosis and treatment. *Sex Transm Dis* 11:100–112, 1984.
Kunin CM: Duration of treatment of urinary tract infections. *Am J Med* 71: 849–854, 1981.
Meares EM Jr: Prostatitis syndromes: New perspectives about old woes. *J Urol* 132:141–147, 1980.
Sourander LB: Urinary tract infection in the aged: An epidemiological study. *Annales Medicinae Internae Fenniae* 55(suppl 45):7–55, 1966.
Yoshikawa TT: Unique aspects of urinary tract infection in the geriatric population. *Gerontology* 30:339–344, 1984.

Chapter 15

Skin and Soft Tissue Infection

This chapter focuses on erysipelas, cellulitis, and infected decubitus ulcer—three soft tissue infections that are especially important in the elderly. However, it should be mentioned that numerous other skin and soft tissue infections may occur in the aged. These infections are impetigo, folliculitis, furuncle, and carbuncle, as well as skin and soft tissue infection that are associated with wounds (trauma, surgery, bites), and severe underlying disease which include such life-threatening soft tissue infections as clostridial myonecrosis, necrotizing fasciitis, synergistic necrotizing cellulitis, progressive bacterial synergistic gangrene, Fournier's gangrene, and streptococcal or staphylococcal myonecrosis. These infectious disease problems are not especially unique to the elderly; therefore, they are not discussed here. The reader is referred to standard infectious disease textbooks for a complete review of these clinical entities.

ERYSIPELAS

General Considerations

Erysipelas is relatively uncommon. However, it is an infection that occurs primarily in the elderly, the very young, and the debilitated. Erysipelas is particularly severe in the elderly (hence its importance), because it usually involves the face and may be complicated by sepsis, ophthalmoplegia, or cavernous sinus thrombosis (1).

Etiology

The most common cause of erysipelas in the elderly is group A beta-hemolytic streptococci. Occasionally, other streptococci may be isolated, and rarely *Staphylococcus aureus* may cause this infection (2). The organisms cause an intense edema, vascular dilatation, and leukocytic cellular infiltration (bacteria are found in tissue spaces and lymphatic channels) in the dermis.

Clinical Manifestations

The lesion of erysipelas occurs primarily in the face, but may also be seen on the extremities, scalp, and abdominal wall. The characteristic dermopathy of erysipelas is an indurated, warm, tender, circumscribed erythematous lesion with a distinct raised (edema) border. The margins may be irregular and serperginous. Occasionally, vesicles and bullae develop. Most patients are systemically ill with an abrupt onset of fever, chills, malaise, and headache (2). If erysipelas progresses to involve the orbit (periorbital cellulitis), symptoms and signs of ophthalmoplegia, increased intraocular pressure, and cavernous sinus thrombosis may be present (3).

Diagnostic Approach

DIFFERENTIAL DIAGNOSIS
Since most cases of erysipelas involve the face, the differential diagnosis includes contact dermatitis, insect bites, exposure, sinusitis, tooth abscess, parotitis, systemic lupus erythematosus, and angioneurotic edema.

LABORATORY TESTS
Blood cultures should be obtained. Culture of the skin including the advancing edge is of little microbiologic value (4). Moreover, the majority of cases are caused by group A beta-hemolytic streptococci.

In patients with periorbital involvement, orbital x-rays should be obtained. Computed tomography of the head may be indicated if alteration of mental status develops.

Treatment

Because of the severity of facial erysipelas in this age group, all elderly patients should be hospitalized. Treatment should begin immediately after blood cultures are obtained. Empiric antibiotic therapy is with aqueous penicillin G, 8–10 million units a day given intravenously in 4 divided doses (2). If the patient improves clinically, and cultures do not

indicate an organism other than streptococci, oral phenoxymethyl penicillin is prescribed, 2 g a day in four divided doses. In penicillin-allergic
patients, vancomycin 1.5–2.0 g a day in two to four divided doses may be
administered intravenously followed by oral erythromycin 2 g a day in
four divided doses when the patient stabilizes clinically. Therapy should
be for 10 days (2).

Erysipelas that involves nonfacial regions may be treated with oral
penicillin on an outpatient basis, providing that the elderly patient is not
clinically ill and is without severe underlying disease(s).

Prevention

Recommendations for preventing erysipelas are not possible, since its
pathogenesis is not clearly understood. Moreover, because the frequency
of erysipelas is relatively low, preventive measures would not be cost
effective.

CELLULITIS

General Considerations

Cellulitis is an acute inflammatory lesion of the skin that begins in the
epidermis and dermis and later involves the deeper subcutaneous tissues.
Although cellulitis occurs in all age groups, there is a greater frequency of
cellulitis of the lower extremity in the older patient (5), most likely related
to trauma, peripheral vascular disease (arterial), diabetes mellitus,
chronic venous insufficiency, and edema.

Etiology

The microbial etiology of cellulitis varies depending on the predisposing
factors of cellulitis (e.g., intravenous needles, lacerations, postoperative
wound, bites, decubitus ulcers) or the presence of certain underlying diseases. Nevertheless, most cases of uncomplicated cellulitis are caused by
group A beta-hemolytic streptococci or S. aureus (4,5). If cellulitis is
associated with human bites, decubitus ulcers, or diabetic foot ulcers, a
mixed flora of anaerobic and aerobic bacteria is not uncommon (6–8). In
elderly patients with leukopenia and/or immunosuppression, aerobic
gram-negative bacilli may be causative pathogens of cellulitis.

Diagnostic Approach

DIFFERENTIAL DIAGNOSIS
Cellulitis associated with lacerations, wounds, or bites, or those cases involving the upper extremities are not difficult to diagnose. Cellulitis of the

lower extremities may be occasionally difficult to distinguish from skin changes due to chronic venous insufficiency, deep vein thrombophlebitis, insect bites, or allergic or contact dermatitis.

LABORATORY TESTS
Blood cultures should be obtained if the patient is ill enough to be hospitalized. Cellulitis associated with draining lesions, abscesses, or pustules should be aspirated, Gram stained, and cultured. Otherwise needle aspiration of the border of the cellulitis is of little diagnostic value (4).

Treatment

For elderly patients with cellulitis who have systemic symptoms (fever, chills, malaise), change in functional status, altered mental status, or facial involvement, hospitalization is recommended. Cellulitis *not* associated with immunosuppression, leukopenia, diabetic foot ulcers, decubitus ulcer, human bites, or postoperative abdominal wounds may be empirically treated with intravenous nafcillin or oxacillin, 6–12 g a day (dose depending on severity of illness) in four to six divided doses. For outpatient treatment, dicloxacillin 1 g orally in four divided doses is recommended. Vancomycin, 1.5 to 2.0 g a day in two to four divided doses, and clindamycin, 600 mg a day in four divided doses, may be substituted for intravenous and oral therapy, respectively, for patients who are allergic to penicillin.

Elderly patients with cellulitis that is associated with mixed aerobic and anaerobic organisms may be treated empirically with intravenous cefoxitin 6–12 g a day. Combination therapy that consists of intravenous clindamycin, 1,800–2,400 mg in three to four divided doses, and an aminoglycoside (gentamicin, tobramycin, or amikacin; see Chapter 5 on antimicrobial therapy: special considerations for dose recommendations) is recommended if the patient is septic or hypotensive. If gram-negative bacilli are suspected or the patient is leukopenic, empiric treatment with a third-generation cephalosporin (e.g., ceftazidime) combined with a broad-spectrum penicillin (e.g., piperacillin) is recommended. Again, if the patient is severely ill, an aminoglycoside should be part of the regimen.

Duration of antimicrobial therapy for cellulitis is generally 10 days.

Prevention

Prevention of cellulitis is primarily through recognition and minimization of the predisposing factors and associated conditions.

DECUBITUS ULCER

General Considerations

Some "purists" prefer the term *pressure sores* instead of decubitus ulcers, since these lesions occur in positions other than the decubitus posture. Nevertheless, we use the traditional term *decubitus ulcer* to encompass all pressure sores or ulcerations. Most cases occur in the elderly patient (9,10). The precise frequency of decubitus ulcer is unknown, although it is estimated to occur in 3 to 5% of hospitalized patients and 6 to 10% of residents in nursing homes (9,11,12). It is estimated that the overall mortality from decubitus ulcers may be as high as 7 to 8% (13). Yet, if bacteremia and sepsis occur with decubitus ulcers, the mortality may approach 40% (14). Thus, our discussion focuses primarily on the infectious complications of decubitus ulcers. For a complete discussion on pathophysiology and general management of decubitus ulcers, the reader is referred to several excellent reviews (15–17).

Etiology

Approximately 95% of all decubitus ulcers occur in the lower part of the body: sacral-coccygeal area, greater trochanter, ischial tuberosity, tuberosity of the calcaneous, and lateral malleolus (15,18). These sites of involvement result from prolonged pressure and shearing force due to chronic recumbent and/or sitting positions. Consequently, decubitus ulcers become constantly exposed to the fecal flora, which includes aerobic gram-negative bacilli and anaerobic bacteria, as well as to the usual skin flora (staphylococci and streptococci). Although whenever decubitus ulcers become infected mixed flora is present, it is often impossible to predict which of the organisms obtained on routine ulcer culture are actual pathogens in a given patient. However, recent studies indicate that with severe decubitus ulcers or worsening lesions, gram-negative bacilli such as *Pseudomonas aeruginosa* and *Providencia* sp. along with anaerobic bacteria are isolated more frequently (18).

Clinical Manifestations

Infection may complicate early or superficial decubitus ulcers (grade 1 or 2 lesions). Grade 1 ulcers involve only the epidermidis. Grade 2 lesions extend to the dermis. If these early lesions become infected, generally evidence of cellulitis is present (redness, heat, and tenderness). However, with more extensive decubitus ulcers (grade 3 or 4), infection is invariably present unless the lesion is meticulously and regularly treated. Grade 3 ulcers extend through the subcutaneous tissue, and grade 4 lesions involve fascia, muscle, and bone. Necrotic tissue that includes skin and muscle is surrounded by purulence and is often associated with a foul smell (anaerobes). Abscess pockets and sinus tracts may be found after appropriate mechanical probing, x-ray studies, and radionuclide scanning.

Patients may also have fever and clinical evidence of bacteremia (sepsis). There may be an associated osteomyelitis (15).

Diagnostic Approach

DIFFERENTIAL DIAGNOSIS
The diagnosis of decubitus ulcers is rarely in doubt when it occurs over the usual pressure sites. However, occasionally such lesions as vasculitis, deep mycotic infection, and a necrotic malignancy may mimic a decubitus ulcer (15).

LABORATORY TESTS
As with all serious infections, blood cultures are essential in the diagnostic evaluation of patients with presumed infected decubitus ulcers. Cultures of the surface of the ulcer have little clinical use. But, cultures of purulent drainage, sinus tracts, abscess pockets, or biopsies of muscle or bone are useful diagnostically. These cultures must be processed both aerobically and anaerobically.

In some cases, an apparent superficial decubitus ulcer may in fact be masking a deeper and more serious infectious process. Under these circumstances, mechanical probing of the ulcer with performance of a sinogram is valuable in discerning a deeper suppurative lesion. Bone x-rays and a radionuclide technetium scan are useful in diagnosing osteomyelitis. In patients suspected of having a suppurative process (e.g., abscess) extending into the pelvis, a body computed tomographic scan should be obtained. A gallium scan may also be helpful.

Treatment

The general treatment principles of decubitus ulcers are to relieve pressure, eliminate risk factors, provide good nutrition, give good local wound care, and treat infections. In patients who are clinically septic; who have osteomyelitis; or who have foul-smelling necrotic tissue, pus, or active cellulitis, systemic antibiotics should be started with drugs that can provide good activity against gram-negative bacilli and anaerobic bacteria, including *Bacteroides fragilis*. A combination of clindamycin and gentamicin has been shown to be effective treatment for sepsis caused by decubitus ulcers (14). Other potentially useful regimens include metronidazole and chloramphenicol for anaerobic bacteria and third-generation cephalosporins and other aminoglycosides for aerobic gram-negative bacilli.

Deep and extensive decubitus ulcers may require surgical intervention, such as extensive débridement, bone resections, and reconstructive plastic procedures. However, extensive surgery in these elderly patients has to be tempered by such factors as risk versus benefits and clinical status as well as by the functional level of the patient.

Controversy exists on the value of applying topical antibiotics or antiseptics on decubitus ulcers. Proponents for topical antiinfective therapy suggest that reducing the quantity of bacteria eliminates one factor that prolongs healing (13,17). Topical agents that have shown some efficacy include silver sulfadiazine, povidone-iodine, metronidazole, and cadexomer iodine (13,19,20). One main objection to topical antiinfectives is the potential of selecting out resistant bacteria.

Prevention

It is obvious that infections related to decubitus ulcers can be prevented by keeping decubitus ulcers from occurring. The single most important preventive measure is the elimination of chronic pressure on any part of the body. In ulcers that have already developed, removal of necrotic tissue, frequent cleansing and dressing of the wound, avoiding treatments that hinder oxygenation of healing tissue, and keeping patients out of urine and feces (due to incontinence) minimize the risk of infection of the decubitus ulcer.

REFERENCES

1. Chow AW: Wound and soft tissue infections, in Yoshikawa TT, Chow AW, Guze LB (eds): *Infectious Disease. Diagnosis and Management.* New York, John Wiley & Sons, 1980, p 223.
2. Yoshikawa TT: Cellulitis and soft tissue infection, in Kass EH, Platt R (eds): *Current Therapy in Infectious Disease,* ed 2. Burlington, Toronto, B.C. Decker, Inc., 1986, p 266.
3. Middleton DB, Ferrante JA: Periorbital and facial cellulitis. *Am Fam Physician* 21:98–103, 1980.
4. Hook EW, III, Hooton TM, Horton CA, et al: Microbiologic evaluation of cutaneous cellulitis in adults. *Arch Intern Med* 146:295–297, 1986.
5. Ginsberg MB: Cellulitis: An analysis of 101 cases and review of the literature. *South Med J* 74:530–533, 1981.
6. Galpin JE, Chow AW, Bayer AS, et al: Sepsis associated with decubitus ulcers. *Am J Med* 61:346–350, 1976.
7. Louie TJ, Bartlett JG, Tally FP, et al: Aerobic and anaerobic bacteria in diabetic foot ulcers. *Ann Intern Med* 85:461–463, 1976.

8. Goldstein EJC, Citron DM, Wield B, et al: Bacteriology of human and animal bite wounds. *J Clin Microbiol* 8:667–672, 1978.
9. Manley MT: Incidence, contributory factors and costs of pressure sores. *S Afr Med J* 53:217–222, 1978.
10. Kostuik JP, Fernie G: Pressure sores in elderly patients. *J Bone Joint Surg* 67(B):1–2, 1985.
11. Peterson DC, Bittmann S: The epidemiology of pressure sores. *Scand J Plast Reconst Surg* 5:62–66, 1971.
12. Garibaldi RD, Brodine S, Matsuyama S: Infections among patients in nursing homes. *N Engl J Med* 305:731–735, 1981.
13. Kucan JO: Bacterial infection in pressure ulcerations and its management. *Geriatr Med Today* 3:87–95, 1984.
14. Chow AW, Galpin JE, Guze LB: Clindamycin for treatment of sepsis caused by decubitus ulcers. *J Infect Dis* 135(suppl):S67–S68, 1977.
15. Reuler JB, Cooney TG: The pressure sore: Pathophysiology and principles of management. *Ann Intern Med* 94:661–666, 1981.
16. Seiler WO, Allen S, Stähelin HB: Decubitus ulcer prevention: A new investigative method using transcutaneous oxygen tension measurement. *J Am Geriatr Soc* 31:786–789, 1983.
17. Seiler WO, Stähelin HB: Decubitus ulcers: Treatment through five therapeutic principles. *Geriatrics* 40:30–43, 1985.
18. Seiler WO, Stähelin HB: Recent findings on decubitus ulcer pathology: implications for care. *Geriatrics* 41:47–58, 1986.
19. Gomolin IH, Brandt JL: Topical metronidazole therapy for pressure sores of geriatric patients. *J Am Geriatr Soc* 31:710–712, 1983.
20. Moberg S, Hoffman L, Grennert M-L, et al: A randomized trial of cadexomer iodine in decubitus ulcers. *J Am Geriatr Soc* 31:462–465, 1983.

SUGGESTED READINGS

Chow AW: Wound and soft tissue infections, in Yoshikawa TT, Chow AW, Guze LB (eds): *Infectious Disease. Diagnosis and Management.* New York, John Wiley & Sons, 1980, p 223.
Ginsberg MB: Cellulitis: An analysis of 101 cases and review of the literature. *South Med J* 74:530–533, 1981.
Reuler JB, Cooney TG: The pressure sore: Pathophysiology and principles of management. *Ann Intern Med* 94:661–666, 1981.
Seiler WO, Stähelin HB: Recent findings on decubitus ulcer pathology: Implications for care. *Geriatrics* 41:47–58, 1986.
Yoshikawa TT: Cellulitis and soft tissue infection, in Kass EH, Platt R (eds): *Current Therapy in Infectious Disease,* ed 2. Burlington, Toronto, B.C. Decker, Inc., 1986, p 266.

Chapter 16

Septic Arthritis and Osteomyelitis

SEPTIC ARTHRITIS

General Considerations

Nongonococcal bacterial arthritis is one of many infectious diseases with an increased incidence in the geriatric population. In fact, between one-third and one-half of patients with this disease are over age 60 (1–5). Moreover, as is the case for many infections in the elderly, pyoarthrosis in this age group is associated with a higher morbidity (loss of joint function) and mortality. This is largely due to a combination of factors, including more virulent pathogens, delays in diagnosis, more serious underlying diseases, preexisting joint disease, and a greater use of immunosuppressive drugs, particularly steroids, in the older age group (1). Thus, despite advances in antimicrobial agents, approximately 50% of elderly persons with infected joints have a poor therapeutic outcome (6).

In general, one or more of the following predisposing risk factors are present in elderly patients with bacterial arthritis: (1) concurrent or recent extraarticular infection; (2) preexisting joint disease (i.e., rheumatoid arthritis, crystalline deposition diseases, degenerative joint disease, prosthetic joint surgery); (3) impaired host defenses (i.e., immunosuppressive drugs, particularly systemic or intraarticular corticosteroids); (4) underlying chronic illness such as diabetes mellitus; and (5) prior antimicrobial therapy (1,5–7). Recent trauma to the joint may also predispose toward the development of pyoarthritis (8).

The first two factors are of key importance in the pathogenesis of bacterial arthritis. Although direct seeding of a joint with bacteria may occur (e.g., from joint surgery) or bacteria may rarely enter a joint space by direct extension from a juxtaarticular osteomyelitis, the most common mechanism by which the synovial space is infected is by hematogenous spread. This fact is critical in understanding the differences in joint pathogens between old and young patients. Preexisting joint disease, common in the elderly, somehow alters host defenses and allows bacterial replication in the joint space once bacteria gain entrance to the joint.

Infection of prosthetic joints in the aged is a different clinical problem from natural joint infections. Although the incidence of these prosthetic infections has fallen from approximately 9% to less than 1% (7,9,10), the dramatic increase in the use of joint prostheses in the elderly makes it an important infection. Furthermore, such infections are typically disastrous and often require removal of the prosthesis, and in some patients reinsertion is not possible. Risks for development of infection in prosthetic joints are as yet ill defined. However, patients who have had an operation performed on the affected joint appear to be at greater risk for infection (9). Moreover, prosthetic joint infections may not only be caused by hematogenous seeding of the prosthesis but also by introduction of pathogens into the joint at the time of operation.

Etiology

The bacteriology of septic arthritis in the elderly differs significantly from younger adults. *Neisseria gonorrhoeae* is the most common cause of joint infection in sexually active adults, but is distinctly rare in the geriatric population. Although gram-positive cocci (*Staphylococcus aureus, Streptococcus pneumoniae,* and other streptococci [usually group A]) account for most cases of nongonococcal bacterial arthritis in both young and old adults, over 20% of pyoarthrosis in the elderly are caused by aerobic gram-negative bacilli (5,6). A small percentage of cases of septic arthritis in the elderly are caused by assorted *Hemophilus, Streptococcus,* and *Bacterioides* species. However, it should be noted that virtually any bacterial species may cause infection of a joint, including *Mycobacterium tuberculosis* (see Chapter 11 on tuberculosis and the discussion below).

There are associations of specific pathogens that cause pyoarthrosis with particular underlying diseases. Septic arthritis due to aerobic gram-negative bacilli tends to occur in patients with severely impaired host defense mechanisms (the very old and the very young) or with urinary tract infection (11). *S. aureus* causes about 80% of pyoarthrosis in patients with rheumatoid arthritis (12,13). Also, this organism is the most common cause of joint infection in patients with diabetes mellitus. In another example, *S. pneumoniae* arthritis is often seen in patients with chronic alcoholism or hypogammaglobulinemia (14).

The causative pathogens of prosthetic joint infections differ somewhat from those that cause natural joint infection. In a recent study of 63 patients (10), *Staphylococcus epidermidis* accounted for 40% and *S. aureus* accounted for 19% of combined cases of early (less than 1 year postoperative) and late prosthetic joint infection. The rest were caused by a variety of pathogens including enterococci, streptococci, and aerobic and anaerobic gram-negative bacilli. This is similar to the results of other series that reported on infections complicating total hip replacement (15–17). The pathogens involved probably reflect that wound contamination at the time of operation is as important as the hematogenous spread in the pathogenesis of prosthetic joint infection. The reason certain patients that are presumably infected at operation develop clinical infection years later is unknown.

Clinical Manifestations

Classically, hematogenously acquired nongonococcal bacterial arthritis has an abrupt onset with significant constitutional symptoms including fever and chills. The infection is typically monoarticular, involving the large weight-bearing joints, usually the knee and less commonly the hip (3,16). The wrist and shoulder may also be involved. Heat, tenderness, effusion, and decreased range of motion are found on physical examination. However, in some elderly patients, fever and chills may be blunted or absent, particularly in the severely immunocompromised or debilitated patient (1–4). Special attention must be paid to patients who have preexisting rheumatic disorders such as rheumatoid arthritis or gout, because the diagnosis of septic arthritis may be delayed or overlooked if joint symptoms due to infection are attributed to exacerbation or reactivation of the underlying rheumatic disease. Thus, we recommend that the diagnosis of septic arthritis be considered in geriatric patients with underlying joint disease if there is (*1*) an acute deterioration in the patient's clinical or functional status; (*2*) fever or chills; (*3*) presence of an extraarticular infection; (*4*) involvement of joints not previously affected by the underlying rheumatic disease; or (*5*) increased pain and effusion in a joint previously affected.

Infections in prosthetic joints may present in a fulminant fashion (i.e., acute onset of pain, fever, swelling). However, a substantial number of patients have persistent pain and loosening of the prosthesis as the only features of the infection (9,10,18).

Tuberculous arthritis in the elderly is a particularly difficult disease to diagnose and treat. In a recent study, a median delay in diagnosis of 8 months in 11 elderly patients with septic arthritis due to *M. tuberculosis* was observed. The initial joint symptoms and signs were nonspecific, and only 50% of patients had evidence of past or present pulmonary tuberculosis (19). Moreover, 50% of the cases had negative tuberculin skin tests or involvement of the wrist joint, in contrast to previous studies that had much lower rates of negative skin test and had disease that only rarely involved the non-weight-bearing joints. Tuberculous arthritis should be considered in patients who have a chronic monoarticular arthritis, particularly if erosive or destructive changes are seen on radiographs.

Diagnostic Approach

DIFFERENTIAL DIAGNOSIS
Diagnostic considerations in bacterial infection of a natural joint include those diseases associated with an acute monoarticular arthritis. These can best be remembered by the acronym CHRIST: *c*rystal deposition diseases; *h*emophilia (or *h*ydroarthrosis); *r*heumatoid variants; *i*nfection; *s*arcoidosis; and *t*rauma.

In cases of prosthetic joint infection that present in an indolent manner, the more common entity of aseptic loosening of the prosthesis should be considered.

SOURCE OF INFECTION
Since hematogenous spread from a distant extraarticular source is the most common mechanism of joint infection, a source of bacteremia should be sought. Certain pathogens suggest specific sources. *S. pneumoniae* pyoarthrosis may result from bacteremia from a pulmonary or pericranial infection, whereas *S. aureus* and group A streptococcal joint infections usually result from bacteremia from a cutaneous infection. Patients with a septic joint caused by gram-negative bacilli should be investigated for a urinary tract infection or gastrointestinal source.

The above comments hold true for cases of prosthetic joint infection that result from bacteremia.

LABORATORY TESTS
Arthrocentesis.   Analysis of synovial fluid from the affected joint is the critical test to making the diagnosis of septic arthritis. Gram stain and culture (aerobic in 5–10% CO_2, anaerobic, mycobacterial, fungal) should be done routinely on all aspirated joint fluid; it should be reiterated that the presence of evidence of coexisting joint disease (e.g., crystals) does not exclude concurrent infection (20). In cases of tuberculous arthritis, culture and histopathologic examination of a synovium biopsy specimen increase the diagnostic yield. In the past, the Gram stain has been reported to be positive in 70 to 90% of patients with bacterial arthritis that were caused by gram-positive cocci and in about 50% of cases that were caused by gram-negative bacilli (5,21). However, in a recent study that examined

23 elderly patients with septic arthritis, the synovial fluid Gram stain was positive in only 3 out of 16 specimens (6).

Inflammatory changes tend to be more marked in synovial fluid from pyoarthritis due to gram-positive cocci compared to gram-negative bacilli, and, in general, synovial fluid leukocytosis is usually more intense in infected joints compared to noninfectious causes of arthritis. Although there is a wide range for synovial white blood cell counts in patients with pyoarthrosis (6,800 to greater than 250,000 white blood cells per cubic millimeter) (5), typically, greater than 90% of white cells are polymorphonucelar cells (PMN). Nevertheless, because of the wide range of synovial leukocyte counts associated with infection, there is overlap with certain noninfectious diseases such as gout and rheumatoid arthritis. Thus, septic arthritis needs to be considered in all cases where purulent fluid is obtained, especially if counts are greater than 50,000 cells per mm^3 (and more so, if greater than 100,000 per mm^3) with over 90% PMN.

Measurement of synovial fluid glucose has less value than Gram stain and leukocyte count, but a difference in glucose concentration between blood and joint fluid exceeding 40 mg/100 ml (synovial fluid glucose being lower) is highly suggestive of bacterial arthritis.

A poor mucin clot and elevated protein concentrations are common in bacterial arthritis, but are nonspecific. Similarly, the limulus lysate test for endotoxin is also nonspecific (22). Other more promising tests include counter-immunoelectrophoresis (for detection of bacterial antigens) or gas liquid chromatography (23) (detection of lactic acid and other products of bacterial metabolism). However, lack of sensitivity in the former and overlap of values in septic and nonseptic joints limit the current usefulness of these tests (7).

The diagnosis of infection in a prosthetic joint is considerably more difficult than in a natural joint infection, particularly in late infection, which may be more insidious (9). Aspiration of the joint (usually under fluoroscopy) is mandatory in all suspected cases. If aspiration is unsuccessful, surgical exploration may be necessary. Aspirated material should be routinely cultured and Gram stained as described above.

Blood Culture and Other Studies. Blood cultures should be obtained routinely; this test is positive in about 50% of cases (5), particularly if gram-positive cocci are involved. Any extraarticular infection source should be searched for carefully and, if present, relevant specimens Gram stained and cultured.

Routine tests such as complete blood count and differential, erythrocyte sedimentation rate (ESR), chest x-ray, and urinalysis are important initial screening tests. Although nonspecific, an elevated ESR is seen routinely in cases of natural and prosthetic joint infection.

Because older patients with bacterial arthritis are likely to have more severe joint infection, serial radiographic evaluation is indicated. Initial or follow-up routine x-rays or tomography (if routine films are normal) may reveal bony erosions, periosteal elevation, narrowing of the joint space consistent with destruction of cartilage, and osteomyelitis (6). Serial gallium or technetium bone scans are also indicated if x-ray films are negative because scans may show signs of osteomyelitis before the radiographs. The initial presence or eventual development of osteomyelitis prolongs therapy (over 6 weeks) and may necessitate early surgery. In cases of prosthetic joint infection, routine radiographs are usually unremarkable or show signs of nonspecific loosening. Radionuclide scanning does not differentiate septic from aseptic loosening.

Tuberculin skin testing should be performed in all cases of inflammatory monoarticular pyoarthrosis in which no bacterial pathogen is isolated.

Treatment

Management of natural joint infections has four components: (1) antimicrobial therapy, (2) drainage, (3) immobilization, and (4) monitoring response.

Fortunately, penicillins and cephalosporins when given parenterally in high doses penetrate well into joint fluid (24). Aminoglycosides do enter joint fluid, but achievable therapeutic concentrations are less predictable than with beta-lactam antibiotics. Moreover, prolonged therapy with aminoglycosides in elderly persons is associated with significant morbidity (i.e., ototoxity and nephrotoxicity). Nevertheless, aminoglycoside levels obtained in synovial fluid are usually at or above the minimal inhibitory concentration of most gram-negative bacillary pathogens that cause septic arthritis (25). Thus, intraarticular administration of antibiotics is not necessary. Moreover, certain drugs may provoke a chemical synovitis.

The duration of therapy is dependent on the pathogen and the clinical response. Streptococcal arthritis generally requires 2 weeks of therapy, whereas staphylococcal arthritis should be treated for 4 to 6 weeks.

Septic arthritis caused by gram-negative bacilli requires prolonged therapy (6 to 8 weeks or longer). Even if the organism is sensitive to a single agent (21), it is recommended that two-drug therapy (usually an aminoglycoside plus a beta-lactam drug) be used, particularly if *Pseudomonas aeruginosa* is isolated. A two-drug regimen has the potential of enhancing the rate of killing of the bacteria by either additive or synergistic effects. Tuberculous arthritis should be treated with isoniazid and rifampin for a minimum of 9 months.

The decision to begin empiric antimicrobial therapy should be based on clinical findings, Gram stain results, and laboratory evaluation of the synovial fluid. Once culture data are known, appropriate adjustments in antibiotics can be made. (See Table 16.1 for specific drug regimens.)

Adequate drainage is essential for management of a septic joint. Benefits of drainage include relief of cartilage-damaging pressure and removal of necrotic debris, enzymes, and toxin. Also, drainage helps prevent a low synovial fluid pH. A low pH inhibits the activity of aminoglycosides (26) and reduces the effectiveness of beta-lactam antibiotics. An added benefit of repeated arthrocentesis is in monitoring response, which is discussed below. The initial drainage should be done by (closed) needle aspirations (27). However, open drainage should be considered when fluid is too thick to aspirate, if the joint is not easily accessible by needle (e.g., hip), early in gram-negative bacillary arthritis (which tends to respond poorly), or when juxtaarticular osteomyelitis and perisynovial abscess are present.

TABLE 16-1 Antimicrobial Therapy for Elderly with Bacterial Arthritis

PATHOGEN	DRUG(S) OF CHOICE[a]	ALTERNATIVE DRUG(S)[a]
Staphylococcus aureus	Nafcillin or oxacillin 8–12 g OR cephalothin 8–12 g	Vancomycin 1.5–2.0 g
Streptococcus (non group D)	Penicillin G, 10–12 million units or first- or second-generation cephalosporin (e.g., cefazolin 3 g)	Vancomycin 1.5–2.0 g OR Chloramphenicol 4–6 g
Escherichia coli	Ampicillin 6 g plus aminoglycoside[b] (e.g., gentamicin 5 mg/kg adjusted for renal function)	Mezlocillin 18 g; or third-generation[c] cephalosporin (e.g., cefoperazone 4 g daily)
Pseudomonas aeruginosa	Amikacin 15 mg/kg plus antipseudomonas penicillin (e.g., piperacillin 18 g)	Ceftazidime[c] 6 g
Unknown or Gram stain equivocal	Oxacillin or nafcillin 8–12 g plus aminoglycoside (e.g., gentamicin 5 mg/kg)[b]	Vancomycin 1.5–2.0 g plus gentamicin 5 mg/kg[b] OR Third-generation cephalosporin (e.g., ceftazidime 6 g)[c]

[a]All drugs should be given intravenously (IV); doses for 24 hours.
[b]Other aminoglycosides such as tobramycin or amikacin in equivalent doses may be used.
[c]Data demonstrating the efficacy of third-generation cephalosorins in this disease are not available. Sensitivities plus joint synovial bactericidal titers are recommended when using these drugs.

Immobilization with splints or traction is required until inflammation appears to resolve, particularly if large weight-bearing joints are involved. During this immobilization period, passive range of motion should be performed to prevent loss of range of motion and minimize contractures. When inflammation appears to have resolved, gradual weight-bearing exercises should be started. In cases of prolonged immobilization, prophylactic measures to prevent thrombophlebitis and pulmonary atelectasis are indicated.

Early in the course of infection, the response to treatment should be monitored, which should consist of daily joint examinations to evaluate the degree of effusion and range of motion as well as articular pain and fever. As the joint effusion diminishes, joint aspiration may be performed less frequently. Synovial fluid obtained after repeat arthrocentesis should be reexamined as described earlier (i.e., Gram stain, culture, leukocyte count, glucose, etc.). A persistently positive culture or Gram stain, an elevated leukocyte count, and a depressed synovial glucose indicate a poor therapeutic result. In such cases, especially when clinical response is slow or poor, we recommend the measurement of joint fluid bactericidal titers to assess the adequacy of antimicrobial activity in the synovial fluid (a titer of 1:8 is adequate). The patient should also be evaluated carefully for the possibility of osteomyelitis and perisynovial abscess. Arthroscopy may be helpful in evaluating difficult cases, but open drainage may eventually be necessary in many of these patients.

Management of infections in prosthetic joints (data are only available for total hip replacement) is somewhat controversial (9). With early infection, surgical wound débridement and prolonged parenteral antimicrobial therapy may be tried. In late infection, the prosthesis and cement must usually be removed concurrently with a course of prolonged antimicrobial therapy. The timing of reinsertion of a new prosthesis is also controversial, although early reinsertion may be possible with the use of antibiotic-impregnated cement (28).

Prevention

Septic arthritis in natural joints can only be prevented by limiting joint trauma and joint disease as well as by preventing bacteremia. Prosthetic joint infection has already been significantly reduced with the increasing experience of surgeons (decreased operating time), clean air operating rooms, and perioperative prophylactic antibiotics (see Chapter 6 on the prevention of infections).

OSTEOMYELITIS

General Considerations

There have been changes in the epidemiology, microbiology, and clinical patterns of osteomyelitis in recent decades (29–31). However, with notable exceptions, there is no increased predilection for osteomyelitis in older persons, and the disease does not differ in old and young individuals. Therefore, osteomyelitis is only briefly discussed with the emphasis placed on differences in clinical presentation in the elderly. For a more detailed discussion on osteomyelitis in general, the reader is referred to several excellent reviews (29–34).

Osteomyelitis can conveniently be divided into three types on the basis of pathogenesis: (1) hematogenous, (2) contiguous, and (3) secondary to vascular insufficiency (29–31). Although typically a disease of children, hematogenous osteomyelitis, in recent years, is being increasingly reported in older adults (32). Osteomyelitis from a contiguous focus of infection (e.g., infected decubitus ulcer, prosthetic joint infection) occurs in older persons presumably because they are most at risk for these exogenous foci of infection. Similarly, older persons are at increased risk for osteomyelitis due to the increased frequency of age-related peripheral vascular disease.

Etiology

Overall, most cases of hematogenous osteomyelitis are caused by S. aureus. However, aerobic gram-negative bacilli, that usually arise from a genitourinary focus, are responsible for an increasing number of cases. The bacteriology of osteomyelitis that result from direct spread from a contiguous focus reflects the bacteriology of the exogenous focus. Although S. aureus is frequently isolated in these infections, it is usually part of a mixed flora. For example, in osteomyelitis from sacral decubiti, multiple aerobic and anaerobic enteric organisms may be involved. Osteomyelitis that complicates peripheral vascular disease is almost always a mixed infection, that frequently yields both aerobic and anaerobic bacteria.

Clinical Manifestations

In children, acute hematogenous osteomyelitis occurs with abrupt fever, systemic toxicity, and local pain and swelling about the involved bone (33). However, in older adults with vertebral osteomyelitis, fever and systemic toxicity may be minimal with malaise and low back pain as the only presenting symptoms (34). On physical examination, localized tenderness is present over the affected vertebra(e). These findings, along with an elevated sedimentation rate and an exogenous source (e.g., urinary tract infection) should heighten the physician's awareness for the presence of vertebral osteomyelitis.

The clinical manifestations of osteomyelitis secondary to contiguous spread of infection depend on the bone(s) involved (30). The femur and tibia are most commonly involved, and these infections result as a complication of trauma or an operation. Initially, patients complain of fever, swelling, and erythema. With recurrent osteomyelitis, systemic toxicity is less common; sinus formation and drainage usually predominate as the clinical features (33).

Clinical features of osteomyelitis due to peripheral vascular disease are variable with a predominance of local symptoms (i.e., pain, swelling, erythema, chronic foot ulcers) (31). Systemic symptoms are relatively uncommon unless septicemia is present.

Tuberculous vertebral osteomyelitis (Pott's disease) in the elderly adult usually involves the lower thoracic spine (in contrast to children in whom the infection occurs primarily in upper thoracic spine) and may produce a characteristic gibbus deformity. Pus may rupture anteriorly and produce a paraspinal "cold" abscess with resultant involvement of the psoas muscle; these patients have fever and abdominal or back pain. Rarely cord compression may ensue and result in paraplegia.

Diagnostic Approach

DIFFERENTIAL DIAGNOSIS
Diagnostic considerations in patients with vertebral tenderness would include fracture or tumor as well as osteomyelitis. In patients with recent trauma or decubitus ulcer, osteomyelitis must be differentiated from overlying soft tissue inflammation or infection.

LABORATORY TESTS
Radiologic Procedures. Early in hematogenous osteomyelitis (less than 10 days after onset) routine x-rays are negative. However, radionuclide scanning (technetium and gallium) may be positive as early as 3 days after disease onset (33), but because scans are nonspecific, clinical correlation is of paramount importance.

Microbiologic Studies. All attempts possible should be made to determine the etiologic pathogens. Cultures of blood and distant sites of infection should always be done. Invasive diagnostic tests (i.e., direct sampling of affected bone) are often indicated, and any needle aspirate of bone or open biopsy material should be cultured both aerobically and anaerobically as well as for fungi and mycobacteria. A biopsy specimen has the added advantage of providing histologic examination of bone. It should be mentioned that swab cultures of wounds or draining sinuses may provide inaccurate information on the pathogens responsible for infection of the bone because of surface colonization by microbes.

Tuberculin Skin Test. This should be done in all cases of vertebral osteomyelitis.

Treatment

There is little information in the literature on optimal antibiotic therapy, such as class of drug(s), duration of therapy, or whether or not antibiotic penetration into bone is even important in the treatment outcome of osteomyelitis (33). Acute hematogenous vertebral osteomyelitis due to bacteria can be treated successfully with 6 weeks of a parenteral antibiotic directed at the offending pathogen (usually determined by culture of needle biopsy material). An operation is usually not necessary unless there is extensive vertebral body destruction with sequestra and abscess formation or signs of cord compression (32). Similar recommendations on antimicrobial therapy can be made for other types of osteomyelitis, though the role of a surgical procedure needs to be determined depending on the clinical situation (necrotic bone and sequestra must be removed). In cases of chronic or recurrent osteomyelitis, prolonged parenteral and oral antimicrobial therapy may be necessary. The role of new potent oral antibiotics such as the quinolones needs to be determined for this disease. Repeated surgical débridement may be necessary in many of these chronic cases.

For tuberculous osteomyelitis, treatment is the same as for tuberculous arthritis.

PREVENTION

Hematogenous osteomyelitis can only be prevented by minimizing or eliminating bacteremia from exogenous infection. Osteomyelitis secondary to contiguous infection in the elderly may be prevented by reducing the incidence of wound infection after orthopedic surgery and prevention of decubitus ulcers. Careful control of diabetes and its complications and reduction of other peripheral vascular disease risk factors may reduce the incidence of osteomyelitis that complicates peripheral vascular disease.

REFERENCES

1. Wilkins WF, Healy LA, Decker JL: Acute infectious arthritis in the aged and chronically ill. *Arch Intern Med* 106:354–364, 1960.
2. Argen RJ, Wilson JR, Wood P: Suppurative arthritis. *Arch Intern Med* 117: 661–666, 1966.
3. Newman JH: Review of septic arthritis throughout the antibiotic era. *Ann Rheum Dis* 35:198–205, 1976.
4. Norman DC, Yoshikawa TT: Responding to septic arthritis. *Geriatrics* 38: 83–91, 1983.
5. Goldenberg DL, Cohen AS: Acute infectious arthritis: a review of patients with nongonococcal joint infections (with emphasis on therapy and prognosis). *Am J Med* 60:369–377, 1976.

6. McGuire NM, Kauffman CA: Septic arthritis in the elderly. *J Am Geriatr Soc* 33:170–174, 1985.
7. Goldenberg DL, Reed JI: Bacterial arthritis. *N Engl J Med* 312:764–771, 1985.
8. Manshady BM, Thompson GR, Weiss JJ: Septic arthritis in a general hospital 1966–1977. *J Rheumatol* 7:523–530, 1980.
9. Hirshman PH, Schurman DJ: Deep infections following total hip replacement, in Remington JS, Schwartz MN (eds): *Current Clinical Topics in Infectious Diseases.* New York, McGraw-Hill, Inc., 1982, vol 3, p 206.
10. Inman RD, Gallegos KV, Brause BD, et al: Clinical and microbial features of prosthetic joint infection. *Am J Med* 77:47–53, 1984.
11. Goldenberg DL, Brandt KD, Cathcart ES, et al: Acute arthritis caused by gram-negative bacilli: A clinical characterization. *Medicine* (Baltimore) 53: 197–208, 1974.
12. Karten I: Septic arthritis complicating rheumatoid arthritis. *Ann Intern Med* 70:1147–1157, 1969.
13. Rimoin DI, Wennberg JE: Acute septic arthritis complicating rheumatoid arthritis. *JAMA* 196:617–621, 1966.
14. Kauffman CA, Watanakunakorn C, Phair JP: Pneumococcal arthritis. *J Rheumatol* 3:409–419, 1976.
15. Conner GC, Steinberg ME, Heppenstall RB, et al: The infected hip after total hip arthroplasty. *J Bone Joint Surg* 66[Am]:1393–1399, 1984.
16. Hunter G, Dandy D: The natural history of the patient with an infected total hip replacement. *J Bone Joint Surg* 59[Br]:293–297, 1977.
17. Fitzgerald RH, Nolan DR, Ilstrup DM, et al: Deep wound sepsis following total hip arthroplasty. *J Bone Joint Surg* 59[Am]:847–855, 1977.
18. Lockshin MD, Brause BD: Infectious arthritis, in Catsonas NJ Jr (ed): *Disease-a-Month.* Chicago-London, Yearbook Medical Publishers, Inc., 1982, vol 28, No 4, p 6.
19. Evanchick CC, Davis DE, Harrington TM: Tuberculosis of peripheral joints: An often missed diagnosis. *J Rheumatol* 13:187–189, 1986.
20. Hamilton ME, Paris TM, Gibson RS, et al: Simultaneous gout and pyoarthrosis. *Arch Intern Med* 140:917–919, 1980.
21. Bayer AS, Chow AW, Louie JS, et al: Gram-negative bacillary septic arthritis: Clinical, radiographic, therapeutic, and prognostic features. *Semin Arthritis Rheum* 7:968–971, 1978.
22. Elin RJ, Knowles R, Barth WF, et al: Lack of specificity of the limulus lysate test in the diagnosis of pyogenic arthritis. *J Infect Dis* 137:507–513, 1978.
23. Brook I, Reza MJ, Bricknell KS, et al: Synovial fluid lactic acid. *Arthritis Rheum* 21:774–779, 1978.
24. Nelson JD: Antibiotic concentrations in septic joint effusions. *N Engl J Med* 284:349–353, 1971.
25. Chow A, Hecht R, Winters R: Gentamicin and carbenicillin penetration into the septic joint. *N Engl J Med* 285:178–179, 1971.
26. Ward TT, Steigbigel RT: Acidosis of synovial fluid correlates with synovial fluid leukocytosis. *Am J Med* 64:933–936, 1978.

27. Goldenberg DL, Brandt KD, Cohen AJ, et al: Treatment of septic arthritis. *Arthritis Rheum* 18:83–90, 1975.
28. Carlsson AS, Göran Josefsson M, Lindberg L: Revision with gentamicin-impregnated cement for deep infections in total hip arthroplasties. *J Bone Joint Surg* 60[Am]:1059–1964, 1978.
29. Waldvogel FA, Medoff G, Swartz MN: Osteomyelitis: A review of clinical features, therapeutic considerations and unusual aspects (Part I). *N Engl J Med* 282:198–205, 1970.
30. Waldvogel FA, Medoff G, Swartz MN: Osteomyelitis: A review of clinical features, therapeutic considerations and unusual aspects (Part II). *N Engl J Med* 282:260–266, 1970.
31. Waldvogel FA, Medoff G, Swartz MN: Osteomyelitis: A review of clinical features, therapeutic considerations and unusual aspects (Part III). *N Engl J Med* 282:316–322, 1970.
32. Waldvogel FA, Vasey H: Osteomyelitis: The past decade. *N Engl J Med* 303:360–370, 1980.
33. Norden CW: Osteomyelitis, in Mandell GL, Douglas GR Jr, Bennett JE (eds): *Principles and Practice of Infectious Diseases,* ed 2. New York, John Wiley & Sons, 1985, p 704.
34. Smith JK, Wiener SL: Osteomyelitis. *Drug Ther/Hospital* 6(Jan):63–67, 1981.

SUGGESTED READINGS

Goldenberg DL, Cohen AS: Acute infectious arthritis: A review of patients with non gonococcal joint infections (with emphasis on therapy and prognosis). *Am J Med* 60:369–377, 1976.

Inman RD, Gallegos KV, Brause BD, et al: Clinical and microbial features of prosthetic joint infection. *Am J Med* 77:47–53, 1984.

McGuire NM, Kauffman CA: Septic arthritis in the elderly. *J Am Geriatr Soc* 33:170–174, 1985.

Norman DC, Yoshikawa TT: Responding to septic arthritis. *Geriatrics* 38:83–91, 1983.

Waldvogel FA, Vasey H: Osteomyelitis: The past decade. *N Engl J Med* 303:360–370, 1980.

Chapter 17

Tetanus

GENERAL CONSIDERATIONS

Although tetanus has decreased at least tenfold over the past 35 to 40 years (the annual average incidence rate for 1982 to 1984 was 0.036 cases/100,000 compared to 0.39 cases/100,000 in 1947) (1), the number of cases in elderly patients has been increasing (1,2). Figure 17.1 illustrates the average crude incidence rates of reported tetanus cases by age group in the United States for the period 1982 to 1984 (1). Of these 234 reported cases, 49, 51, and 32 cases were in the age groups of 60 to 69, 70 to 79, and

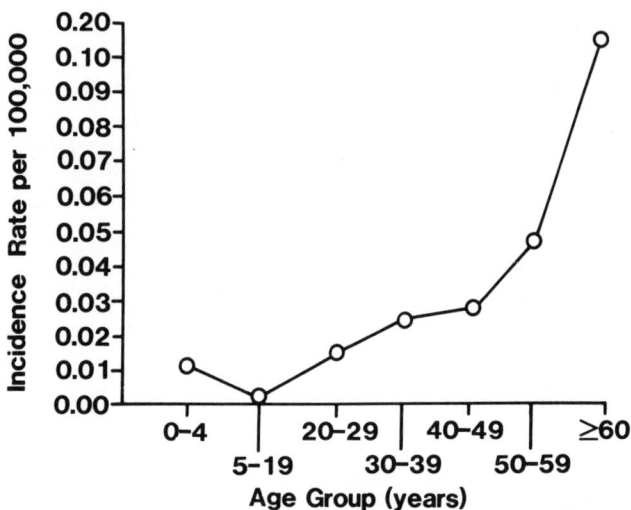

Figure 17.1. Average incidence rates per 100,000 of tetanus cases by specific age groups reported in the United States, 1982–1984.

80 or older, respectively; or expressed as a group, 59% of all cases of tetanus were in persons 60 years or older (1).

The overall case-fatality rate for tetanus in the early 1900s was as high as 70% (2). This mortality has fallen to an overall case-fatality rate of 26% in 1982 to 1984 (1). However, for patients 60 years or older, the mortality was 52% (13% for those under 60 years).

The fundamental reason for the unusually high attack and fatality rates of tetanus in the aged is the lack of immunity to this infection. Inadequate immunization status in the elderly has been clearly documented. One study showed that 47% of persons in a senior citizen center (mean age 68 years) and 71% of convalescent hospital subjects (mean age 82 years) lacked protective levels of tetanus antibodies in their serum ($\geqslant 0.01$ unit/ml) (3). It also has been shown that the serum antibody response to tetanus toxoid may be less in the elderly compared to younger adults (4).

ETIOLOGY

Tetanus is caused by *Clostridium tetani,* a motile, gram-positive, anaerobic, nonencapsulated, spore-forming bacillus (5). The organism is ubiquitous in soil and in the feces of humans and many domestic animals. In its vegetative form, *C. tetani* elaborates the neurotoxin, tetanospasmin, which is responsible for the clinical disease. The toxin is extremely potent and binds to and has an effect on several areas of the nervous system, such as anterior horn cells of the spinal cord, motor nerve endings of muscle fibers, and myoneurojunction of the sympathetic nervous system.

C. tetani remains in its spore form in the environment. These spores are resistant to extremes of temperature, as well as several chemical disinfectants, and are not capable of producing toxin. Once the spores are introduced into the tissue (by puncture wounds, cuts, or burns), proper anaerobic conditions need to exist in order for the spores to germinate into their vegetative form. After germination occurs, the bacteria release their toxin, which is disseminated hematogenously or via lymphatics.

CLINICAL MANIFESTATIONS

The incubation period for tetanus varies from 3 days to 3 weeks, with most patients exhibiting symptoms between the fifth and tenth day (6,7). Generally, the shorter the incubation period, the more severe are the clinical manifestations. There are three clinical forms of tetanus in adults: generalized, local, and cephalic. Approximately 80 to 90% of cases of tetanus in the United States are generalized. The clinical manifestations of tetanus in the elderly are not different from those of younger adults, but are more severe.

Generalized Tetanus

The most common symptom is jaw and facial muscle tightness, which may or may not be accompanied by constitutional symptoms. As the diseases progresses, frank trismus occurs in 75% of patients (7), which is frequently accompanied by stiffness of the neck, difficulty in swallowing, rigidity of abdominal muscles, and fever. Profound muscle rigidity of the jaw and facial muscles produces a characteristic facial expression called *risus sardonicus.* These initial clinical features are followed by waves of persistent muscle contractions and spasms that involve the extremities and back, which result in opisthotonos. Laryngeal spasms may occur which results in asphyxiation. Autonomic dysfunction, primarily sympathetic overactivity, is more common in the elderly and is manifested by major fluctuations in blood pressure (hypertension and hypotension), tachycardia, sweating, hyperthermia, and cardiac arrhythmias (8–10). Bladder and bowel function may also be impaired. All of these manifestations may persist as long as several months, but usually taper in intensity over 4 to 6 weeks.

Complications of tetanus include aspiration pneumonia, fractures of the long bones and spine, stress ulcer, pulmonary embolism, undernutrition, fluid and electrolyte disturbances, rhabdomyolysis, decubitus ulcer, catheter-related bladder infection, and intravenous catheter infections.

Local Tetanus

Local tetanus is an uncommon form of tetanus that is manifested by rigidity and persistent contractions of muscles in the same anatomic site as the injury that produced tetanus. It may develop into generalized tetanus if untreated, but most often it is a relatively mild disease, which has a mortality of 10% (7).

Cephalic Tetanus

Cephalic tetanus an unusual and also an uncommon form of tetanus. It results from injuries to the head, face, or neck region or from chronic otitis media (*C. tetani* infection). The clinical findings are characterized by dysfunction of cranial nerves III, IV, VI, IX, X, and XII. Cephalic tetanus may evolve into the generalized form of the disease. The prognosis for cephalic tetanus is poorer than for local tetanus.

DIAGNOSTIC APPROACH

Differential Diagnosis

The differential diagnosis of generalized tetanus is extensive. The conditions that would mimic trismus include dental abscess, mandibular fracture, mumps, tonsillitis, retropharyngeal abscess, or mandibular osteomyelitis. The generalized muscle spasms and posture may resemble phenothiazine reactions, hypocalcemic tetany, seizures, narcotic withdrawal, strychnine poisoning, rabies, or hysterical reactions (11).

Laboratory Tests

Tetanus is a *clinical* diagnosis. Occasionally, the organism may be identified or isolated from the wound site by Gram stain or anaerobic culture. Nevertheless, laboratory tests to monitor for the complications of tetanus should be done. These tests include electrocardiogram, chest x-ray, arterial blood gases, electrolytes, complete blood count, renal function tests, muscle enzymes, and appropriate cultures when secondary infection is suspected.

TREATMENT

A favorable outcome for tetanus patients is dependent on meticulous medical and nursing care. All elderly patients with suspected tetanus should be placed in an intensive care unit (12), preferably in an isolated and quite room. Therapy is directed toward (*1*) neutralizing unbound toxin; (*2*) adequate ventilatory support; (*3*) controlling muscle spasms; and (*4*) preventing and/or treating complications.

Neutralizing Unbound Toxin

Human tetanus immune globulin (TIG), 3,000–6,000 units intramuscularly, should be administered in several sites with part of the TIG used to infiltrate around the wound site. Débridement of the wound should be carried out (to remove toxin-producing organisms and their anaerobic environment) several hours *after* the patient has received TIG (surgical manipulation may release free tetanospasmin). Tetanus toxoid should be administered (Tetanus infection does not necessarily confer immunity to subsequent tetanus since the neurotoxin may be too low in concentration to effect an immune response) and repeated in 4 to 6 weeks and again in 6 months. Aqueous penicillin G, 1 million units intravenously every 6 hours should be administered for 5 to 7 days to eliminate any remaining viable, vegetative forms of *C. tetani*.

Ventilatory Support

Virtually all patients with tetanus experience some type of respiratory complication. Therefore, the importance of early airway management cannot be overemphasized, especially in the elderly, who frequently have a decreased pulmonary reserve capacity. Intubation of the trachea often is required; following intubation, tracheostomy should be performed as soon as possible (11). Most patients should be placed on a volume-limited respirator. Meticulous and aseptic airway care as well as prompt treatment of aspiration pneumonia or atelectasis are critical for a good prognosis.

Control of Muscle Spasms

Diazepam given in the form of intermittent intravenous bolus (2–20 mg every 1 to 8 hours) or continous intravenous infusion (2–10 mg per hour) has been effective in controlling painful muscle spasms, anxiety, and nightmares (13,14). Chlorpromazine 25–50 mg given intravenously every 6 hours as needed may be required if patients fail to respond to diazepam. Meprobamate, administered orally, 400 mg every 3 to 4 hours, and secobarbital (or pentobarbital) 50–100 mg intramuscularly every 6 hours can also be used for muscle contractions and sedation, respectively.

Dantrolene is a drug that acts peripherally to cause muscle relaxation. It has been used in one patient with tetanus (15). The dose is 1–2 mg/kg given intravenously or orally every four hours. Hepatitis is a potential complication. This drug's role in treating tetanus is still undefined (11).

If tetanus contractions cannot be controlled, especially if ventilation is compromised, muscle paralysis should be effected with a nondepolarizing neuromuscular blocker such as D-tubocurarine by intravenous drip (mix in 5% dextrose solution to a concentration of 1 mg/ml). It is infused at a rate necessary to cause paralysis (up to 15 mg/hr) (6). *It is absolutely imperative that with neuromuscular blockade, the patient is ventilated adequately by mechanical means.*

Prevention or Treatment of Complications

The patient's pulmonary status should be followed carefully for possible atelectasis, pneumonia, or pulmonary embolism. Prophylactic subcutaneous heparin, 5,000 units every 12 hours, is recommended unless the patient has a bleeding or coagulation disorder. Frequent tracheal suction and prompt treatment of pneumonia with appropriate antibiotics are essential.

Autonomic dysfunction should be treated only if the symptoms compromise the patient's overall management and survival. In elderly patients, vigorous pharmacologic treatment (e.g., beta-blockers) of hypertension, hypotension, tachycardia, or bradycardia may be more hazardous than the underlying clinical problem. Cardiac arrhythmias (e.g., ventricular irritability) should be treated.

Antacids or hydrogen-ion blocking agents should be given to minimize stress ulcers. Frequent turning and proper skin care are essential to prevent decubitus ulcers. Because of the extreme muscle contractions and excessive sympathetic activity, high caloric expenditure occurs. Therefore, careful nutritional intake as well as proper fluid and electrolyte balance are important. Intravenous hyperalimentation may be required. Attention should be paid to avoid urinary retention and fecal impaction.

PREVENTION

Prevention of tetanus is nearly 100% if the elderly are adequately immunized with tetanus toxoid (see Chapter 6 on prevention of infections) (14). Tetanus immune globulin is indicated for those persons with tetanus-prone wounds (1) whose tetanus immunization status is uncertain or (2) who have received less than three previous immunization doses (17). Tetanus-prone wounds have the following features or associated factors: (*1*) wound of more than 6 hours, (*2*) wounds that are stellate, more than 1 centimeter in depth, or caused by avulsion or abrasion, (*3*) wounds caused by a missile or by crushing, burning, or frostbite, and (*4*) wounds that are contaminated (e.g., dirt, feces, soil, saliva), appear infested, or have devitalized tissue (18). All wounds should be cleaned and debrided as indicated.

REFERENCES

1. Division of Immunogenetics, Centers for Disease Control: Tetanus— United States, 1982–1984. *MMWR* 34:602–611, 1985.
2. Faust RA, Vickers OR, Cohn I Jr: Tetanus: 2,449 cases in 68 years at Charity Hospital. *J Trauma* 16:704–712, 1976.
3. Weiss BP, Strassburg MA, Feeley JC: Tetanus and diphtheria immunity in an elderly population in Los Angeles County. *Am J Public Health* 73:802–804, 1983.
4. Yeni P, Carbon C, Tremolieres F, et al: Serum levels of antibody to toxoid during tetanus and after specific immunization of patient with toxoid. *J Infect Dis* 145:278, 1982.
5. Martin RR: Clostridium tetani (tetanus), in Mandell GL, Douglas GR, Jr., Bennett JE (eds): *Principles and Practice of Infectious Diseases,* ed 2. New York, John Wiley & Sons, 1985, p 1355.
6. Bornstein DL: Tetanus, in Kass EH, Platt R: *Current Therapy in Infectious Disease* ed 2. Burlington, Ontario, B.C. Decker Inc., 1986, p 378.
7. Alfery DD, Rauscher AL: Tetanus: A review. *Crit Care Med* 7:176–181, 1979.
8. Kerr JH, Corbett JL, Prys-Roberts C, et al: Involvement of the sympathetic nervous system in tetanus: Studies of 82 cases. *Lancet* 2:236–241, 1968.
9. Kanarek DJ, Kaufman B, Zwi S: Severe sympathetic hyperactivity associated with tetanus. *Arch Intern Med* 132:602–604, 1973.
10. Kerr JH, Travis KW, O'Rourke RA, et al: Autonomic complications in a case of severe tetanus. *Am J Med* 57:303–310, 1974.
11. Bleck TP: Pharmacology of tetanus. *Clin Neuropharmacol* 9:103–120, 1986.

12. Trujillo MJ, Castillo A, España JV, et al: Tetanus in the adult. Intensive care and management experience with 233 cases. *Crit Care Med* 8:419-423, 1980.
13. Vassa NT, Yajnik VH, Joshi KR, et al: Comparative clinical trial of diazepam with other conventional drugs in tetanus. *Postgrad Med J* 50:755-758, 1974.
14. Dasta JF, Brier KL, Kidwell GA, et al: Diazepam infusion in tetanus: Correlation of drug levels with effect. *South Med J* 74:278-280, 1981.
15. Tidyman M, Prichard JG, Dreamer RL, et al: Adjunctive use of dantrolene in severe tetanus. *Anesth Analg* 64:538-540, 1985.
16. Immunization Practices Advisory Committee: Diphtheria, tetanus, and pertussis: Guidelines for vaccine prophylaxis and other preventive measures. *MMWR* 34:405-426, 1985.
17. Adams SL: Tetanus immunization for nursing home residents. *JAMA* 256: 526, 1986.
18. American College of Surgeon Committee on Trauma: Prophylaxis against tetanus in wound management. *Bull Am Coll Surg* 69:22-23, 1984.

SUGGESTED READINGS

Bleck TP: Pharmacology of tetanus. *Clin Neuropharmacol* 9:103-120, 1986.
Division of Immunogenetics, Centers for Disease Control: Tetanus—United States, 1982-1984. *MMWR* 34:602-611, 1985.
Immunization Practices Advisory Committee: Diphtheria, tetanus, and pertussis: Guidelines for vaccine prophylaxis and other preventive measures. *MMWR* 34:405-426, 1985.
Martin RR: Clostridium tetani (tetanus), in Mandell GL, Douglas GR Jr, Bennett JE (eds): *Principles and Practice of Infectious Diseases,* ed 2. New York, John Wiley & Sons, 1985, p 1355.
Weiss BP, Strassburg MA, Feeley JC: Tetanus and diphtheria immunity in an elderly population in Los Angeles County. *Am J Public Health* 73:802-804, 1983.

Chapter 18

Sepsis

GENERAL CONSIDERATIONS

Sepsis and septicemia describe a clinical syndrome caused by the presence of microorganisms (bacteria, fungi, rickettsiae, viruses, etc.) or microbial toxins (e.g., endotoxin) in the blood. Since most cases of sepsis in the geriatric age group are caused by bacterial infections, the discussion in this chapter focuses only on the diagnosis and treatment of bacteremic forms of this syndrome.

Bacterial sepsis in the adult is caused predominantly by aerobic or facultative anaerobic gram-negative bacilli. Gram-negative bacillary sepsis (also called gram-negative bacteremia) is increasing in frequency in the United States (1), and its incidence increases with age, especially after the age of 60 (2,3). Forty percent of all cases of sepsis occurs in the elderly (4). More importantly, the elderly patient with sepsis suffers a significantly higher mortality when compared to younger adults, which may approach 70% (5). Approximately 60% of all deaths related to sepsis occur in the elderly (4). Inexplicably, when sepsis has been described in the elderly from studies focusing exclusively on an aged population, the overall mortality is approximately 25% (6–9). This difference most likely reflects the severity of illness in the study sample, since most patients in studies that involved exclusively elderly patients did not include those who were in shock. However, age is only one factor that influences mortality. Nevertheless, if patients have a nonfatal underlying disease (i.e., degenerative joint disease), age then has an adverse effect on survival (10). Mortality does not significantly differ with age if all patients have severe underlying diseases (e.g., rapidly fatal diseases such as leukemia or far-advanced cancer; ultimately fatal diseases such as end-stage renal disease, chronic cirrhosis, or collagen-vascular disease) (10). The presence of hypotension or shock may double or triple the mortality (3,11). Other factors having a negative impact on survival include the following: nosocomial episodes of bacteremia, polymicrobial bacteremia, bacteremia caused by *Pseudomonas aeruginosa* or antibiotic-resistant organisms, and bacteremia associated with pneumonia (3).

ETIOLOGY

The majority of bacterial sepsis in the elderly occur from infections arising from the urinary tract. Other important sites of infections include lungs, abdominal viscera, skin, and soft tissues (Table 18.1) (6–10). Thus, it is not surprising that gram-negative bacilli are involved in 60 to 70% of bacteremic cases in the old (Table 18.2) (6–12,13). The most common pathogen is *Escherichia coli* followed by *Klebsiella* and *Proteus* species. Streptococci (primarily *S. pneumoniae* and enterococci) and *Staphylococcus aureus* are the dominant gram-positive bacteria that cause sepsis in the aged (6–12). These gram-positive pathogens are usually isolated from infections that involve the lungs, heart valves, skin, and soft tissues. Anaerobic bacteria have been isolated in a significant number of elderly patients in whom intraabdominal infection and decubitus ulcers were the primary source of bacteremia (8).

TABLE 18.1 Studies on Sepsis in the Elderly

PARAMETER	STUDY (REFERENCE NUMBER)			
	(6)	(7)	(8)	(9)
Total number of cases	100	39	351	50
Community acquired	100	NS[a]	NS	43
Nosocomial	0	NS	NS	7
Female:male	62:38	21:18	NS	30:20
Mean age, years	74	81	NS	NS[b]
Source: number of cases (%)				
Urinary tract	34 (34)	11 (28)	115 (33)	12 (24)
Biliary tract	20 (20)	6 (15)	NS[c]	4 (8)
Abdominal	8 (8)	NS	59 (17)	NS
Lungs	13 (13)	2 (5)	NS	11 (22)
Skin/soft tissue[d]	NS	2 (5)	55 (16)	6 (12)
Other sites	14 (14)	1 (3)	122 (35)	7 (14)
Unknown	11 (11)	NS	NS	10 (20)
Mortality, %	26	15	NS	24

[a]NS, not stated.
[b]All patients 65 years or older: 13 (65–74); 20 (75–84), and 17 (85 and older).
[c]Grouped under abdominal infections.
[d]Includes decubitus ulcers.

TABLE 18.2   Pathogens Causing Sepsis in the Elderly

	STUDY (REFERENCE NUMBER)			
	(6)	(7)	(8)	(9)
Total number cases	100	39	452[b]	50
Organisms[a]				
Gram-positive cocci	29	11	93[c]	28
Streptococcus pneumoniae	9	7	NS[e]	6
Enterococcus	7	0	27	0
Other streptococci	6	4	NS	10
Staphylococcus aureus	6	0	32	10
Other cocci	1	0	NS	2
Gram-negative bacilli	70	25	275[c]	22[d]
Escherichia coli	43	19	108	8
Klebsiella sp.	16	1	72[f]	4
Proteus sp.	5	6	41	1
Polymicrobic[g]	10	3	55	6
Anaerobic bacteria	4	3	73	—[d]

[a]Number of organisms may exceed total number of cases because of polymicrobial cases.
[b]Total number of blood isolates (from 351 patients).
[c]Only stated as gram-positive or gram-negative.
[d]Anaerobic organisms included (2 *Bacteroides fragilis*).
[e]Not stated.
[f]Includes *Serratia* and *Enterobacter* species.
[g]Individual isolates tabulated in other categories.

CLINICAL MANIFESTATIONS

Pathophysiology

The pathophysiology of gram-negative bacteremia is complex. One important virulence factor common to all species of gram-negative bacilli is endotoxin, a complex lipopolysaccharide (LPS) in the cell wall of the organism. LPS consists of long chain oligosaccharides and a core glycolipid that contains lipid A (1). It is lipid A that initiates the series of cascading, physiologic reactions that are responsible for the clinical manifestations of sepsis. These physiologic events involve the following systems or subsystems: complement, kallikrein-kinin, coagulation, fibrinolysis, endorphins, histamine, and prostaglandins (1). The outcome of these reactions is loss of vascular tone (vasodilation), excessive vascular permeability, intravascular coagulation, endothelial damage, and inflammation, which result in hypoperfusion of organs and tissues (i.e., shock).

Clinical Features

The classic manifestations of sepsis are fever, chills, and hypotension. Patients may have evidence of end organ failure, for example, oliguria or congestive heart failure. However, in the septic geriatric patient, clinical manifestations may be quite atypical. Altered mentation, delirium, malaise, weakness, nausea, vomiting, falls, or tachypnea are common complaints in the elderly patient with bacteremia (7,9,11,12). Elderly patients may not manifest fever with bacteremia (13,14) or may even be hypothermic (7,9). This is significant because a lack of fever response is associated with a poorer prognosis in all patients with bacteremia (10,15). Hypotension is also more common in the aged with bacteremia, and results in multiple organ dysfunction and higher death rate.

DIAGNOSTIC APPROACH

Differential Diagnosis

The differential diagnosis of sepsis includes any infectious disease that might occur in the elderly, as well as such noninfectious disorders as congestive heart failure, cardiogenic shock, dehydration, hypoadrenalism, electrolyte disorders, drug reactions, or acute blood loss.

Laboratory Tests

MICROBIOLOGIC STUDIES

Blood culture is the most important test for the diagnosis of bacterial sepsis. Two sets of blood cultures should be taken immediately, and another two sets should be obtained 30 minutes later from another site.

Urinalysis and urine culture are important tests, since urinary tract infections are the most common cause of sepsis in the elderly. All available body fluids (e.g., pleural, joint, cerebrospinal), pus, drainage sites, and tissue specimens should be Gram stained and sent for aerobic and anaerobic cultures. Serologic studies (e.g., Legionella titers) should be obtained as indicated.

X-RAYS AND SCANS

A chest x-ray should be done on all septic elderly patients to exclude pneumonia. If the patient has any abdominal symptoms or signs, a plain x-ray of the abdomen may be helpful. Otherwise, ultrasonography, radionuclide scans (e.g., liver scan), and/or computed tomography of the abdomen should be obtained if the primary source of sepsis is not clinically evident, since biliary sepsis and intraabdominal abscesses are common causes of fever and bacteremia in the elderly (see Chapter 13 on intraabdominal infections).

BLOOD TESTS

A complete blood count, electrolytes, coagulation tests, renal and liver function tests, as well as arterial blood gases should be part of the initial laboratory studies on all septic patients. These tests help determine the severity of the patient's clinical status and the need for adjunctive supportive care (e.g., fluid, electrolytes, transfusion). In patients with hypotension, poor urinary output, or metabolic acidosis, a blood lactate level should be determined. Lactate (or lactic acid) levels correlate well with the degree of anaerobic metabolism and are reliable indicators of prognosis (high lactate correlates with poor prognosis) (11).

TREATMENT

Correction of Hypoperfusion

VOLUME STATUS

If the elderly patient's intravascular volume status is not clear, or if the patient has a tenuous cardiovascular condition, a pulmonary artery (Swan-Ganz) catheter should be inserted. The patient's pulmonary capillary wedge pressure assists in determining his/her fluid status. Most patients with hypotension are volume depleted and require *careful* but rapid fluid resuscitation. It remains controversial whether crystalloid solutions (e.g., normal saline or Ringer's lactate) or colloids (albumin, hydroxyethyl starch, plasma, or blood) should be used to replenish the intravascular volume. In one study of elderly patients with septic shock, patients who received colloids required less volume than patients who received crystalloids to reach the same hemodynamic end points (16). Therefore, we recommend giving colloid solutions *initially* (including blood if the patient is anemic), 500–1000 ml over 1 to 4 hours depending on the severity of hypotension and level of hypovolemia. The capillary wedge pressure and/or clinical response (improved mentation, increased blood pressure, increased urine output) should be the guide to additional fluid replacement. Crystalloid solution should be used initially if colloids are not available or are contraindicated (overt congestive heart failure), or if there is an electrolyte imbalance.

VASOACTIVE DRUGS

If hypoperfusion (hypotension) is still clinically evident *after* intravascular fluid repletion has been accomplished, vasoactive agents should be started. Dopamine is the drug of choice. A dose of 400 mg is mixed in 250 ml of 5% dextrose solution and begun at a rate of 5–10 µg/kg body wt/min and increased to the lowest dose that maintains adequate perfusion. As the dose is increased above 25 µg/kg/min, alpha-adrenergic effects dominate, and vasoconstriction of renal and other arterial beds begin to occur. If dopamine is unsuccessful, dobutamine in doses of 2–15 µg/kg/min may be tried to reverse the hypoperfusion state. However, a lack of response to dopamine may occur in patients with severe acidosis or hypovolemia.

CORTICOSTEROIDS

The use and value of large doses of corticosteroids in the management of septic shock remains highly controversial (1,11,17). However, although the adverse effects of one or two pharmacologic doses of corticosteroids is relatively minimal, we suggest that the use of corticosteroids be reserved for elderly patients with sepsis who fail to respond to fluid repletion and vasoactive drugs within 1 to 2 hours. A single dose of methylprednisolone 30 mg/kg should be given intravenously. A second dose may be repeated in 12 to 24 hours if there is no response.

NALOXONE

Naloxone blocks the analgesic and hypotensive effects of endorphins. Because endorphins are felt to be important in the pathophysiology of gram-negative sepsis, some investigators have shown in animal models that naloxone blocks or reverses the hypotensive effects of endotoxin (18,19). Although isolated case reports on the use of naloxone in patients with sepsis have shown some salutary responses (20), a careful prospective, randomized, double-blind, placebo-controlled trial failed to demonstrate a superiority of naloxone over the placebo in ameliorating hypotension in septic shock (21). Therefore, this form of treatment of sepsis cannot currently be recommended.

ANTISERUM

An investigational form of treatment of gram-negative bacteremia is using antiserum that contains antibodies to endotoxin produced by immunizing human volunteers. Preliminary clinical trials that treated patients with gram-negative sepsis with endotoxin antiserum resulted in decreased morbidity compared to controls (22).

Antimicrobial Therapy

Antimicrobial therapy for the elderly with sepsis should be initiated empirically as soon as possible after all necessary microbiologic studies are obtained. In acutely ill, hypotensive patients, unnecessary delays in antibiotic administration may compromise chances for survival.

The choices of drugs for sepsis are many and should be based on the answers to the following questions:

1. What is the presumed primary site of infection?
2. Is the sepsis community-acquired or nosocomial?
3. Has the patient been on antibiotics within the past 2 to 3 weeks?
4. What underlying diseases does the patient have? Is he/she leukopenic and/or immunosuppressed?
5. Does the patient have renal failure? Is he/she allergic to any antibiotics?

Table 18.3 provides dose recommendations for empiric antimicrobial therapy based on many of the above factors. All drugs should be administered intravenously, usually in maximum doses. (Please refer to Chapter 5 on antimicrobial therapy for specific recommended doses.) It should be emphasized that once a specific pathogen or pathogens has (have) been isolated, the antibiotics should be appropriately changed. Therapy should be for a minimum of 10 days.

Supportive Care

All abscesses should be drained and all necrotic tissue debrided. An operation should be performed as indicated (e.g., cholecystectomy, appendectomy).

Pulmonary care that includes adequate oxygenation should be monitored carefully. Adult respiratory distress syndrome (ARDS) as well as aspiration is a common complication of septic shock. Elderly patients with poor ventilatory capacity may require intubation and mechanically assisted ventilation.

Cardiac failure is more common in the elderly who suffer from sepsis; therefore, careful fluid management is essential. Arrhythmias should be properly treated.

It is critical to monitor urine output and renal function. Again, careful fluid and electrolyte management and intermittent doses of furosemide (40–120 mg intravenously) may be required to maintain proper fluid and electrolyte balance. Severe metabolic acidosis may require $NaHCO_3$ therapy. If renal failure supervenes, dialysis may be required to alleviate acidosis and associated fluid retention and hyperkalemia.

Intravascular coagulation is difficult to manage. Only after the infection and shock are controlled will intravascular coagulation cease. If severe bleeding occurs, fresh frozen plasma, whole blood, and/or platelets may be required. Whether heparin is helpful or harmful for the treatment of intravascular coagulation is controversial.

TABLE 18.3 Recommendations for Empiric Antimicrobial Therapy for Sepsis in the Elderly

PRIMARY SITE OF INFECTION	DRUG(S) OF CHOICE	ALTERNATIVE DRUGS
I. Community acquired		
A. No hypotension; no prior antibiotics		
Urinary tract infection		
No catheter	Any cephalosporin	Trimethoprim-sulfamethoxazole (TMP-SMZ)
Chronic catheter	Ampicillin plus third-generation cephalosporin	(1) Vancomycin plus third-generation cephalosporin
		OR
		(2) TMP-SMZ plus third-generation cephalosporin
Pneumonia	(1) Cefuroxime	(1) TMP-SMZ plus piperacillin[a]
	OR	OR
	(2) Third-generation cephalosporin	(2) Vancomycin plus piperacillin
Cholecystitis	(1) Cefoxitin	TMP-SMZ plus piperacillin
	OR	
	(2) Third-generation cephalosporin	
Intraabdominal sepsis, decubitus ulcer, or *unknown*	Cefoxitin	(1) Third-generation cephalosporin
		OR
		(2) TMP-SMZ plus clindamycin
		OR
		(3) TMP-SMZ plus metronidazole
		OR
		(4) Clindamycin (or metronidazole) plus piperacillin

B. Hypotension; prior antibiotics; leukopenia

Urinary tract (catheter or no catheter)	Ampicillin plus aminoglycoside	(1) Vancomycin plus aminoglycoside OR (2) TMP-SMZ plus aminoglycoside OR (3) Third-generation cephalosporin plus piperacillin
Pneumonia	(1) Cefuroxime plus aminoglycoside OR (2) Piperacillin plus aminoglycoside	(1) Clindamycin plus aminoglycoside OR (2) Piperacillin plus third-generation cephalosporin
Cholecystitis	(1) Cefoxitin plus aminoglycoside OR (2) Ampicillin plus clindamycin plus aminoglycoside	(1) Piperacillin plus third-generation cephalosporin OR (2) Third-generation cephalosporin plus aminoglycoside
Intraabdominal sepsis, decubitus ulcer, or *unknown*	(1) Metronidazole (or clindamycin) plus ampicillin plus aminoglycoside	Third-generation cephalosporin plus piperacillin

II. Hospital acquired
Same regimens as for community acquired, section B.

---

[a]Mezlocillin or azlocillin may also be used.

221

PREVENTION

Sepsis can only be prevented by early recognition and treatment of all significant infections. Minimizing unnecessary hospitalization of elderly persons, and limiting the use of indwelling bladder catheters and intravenous catheters as well as long-term antibiotics significantly decreases the frequency of nosocomial bacteremia.

In the future, it is possible that a vaccine against gram-negative infections could be developed (23).

REFERENCES

1. Jacobson MA, Young LS: New developments in the treatment of gram-negative bacteremia. *West J Med* 144:185–194, 1986.
2. Kreger BE, Craven DE, Darling PC, et al: Gram-negative bacteremia. III. Reassessment of etiology, epidemiology and ecology in 612 patients. *Am J Med* 68:332–343, 1980.
3. Bryan CS, Reynolds KL, Brenner ER: Analysis of 1,186 episodes of gram-negative bacteremia in non-university hospitals: The effects of antimicrobial therapy. *Rev Infect Dis* 5:629–638, 1983.
4. Holloway WJ: Management of sepsis in the elderly. *Am J Med* 30(suppl B):143–148, 1986.
5. Hodgin UG, Sanford JP: Gram-negative bacteremia. An analysis of 100 patients. *Am J Med* 39:952–960, 1965.
6. Esposito AL, Gleckman RA, Cram S, et al: Community-acquired bacteremia in the elderly: analysis of one hundred consecutive episodes. *J Am Geriatr Soc* 28:315–319, 1980.
7. Madden JW, Croker JR, Beynon GPJ: Septicemia in the elderly. *Postgrad Med J* 57:502–506, 1981.
8. Shimada K: Geriatric sepsis, in *Sixth International Cefoperazone Symposium.* Princeton, N.J., Excerpta Medica, 1983, p 264.
9. Windsor ACM: Bacteremia in a geriatric unit. *Gerontology* 29:125–130, 1983.
10. Bryant RE, Hood AF, Hood CE, et al: Factors affecting morbidity of gram-negative rod bacteremia. *Arch Intern Med* 127:120–128, 1971.
11. Houston MC: Special considerations in the management of septic shock in the elderly. *Geriatr Med Today* 5:65–77, 1986.
12. Holloway WA, Reinhardt J: Septic shock in the elderly. *Geriatrics* 39:48–54, 1984.
13. Gleckman R, Hibert D: Afebrile bacteremia: A phenomenon in geriatric patients. *JAMA* 248:1478–1481, 1981.
14. Finklestein MS, Petkun WM, Freedman ML, et al: Pneumococcal bacteremia in adults: Age-dependent differences in presentation and in outcome. *J Am Geriatr Soc* 31:19–27, 1983.
15. Weinstein MP, Murphy JR, Reller LB et al: The clinical significance of positive blood cultures: A comprehensive analysis of 500 episodes of bacteremia and fungemia in adults. II. Clinical observations with special reference to factors influencing prognosis. *Rev Infect Dis* 5:54–70, 1983.

16. Rackow EC, Falk JL, Fein IA, et al: Fluid resuscitation in circulatory shock. A comparison of the cardiorespiratory effects of albumin, hetastarch and saline solutions in patients with hypovolemic and septic shock. *Crit Care Med* 11:823–850, 1983.
17. Craven DE, McCabe WR: Gram-negative bacteremia, in Kass EH, Platt R (eds): *Current Therapy in Infectious Diseases* ed 2. Toronto, B.C. Becker, Inc., 1986, p 331.
18. Faden AI, Holaday JW: Experimental endotoxic shock: The pathophysiologic function of endorphins and treatment with opiate antagonists. *J Infect Dis* 142:229–238, 1980.
19. Hinshaw LB, Beller BK, Chang AC, et al: Evaluation of naloxone for therapy of *Escherichia coli* shock—species differences. *Arch Surg* 119:1410–1418, 1981.
20. Groeger JS, Carlon BC, Howland WS: Naloxone in septic shock. *Crit Care Med* 11:650–654, 1983.
21. DeMaria A, Heffernan JJ, Grindlinger GA, et al: Naloxone versus placebo in treatment of septic shock. *Lancet* 1:1363–1365, 1985.
22. Ziegler EJ, McCutchan JA, Fierer J, et al: Treatment of gram-negative bacteremia and shock with human antiserum to mutant *Escherichia coli* core lipopolysaccharide. *N Engl J Med* 307:1225–1230, 1982.
23. Braude AI, Ziegler EJ, McCutchan JA, et al: Immunization against nosocomial infection. *Am J Med* 70:463–466, 1981.

SUGGESTED READINGS

Bryan CS, Reynolds KL, Brenner ER: Analysis of 1,186 episodes of gram-negative bacteremia in non-university hospitals: The effects of antimicrobial therapy. *Rev Infect Dis* 5:629–638, 1983.

Esposito AL, Gleckman RA, Cram S, et al: Community-acquired bacteremia in the elderly: Analysis of one hundred consecutive episodes. *J Am Geriatr Soc* 28:315–319, 1980.

Houston MC: Special considerations in the management of septic shock in the elderly. *Geriatr Med Today* 5:65–77, 1986.

Jacobson MA, Young LS: New developments in the treatment of gram-negative bacteremia. *West J Med* 144:185–194, 1986.

Madden JW, Croker JR, Beynon GPJ: Septicemia in the elderly. *Postgrad Med J* 57:502–506, 1981.

Windsor ACM: Bacteremia in a geriatric unit. *Gerontology* 29:125–130, 1983.

Chapter 19

Herpes Zoster

GENERAL CONSIDERATIONS

Herpes zoster is a cutaneous vesicular eruption that is often followed by radicular pain. Herpes zoster results from recrudescence of the varicella-zoster (VZ) virus. It occurs with increasing frequency with advancing age. In the classic study by Hope-Simpson (1), the incidence of herpes zoster from childhood to 50 years was 2.5 cases per 1,000 patients. This incidence doubled for individuals aged 50 years and quadrupled for those aged 80 years and older. Similar results have been confirmed in more recent studies (2). In addition to old age, other such factors as lympho-reticular malignancies, immunosuppression, local irradiation, and collagen-vascular diseases increase the susceptibility of a person to herpes zoster (3,4). Patients with Hodgkin's disease are particularly at risk to herpes zoster, with an incidence as high as 25% (5).

The higher incidence of herpes zoster in the elderly appears to be related to a decline in cell-mediated immune response to the VZ virus with age (6–8). Humoral immunity (antibodies to VZ virus) has a lesser role in the containment of VZ virus infection. However, circulating immune complexes have been demonstrated in sera from 50% of healthy persons with localized zoster, suggesting that tissue damage from immune-complex deposition may be another pathogenetic mechanism for this infection (9).

ETIOLOGY

Herpes zoster is caused by the herpes virus, varicella-zoster; VZ virus is also the etiology of chickenpox (varicella) (10). Although varicella may be contracted from patients with active herpes zoster, herpes zoster is not contracted from patients with chickenpox (11). For the pathogenesis of herpes zoster it is postulated that the sensory ganglia are infected during the primary infection of varicella. After a latency period, viral replication occurs, and the VZ virus moves antidromically along the nerve to the skin (12). VZ virus has been demonstrated in the sensory ganglia in patients with active herpes zoster. However, the virus has never been isolated from the ganglia at autopsies of individuals without a recent history of herpes zoster (10). Moreover, isolated cases of herpes zoster appear to resemble reinfection rather than reactivation (12). Nevertheless, the prevailing opinion remains that herpes zoster is caused by reactivation of the latent VZ virus.

CLINICAL MANIFESTATIONS

Herpes zoster typically begins with an abrupt onset of pain along a specific dermatome. The pain is described as burning, stabbing, lancing, or aching, and it may be constant or intermittent (14,15). At times this pain is mistaken for acute myocardial infarction, acute cholecystitis, acute surgical abdomen, herniated invertebral discs, kidney stones, headache, or glaucoma (15,16). Within 3 to 4 days after the onset of pain, the rash begins to appear. It starts as a macular erythematous rash that progresses to papules on a red base and eventually turns into the classic vesicles. Within several days, the vesicles become pustular; the lesions then dry, crust, and eventually clear within 10 to 14 days (15,16). The vesicles are typically clustered and vary in size.

The eruption is invariably unilateral, rarely crossing the midline. The thoracic dermatome is involved in 50 to 60% of cases; the trigeminal nerve (1–15%) as well as the cervical (10–15%), lumbar (10–15%), and sacral dermatome (1–3%) are involved.

Complications during the active inflammatory stage of the disease include dissemination, motor paralysis, encephalitis, severe ocular involvement (keratitis, uveitis, iridocyclitis, glaucoma), and seventh cranial nerve infection (Ramsey-Hunt syndrome: facial paralysis, earache, deafness, and vertigo) (17–19).

Postherpetic neuralgia, which is usually defined as the persistence of pain 1 month after the herpes zoster rash has healed (20), is the most common complication of herpes zoster. It occurs in up to 50% of elderly patients age 60 years or older (up to 75% in those 70 years or older), and it is rarely found in persons with herpes zoster under the age of 30 (15). The neuralgia may persist for several months to several years.

DIAGNOSTIC APPROACH

Differential Diagnosis

During the preeruption period of herpes zoster, the prodromal pain may not be easily differentiated from other somatic or visceral causes of pain, that is, cardiac, pulmonary, abdominal, or renal. Thus, such disorders as ischemic heart disease, cholecystitis, appendicitis, diverticulitis, renal colic, pleurisy, or ulcer disease must be considered in the differential diagnosis.

The vesicular eruption may occasionally be mistaken for herpes simplex, echovirus, coxsackievirus, and dermatitis herpetiformis.

Laboratory Tests

Early in the vesicular phase, virus may be isolated from the vesicle fluid. The virus may be quickly seen by cytologic examination using the Tsanck test. However this test does not differentiate VZ virus from other herpes viruses. Culture for the virus can only be done in a laboratory that is equipped to maintain cell cultures routinely. Counterimmunoelectrophoresis of vesicle fluid for viral antigen appears to be a sensitive, specific, and relatively rapid method of making a laboratory diagnosis of herpes zoster (21).

Serologic tests are not useful for the immediate diagnosis of herpes zoster, since antibody titers may be present in persons without active disease.

TREATMENT

Therapy for herpes zoster in the elderly has not been well established, although the therapeutic goal and approach for herpes zoster in the elderly is different than that for the young. Furthermore, if the individual is immunosuppressed, the management also differs.

Normal Elderly

In elderly persons 60 years or older who do *not* have disorders predisposing to herpes zoster or who are not taking medications (or treatment) that cause immunosuppression, the primary goal in treatment is prevention of postherpetic neuralgia. Local skin care for vesicular lesions using cool Burow's (aluminum acetate) wet-to-wet compresses for 30 minutes, three times a day followed by gentle air drying enhances crusting of lesions. Initial pain should be controlled with mild analgesics. More severe pain may require codeine preparations, which place the elderly patient at risk for constipation.

Although still somewhat controversial, limited data suggest that systemic corticosteroids, when given during the active stage of herpes zoster, may significantly reduce the incidence of postherpetic neuralgia (22,23). These studies do have some serious flaws, such as lack of statistical analysis (22) and placebo controls (23,24). Nonetheless, in elderly patients who are not immunosuppressed, the administration of corticosteroids, which are tapered over 3 or 4 weeks, does not appear to place the patient at great risk for dissemination of the VZ virus. An oral dose of prednisone 60 mg a day for 1 week, followed by doses of 30 mg a day and 15 mg a day for each of the next 2 weeks, respectively, is one regimen that has been used successfully (25). Additionally, any elderly patient with Ramsay-Hunt syndrome, zoster encephalitis or myelitis, motor paralysis, or severe ocular infection should receive systemic corticosteroid therapy (16). Recently, adenosine monophosphate has been shown to be effective in preventing postherpetic neuralgia (26).

Once postherpetic neuralgia is established, it is extremely difficult to manage. As mentioned earlier, potent narcotic drugs become problematic in the old. A variety of therapies including transcutaneous stimulation, acupuncture, biofeedback, and nerve blocks have met with only limited success (20,27). For dull persistent pain, tricyclic drugs have had variable but encouraging success. Amitriptyline should be started at 25 mg at bedtime and can be gradually increased to 75 mg a night depending on response and side effects (28). For lancinating tic-like pain, carbamazepine may be useful; a dose of 100 mg four times a day may be tried for 4 weeks. Other therapeutic regimens for postherpetic neuralgia include chorprothixene 50–100 mg intravenously followed by oral doses of 50 mg every 6 hours for 7 to 10 days (29), and subcutaneous injection of triamcinolone (14).

Immunosuppressed Elderly

Elderly patients with immunosuppression from either diseases and/or drugs require treatment directed toward prevention of both viral spread and postherpetic neuralgia. In these patients, use of corticosteroids to prevent postherpetic neuralgia may further compromise their host defenses against VZ virus replication and dissemination. Therefore, in these patients, antiviral therapy is the cornerstone of therapy. Acyclovir is currently the treatment of choice for acute herpes zoster infection in the immunosuppressed host (30). Intravenous acyclovir in a dose of 500 mg per square meter of body surface is given every 8 hours as a 1-hour infusion for 7 days (30). However, a recent study suggested that oral and intravenous acyclovir are equally effective for herpes zoster in patients over 65-years old (31). Vidarabine has also been effective in treating herpes zoster in immunosuppressed patients (32), but is not as effective as acyclovir (30). However, neither drug prevents postherpetic neuralgia in either nonsuppressed or immunosuppressed patients (33).

The postherpetic neuralgia in these elderly patients cannot be expected to be prevented and, therefore, should be treated as outlined earlier. Table 19.1 summarizes therapeutic recommendations for elderly patients with herpes zoster.

TABLE 19.1 Treatment of Herpes Zoster in the Elderly

PATIENT'S IMMUNE STATUS	ANTIVIRAL THERAPY	PREVENTION OF POSTHERPETIC NEURALGIA
Normal	No	Prednisone for 3 weeks
Immunosuppressed	Acyclovir for 7 days	No

PREVENTION

Prevention of herpes zoster is likely to be available in the near future. A live attenuated varicella vaccine using the OKA-strain of VZ virus is currently being tested in the United States in order to determine its efficacy in preventing serious varicella infections, especially in the immunosuppressed host (34,35). Although this vaccine's role in preventing herpes zoster is unknown, one preliminary study indicated that when it was given to healthy elderly who had reduced lymphoproliferative immune response to VZ virus antigen (but had normal antibodies to the virus), this vaccine induced a change from negative to a positive cell-mediated immune response to VZ virus antigen in 85% of the volunteers (36). The clinical relevance of this change was not evaluated. However, it suggests that immune response to VZ virus antigen was augmented, which may indicate host resistance to this infection.

REFERENCES

1. Hope-Simpson RE: The nature of herpes zoster. A long-term study and a new hypothesis. *Proc Roy Soc Med* 58:9–20, 1965.
2. Ragozzino MW, Melton LJ III, Kurland LT, et al: Population-based study of herpes zoster and its sequelae. *Medicine* 61:310–316, 1982.
3. Glaser RB: Clinical aspects of herpes zoster. *West J Med* 139:718–720, 1983.
4. Damtew B, Frengley D: Herpes zoster: a scourge of old age. *Geriatr Med Today* 5:22–34, 1986.
5. Schimpff S, Serpick A, Stoler B, et al: Varicella-zoster infection in patients with cancer. *Ann Intern Med* 76:241–254, 1983.
6. Miller AE: Selective decline in cellular immune response to varicella-zoster in the elderly. *Neurology* 30:582–587, 1980.
7. Berger R, Florent G, Just M: Decrease of the lymphoproliferative response to varicella-zoster virus antigens in the aged. *Infect Immunity* 32:24–27, 1981.
8. Burke BL, Steele RW, Beard DW, et al: Immune responses to varicella-zoster in the aged. *Arch Intern Med* 142:291–293, 1982.
9. Nielson H, Olholm P, Feldt-Rasmussen U, et al: Circulating immune complexes and complement-fixing antibodies in patients with varicella-zoster

infection: relationship to debut of the disease. *Scand J Infect Dis* 12:21-26, 1980.

10. Weller TH: Varicella and herpes zoster. Changing concepts of the natural history, control, and importance of a not-so-benign virus. *N Engl J Med* 309:1363-1368, 1983.

11. Loeser JD: Herpes zoster and postherpetic neuralgia. *Pain* 25:149-164, 1986.

12. Pallett AP, Nicholls MWN: Varicella-zoster: Reactivation or reinfection? *Lancet* 1:160, 1986.

13. Miller LH, Brunell PA: Zoster, reinfection or activation of latent virus? *Am J Med* 49:480-483, 1970.

14. Becker LE: Herpes zoster: A geriatric disease. *Geriatrics* 34:41-47, 1979.

15. Harnisch JP: Zoster in the elderly: Clinical, immunologic and therapeutic considerations. *J Am Geriatr Soc* 32:789-793, 1984.

16. Reuler JB, Chang MK: Herpes zoster: Epidemiology, clinical features and management. *South Med J* 97:1149-1156, 1984.

17. Jemsek J, Greenberg SB, Taber L, et al: Herpes zoster-associated encephalitis: Clinicopathologic report of 12 cases and review of the literature. *Medicine* 62:81-97, 1983.

18. Womack LW, Liesegang TJ: Complications of herpes zoster ophthalmicus. *Arch Ophthalmol* 101:42-45, 1983.

19. Lass JH: Herpes zoster: Protecting older patients' vision. *Geriatrics* 39:79-94, 1984.

20. Watson PN, Evans RJ: Postherpetic neuralgia: a review. *Arch Neurol* 43:836-840, 1986.

21. Frey HM, Steinberg SP, Gershon AA: Rapid diagnosis of varicella-zoster virus infections by countercurrent immunoelectrophoresis. *J Infect Dis* 143:274-280, 1981.

22. Eaglestein WH, Katz R, Brown JA: The effects of early corticosteroid therapy in the skin eruption and pain of herpes zoster. *JAMA* 211:1681-1683, 1970.

23. Keczkes K, Basheer AM: Do corticosteroids prevent postherpetic neuralgia? *Br J Dermatol* 102:551-555, 1980.

24. Levinson W, Shaw JC: Treatment of herpes zoster with corticosteroids—fact or faith? *West J Med* 142:117-118, 1985.

25. Elliott FA: Treatment of herpes zoster with high doses of prednisone. *Lancet* 2:610-611, 1984.

26. Sklar SH, Blue WT, Alexander EJ, et al: Herpes zoster. The treatment and prevention of neuralgia with adenosine monophosphate. *JAMA* 253:1427-1430, 1985.

27. Price RW: Herpes zoster. An approach to systemic therapy. *Med Clin North Am* 66:1105-1118, 1982.

28. Watson CP, Evans RJ, Read K, et al: Amitriptyline vs. placebo in postherpetic neuralgia. *Neurology* 320:671-673, 1982.

29. Farber GA, Burks JW: Chlorprothixene therapy for herpes zoster neuralgia. *South Med J* 67:803-812, 1974.

30. Shepp DH, Dandliker DS, Meyers JD: Treatment of varicella-zoster infection in severely immunocompromised patients. A randomized comparison of acyclovir and vidarabine. *N Engl J Med* 314:203-212, 1986.

31. Peterslund NA, Esmann V, Ipsen J, et al: Oral and intravenous acyclovir are equally effective in herpes zoster. *J Antimicrob Chemother* 14:185–189, 1984.
32. Whitley RJ, Soong S-J, Dolin R, et al: Early vidarabine therapy to control the complications of herpes zoster in immunosuppressed patients. *N Engl J Med* 307:971–975, 1982.
33. Nicholson KG: Antiviral therapy. Varicella-zoster virus infections, herpes labialis and mucocutaneous herpes and cytomegalovirus infections. *Lancet* 2:677–681, 1984.
34. Gershon AA: Live attenuated varicella vaccine. *J Infect Dis* 151:859–862, 1985.
35. Hilleman MR: Newer directions in vaccine development and utilization. *J Infect Dis* 151:407–419, 1985.
36. Berger R, Leuseher D, Just M: Enhancement of varicella-zoster immune responses in the elderly by boosting with varicella vaccine. *J Infect Dis* 149:647, 1984.

SUGGESTED READINGS

Berger R, Leuseher D, Just M: Enhancement of varicella-zoster immune responses in the elderly by boosting with varicella vaccine. *J Infect Dis* 149: 647, 1984.
Burke BL, Steele RW, Beard DW, et al: Immune responses to varicella-zoster in the aged. *Arch Intern Med* 142:291–293, 1982.
Gershon AA: Live attenuated varicella vaccine. *J Infect Dis* 151:859–862, 1985.
Hope-Simpson RE: The nature of herpes zoster. A long-term study and a new hypothesis. *Proc Roy Soc Med* 58:9–20, 1965.
Levinson W, Shaw JC: Treatment of herpes zoster with corticosteroids—fact or faith? *West J Med* 142:117–118, 1985.
Reuler JB, Chang MK: Herpes zoster: Epidemiology, clinical features and management. *South Med J* 97:1149–1156, 1984.
Shepp DH, Dandliker DS, Meyers JD: Treatment of varicella-zoster infection in severely immunocompromised patients. A randomized comparison of acyclovir and vidarabine. *N Engl J Med* 314:203–212, 1986.
Watson PN, Evans RJ: Postherpetic neuralgia: a review. *Arch Neurol* 43:836–840, 1986.
Weller TH: Varicella and herpes zoster. Changing concepts of the natural history, control, and importance of a not-so-benign virus. *N Engl J Med* 309: 1363–1368, 1983.

Part 3

SPECIFIC PATHOGENS

Chapter 20

Staphylococcal Infections

GENERAL CONSIDERATIONS

Staphylococcus aureus infections were major causes of morbidity and mortality before the availability of effective antimicrobial agents. With the development of semisynthetic penicillinase-resistant penicillins and first-generation cephalosporins, many clinicians assumed that the role of *S. aureus* as a major pathogen would markedly decrease. However, this has not been the case, particularly in the very young, the old, and those with compromised host defenses. Moreover, *S. aureus* is no longer susceptible to penicillin G. Of even more concern is the rising incidence of methicillin-resistant *S. aureus* (MRSA) (1,2)—a pathogen that is frequently isolated in the elderly.

Coagulase-negative staphylococci include at least 14 species (3); however, only two species are clinically relevant, *S. saprophyticus,* an important cause of many urinary tract infections in young women (4), and *S. epidermidis,* a pathogen responsible for infections of prosthetic devices, many of which are inserted in the elderly (5).

MICROBIOLOGY, EPIDEMIOLOGY, AND HOST-PARASITE INTERACTION

S. aureus

Staphylococci belong to the family Micrococcaceae. They are aerobic and facultatively anaerobic cocci that are gram positive, catalase positive, and oxidase negative. The major characteristics that differentiate *S. aureus* from other staphylococci are that it is coagulase positive and that it ferments mannitol. *S. aureus* produces and elaborates several types of extracellular products, which display either enzymatic or nonenzymatic activities. The role(s) of these extracellular proteins is (are) not totally known, although some appear to be clearly important in the biologic characteristics of the organism as well as the pathogenesis of some of the clinical syndromes caused by *S. aureus,* for example, exfoliatin, enterotoxin, erythrogenic toxin, hyaluronidase, beta-lactamase, and coagulase (6).

S. aureus bacteremia occurs with disproportionately high frequency in the aged. In one study of 77 cases of *S. aureus* bacteremia, 33 (43%) occurred in patients between the seventh and ninth decades (7). Another study of 400 episodes of *S. aureus* bacteremia reported a 21.5% incidence in persons 65 years and older (8). In a study of 44 patients with MRSA bacteremia, 53% were in patients 60 years or older (9). The organism commonly resides on the skin and anterior nares of humans. Approximately 15 to 35% of the population may be chronic or persistent nasal carriers of *S. aureus,* and 15 to 50% may be intermittent carriers (6). However, the proportion of the geriatric population that are intermittent or persistent carriers of *S. aureus* is unknown.

Many disease states or conditions that are associated with increased frequency of *S. aureus* infections occur with high frequency in the elderly. These include hematologic malignancies, diabetes mellitus, uremia (especially hemodialysis), open fractures, anatomically damaged joint spaces, prosthetic devices, and vascular access sites or devices (6,10). Factors that appear to be important in increasing the host susceptibility to *S. aureus* infection include disruption of skin and epithelial surfaces, granulocytopathies, and immunosuppression. The major host defense mechanism against *S. aureus* appears to be granulocyte phagocytosis, although macrophages, complement, and immune mechanisms probably also play a role in eradicating this pathogen (11).

S. epidermidis

In contrast to *S. aureus, S. epidermidis* is coagulase negative and does not ferment mannitol. *S. epidermidis* is capable of producing extracellular enzymes, but its role in the pathogenesis of diseases is not clear.

The association between aging and susceptibility to *S. epidermidis* appears to be related to the predisposing factors or conditions to *S. epidermidis* infection. Such devices as prosthetic heart valves, prosthetic hips and knee joints, central nervous system shunts, and vascular grafts or shunts are commonly placed in older patients—these foreign bodies are the major predisposing conditions for *S. epidermidis* infections. In addition, immunosuppression, granulocytopenia, and disruption of cutaneous surfaces facilitate infection by this organism (3,5).

S. epidermidis is part of the normal microflora of the skin and is easily shed from the cutaneous surfaces to contaminate the air, other persons, or inanimate environmental surfaces (5). Thus, *S. epidermidis* infections occur by contamination of a surgical site or breaks in natural barriers to infection.

CLINICAL SYNDROMES

S. aureus

S. aureus infects virtually any body site. Moreover, bacteremia from a primary *S. aureus* infection is common and can lead to secondary sites of infection as well as to metastatic abscesses.

INTRAVASCULAR INFECTIONS
Intravascular infections are the most common causes of *S. aureus* bacteremia (7–9). Frequent sites of intravascular infections include arteriovenous fistulas and intravenous catheters. The majority of these infections are nosocomially acquired.

SKIN AND SOFT TISSUE INFECTIONS
Skin and soft tissue infections make up the second most frequent cause of *S. aureus* bacteremia (7–9). In the elderly, these would include wound infections, burns, cellulitis, furuncles, and carbuncles.

SKELETAL INFECTIONS
S. aureus is a major pathogen that causes osteomyelitis and septic arthritis in the elderly (see Chapter 16 on septic arthritis and osteomyelitis). Additionally, *S. aureus* and *S. epidermidis* are the major etiologic pathogens for wound sepsis following total hip arthroplasty (14).

CARDIAC VALVE INFECTIONS
Both natural and prosthetic valve infections in the aged may be caused by *S. aureus* (see Chapter 12 on infective endocarditis).

CENTRAL NERVOUS SYSTEM INFECTIONS
Central nervous system (CNS) infections caused by *S. aureus* occur in the geriatric age group. The majority of cases of CNS infections in the elderly is meningitis that occurs either spontaneously or following craniotomy or head injury (15).

PLEUROPULMONARY INFECTIONS

Pneumonia in the elderly may be caused by *S. aureus* (see Chapter 10 on pneumonia). Empyema and lung abscess are also common infections caused by *S. aureus*.

OTHER INFECTIONS

S. aureus may cause other infections, that is, food-borne gastroenteritis, invasive enterocolitis, impetigo, myositis, toxic epidermal necrolysis, blepharitis, conjunctivitis, keratitis, corneal ulcers, pericarditis, epidural abscess, genitourinary infections, and toxic shock syndrome. However, these *S. aureus* infections are not especially important or unique to the elderly.

S. epidermidis

The major infections associated with *S. epidermidis* involve foreign bodies, that is, prosthesis insertion. However, *S. epidermidis* may be a significant pathogen in urinary tract infections of the elderly (16) as well as the occasional cause of intraabdominal abscesses (17). Additionally, *S. epidermidis* has been isolated with unusual frequency from patients who are immunosuppressed and/or granulocytopenic (12,13), conditions that occur in the elderly who receive chemotherapy for malignancy. The mortality in these older patients with bacteremia may be as high as 49% (18).

PROSTHETIC HEART VALVE INFECTIONS

Insertion of prosthetic heart valves is now a common occurrence among elderly patients. Consequently, infection of these valves is a serious complication in the elderly. *S. epidermidis* is the single most common pathogen that causes prosthetic valve endocarditis (19).

PROSTHETIC JOINT INFECTIONS

Prosthetic joints, particularly the hip, are common in the elderly, who frequently suffer from fractures and osteoarthritis. Infections of these devices is devastating to the patient and is extremely costly to manage. *S. epidermidis* and *S. aureus* as well as aerobic gram-negative bacilli are common etiologic pathogens (14). (See also Chapter 16 on septic arthritis and osteomyelitis.)

CENTRAL NERVOUS SYSTEM SHUNTS

Some elderly persons may develop normal pressure hydrocephalus, which is best treated by a shunting procedure, for example, ventriculojugular or ventriculoperitoneal shunts. These foreign bodies are infected most often with *S. epidermidis* (20).

OTHER SITES

Other *S. epidermidis* infections that may occur in the elderly include those that involve arteriovenous grafts or shunts, peritoneal dialysis catheters, and Hickman-Broviac catheters (21–23).

DIAGNOSTIC APPROACH

S. aureus

All involved tissues, body fluids, or purulent material should be immediately examined by a Gram stain. The finding of large gram-positive cocci in clusters is presumptive evidence for presence of staphylococci. These same clinical specimens should also be sent for culture. The isolation of *S. aureus* in culture media is relatively easy, and identification should be possible within 48 hours.

Blood cultures are essential, not only for diagnostic purposes, but also to determine if bacteremia with secondary seeding to other sites may have occurred. A serologic test for *S. aureus* is available, such as the teichoic acid antibody test. However, its clinical use as a diagnostic tool has been in question because of its relatively low sensitivity (6).

Appropriate x-rays and scans should be obtained depending on the site(s) of infection.

S. epidermidis

The diagnostic evaluation is the same as described for *S. aureus*. However, there is currently no serologic test for *S. epidermidis.*

One important point should be underscored with reference to isolation of *S. epidermidis* from the blood or body fluids that are normally sterile. Oftentimes, isolation of this organism is considered as a contaminant and disregarded as a cause of infection. It should be stated that if *S. epidermidis* is isolated from the blood or potential site of infection from an elderly patient with a prosthesis or foreign body, the organism must be considered as a pathogen until it is proven otherwise.

TREATMENT

S. aureus

Most *S. aureus* are resistant to penicillin G or other penicillin analogues that are susceptible to beta-lactamase (penicillinase). Therefore, for most cases of serious *S. aureus* infections in the elderly, intravenous oxacillin or nafcillin should be administered in doses of 6 to 12 g a day in four to six divided doses. First-generation cephalosporins, for example, cephalo-thin or cefazolin, are also effective against most strains of *S. aureus.* For the elderly, we recommend cefazolin 2–4 g a day (dose depending on severity of disease) in two to four divided doses. Elderly persons who are allergic to penicillin may be treated effectively with intravenous van-comycin 1.5–2.0 g a day in two to four divided doses. Duration of therapy varies depending on site of infection, severity of disease, and clinical re-sponse of the patient. Infections that involve the heart valve and bones generally require 4 to 6 weeks of antibiotic therapy; most other *S. aureus* infections require 10 to 14 days of therapy.

For *S. aureus* infections that can be managed on an outpatient basis, dicloxacillin or cloxacillin is recommended in doses of 2–4 g a day or 1–2 g a day, respectively, in four divided doses.

Occasionally, methicillin-resistant *S. aureus* (MRSA) strains are iso-lated. These organisms are uniformly resistant to methicillin, oxacillin, nafcillin, and most cephalosporins. Vancomycin is the drug of choice for MRSA infections (9), in doses described above. Additionally, the newer carbapenem, imipenem, is an effective antibiotic against MRSA and may be considered as an alternative agent for infections caused by this pathogen (24). The recommended dose is 2 to 4 g a day in four divided doses.

S. epidermidis

S. epidermidis may show resistance to methicillin (up to 25% of all strains). The drug of choice for these resistant strains is vancomycin (same dose as described for *S. aureus* infection). Therefore, in severely ill patients or patients with deep-seated *S. epidermidis* infections, vancomycin should be initiated empirically until culture and sensitivity data become available. In patients with central nervous system shunt infections, it has been recommended that rifampin (600–1,200 mg a day) be added to van-comycin (25). The rationale is twofold: (*1*) vancomycin's penetration into the cerebrospinal fluid (CSF) may be unpredictable (rifampin has in vitro activity against *S. epidermidis* and penetrates well into the CSF); and (*2*) tolerance (this organism is inhibited but not killed by an antibiotic) occasionally is seen with strains of *S. epidermidis* (rifampin enhances kill-ing of the organism). Similar recommendations, such as vancomycin and rifampin, have been prescribed for *S. epidermidis* prosthetic valve en-docarditis (19).

Strains of *S. epidermidis* that are susceptible to penicillin G should be treated with this agent. Likewise, strains susceptible to methicillin should be treated with oxacillin or nafcillin or a first-generation cephalosporin.

Despite effective antimicrobial therapy, most prosthetic devices have to be surgically removed to effect a microbiologic cure. Under these circumstances, chemotherapy is continued for 2 to 4 weeks. However, in some instances, a very fragile elderly patient may not tolerate a surgical intervention; thus, prolonged antibiotic therapy (6 weeks or more) may be the only alternative available for treatment.

PREVENTION

S. aureus

Prevention of S. aureus infections is not always possible, since often the primary site of infection is never diagnosed. Careful observation of infection control principles and aseptic surgical techniques are imperative in reducing the risk of S. aureus infections. Chronic carriers of S. aureus organisms should be discouraged from coming into close contact with elderly persons who are particularly susceptible to staphylococcal infections. Active treatment to eliminate the carrier state of S. aureus is generally unsuccessful.

S. epidermidis

As with S. aureus, adhering to basic principles of infection control and aseptic surgical techniques is paramount in preventing or reducing S. epidermidis infection of prosthetic devices. Preoperative chemoprophylaxis for cardiovascular surgery and for orthopedic surgery that involves prosthetic devices is recommended for the elderly (see Chapter 6 on prevention of infections).

REFERENCES

1. Keane CT, Cafferkey MT: Re-emergence of methicillin-resistant *Staphylococcus aureus* causing severe infection. *J Infect* 9:6-16, 1984.
2. Cafferkey MT, Coleman D, McGrath B, et al: Methicillin-resistant *Staphylococcus aureus* in Dublin 1971-84. *Lancet* 2:705-708, 1985.
3. Kloos WE: Coagulase-negative staphylococci. *Clin Microbiol Newsletter* 4:75-79, 1982.
4. Hovelius B, Mardh P-A: *Staphylococcus saprophyticus* as a common cause of urinary tract infections. *Rev Infect Dis* 6:318-337, 1984.
5. Lowy FD, Hammer SM: *Staphylococcus epidermidis* infections. *Ann Intern Med* 99:834-839, 1983.
6. Yoshikawa TT: Staphylococcal infections, in Yoshikawa TT, Chow AW, Guze LB (eds): *Infectious Diseases. Diagnosis and Management.* New York, John Wiley & Sons, 1980, p 322.
7. Michel MF, Priem CC, Verbrugh HA, et al: *Staphylococcus aureus* bacteremia in a Dutch teaching hospital. *Infection* 13:267-272, 1985.

8. Gransden WR, Eykyn SJ, Phillips I: *Staphylococcus aureus* bacteraemia: 400 episodes at St. Thomas's Hospital. *Br Med J* 288:300–303, 1984.

9. Cafferkey MT, Hone R, Keane CT: Antimicrobial chemotherapy of septicemia due to methicillin-resistant *Staphylococcus aureus. Antimicrob Agents Chemother* 28:819–823, 1985.

10. Yoshikawa TT: Aging, infections and diabetes mellitus, in Cuhna B (ed): *Infectious Diseases of the Elderly.* John Wright, Inc., in press.

11. Leijh PCJ, Van Zwet TL, Van Furth R: Effect of concanavalin A on intracellular killing of *Staphylococcus aureus* by human phagocytes. *Clin Exp Immunol* 58:557–565, 1984.

12. Winston DJ, Dudnick DV, Chapin M, et al: Coagulase-negative staphylococci bacteremia in patients receiving immunosuppressive therapy. *Arch Intern Med* 143:32–36, 1983.

13. Wade JC, Schimpff, Newman KA et al: *Staphylococcus epidermidis:* An increasing cause of infections in patients with granulocytopenia. *Ann Intern Med* 97:503–508, 1982.

14. Fitzgerald RH, Nolan DR, Ilstrup DM, et al: Deep wound sepsis following total hip arthroplasty. *J Bone Joint Surg* 59-A:847–855, 1977.

15. Fong IW, Ranalle P: *Staphylococcus aureus* meningitis. *Q J Med* 53:289–299, 1984.

16. Leighton PM, Little JA: Identification of coagulase-negative staphylococci isolated from urinary tract infections. *Am J Clin Pathol* 85:92–95, 1986.

17. Harris LF: Nosocomial intraabdominal abscesses caused by coagulase-negative staphylococci. *J Infect Dis* 152:1091–1092, 1985.

18. Ponce De Leon S, Wenzel RP: Hospital-acquired blood stream infections with *Staphylococcus epidermidis.* Review of 100 cases. *Am J Med* 77:639–644, 1984.

19. Karchmer AW, Archer GL, Dismukes UE: *Staphylococcus epidermidis* causing prosthetic valve endocarditis: Microbiological and clinical observations as guides to therapy. *Ann Intern Med* 98:447–455, 1983.

20. Shoenbaum SC, Gardner P, Shillito J: Infections of cerebrospinal fluid shunts: Epidemiology, clinical manifestations and therapy. *J Infect Dis* 131:543–552, 1975.

21. Liekwig WG Jr, Greenfield LJ: Vascular prosthetic infections: Collected experience and results of treatment. *Surgery* 81:335–342, 1977.

22. Kubin J, Rogers WA, Taylor HM, et al: Peritonitis during continuous ambulatory peritoneal dialysis. *Ann Intern Med* 92:773, 1980.

23. Pessa ME, Howard RJ: Complications of Hickman-Broviac catheters. *Surg Gynecol Obstet* 161:257–260, 1985.

24. Fan W, Del Busto R, Love M, et al: Imipenem-cilastatin in the treatment of methicillin-sensitive and methicillin-resistant *Staphylococcus aureus* infections. *Antimicrob Agents Chemother* 29:26–29, 1986.

25. Gombert ME, Landesman SH, Corrado ML, et al: Vancomycin and rifampin therapy for *Staphylococcus epidermidis* meningitis associated with CSF shunts: Report of three cases. *J Neurosurg* 55:633–636, 1981.

SUGGESTED READINGS

Cafferkey MT, Hone R, Keane CT: Antimicrobial chemotherapy of septicemia due to methicillin-resistant *Staphylococcus aureus. Antimicrob Agents Chemother* 28:819–823, 1985.

Karchmer AW, Archer GL, Dismukes UE: *Staphylococcus epidermidis* causing prosthetic valve endocarditis: Microbiological and clinical observations as guides to therapy. *Ann Intern Med* 98:447–455, 1983.

Lowy FD, Hammer SM: *Staphylococcus epidermidis* infections. *Ann Intern Med* 99:834–839, 1983.

Michel MF, Priem CC, Verbrugh HA, et al: *Staphylococcus aureus* bacteremia in a Dutch teaching hospital. *Infection* 13:267–272, 1985.

Shoenbaum SC, Gardner P, Shillito J: Infections of cerebrospinal fluid shunts: Epidemiology, clinical manifestations and therapy. *J Infect Dis* 131:543–552, 1975.

Chapter 21

Streptococcal Infections

GENERAL CONSIDERATIONS

A variety of streptococcal infections occur with extremely high frequency in the aging population. Interestingly, many of the species of streptococci have an unusually high predilection for the very young and the very old. This association for those at the extremes of the age spectrum suggests that altered host defenses may be a predisposing factor.

Streptococci that are particularly relevant to the older population include *Streptococcus pneumoniae;* group D streptococci, which includes the enterococci (*S. faecalis* is most common) and nonenterococcal *S. bovis;* group B streptococci (*S. agalactiae*); and group G streptococci. Some recent studies suggest that group A streptococci (*S. pyogenes*) and group C streptococci may have an important role in infections in the elderly, but data are too scant to make any valid conclusions (1–4).

MICROBIOLOGY, EPIDEMIOLOGY, AND HOST-PARASITE INTERACTION

Streptococcal Microbiology

Streptococci are aerobic and facultatively anaerobic gram-positive organisms that are spherical or ovoid and nonmotile. They are differentiated easily from staphylococci by their negative catalase reaction. They are grown best on sheep blood agar; alpha- (incomplete, greenish), beta- (complete, clear), or gamma- (none) hemolysis may be seen. Presumptive identification of streptococci is quickly feasible by readily available chemical tests. Definitive serogrouping can be done by formal Lancefield precipitation reactions.

S. pneumoniae

S. pneumoniae (pneumococci) are gram-positive cocci that appear in pairs or in short chains. On blood agar, they are alpha-hemolytic (like viridans streptococci). S. pneumoniae show a zone of inhibition, a diameter of at least 15 mm when exposed to an optochin disk (ethylhydrocupreine), and demonstrate a Quellung reaction with appropriate capsular antiserum. There are over 80 capsular serotypes of S. pneumoniae, with 23 of the more clinically relevant serotypes contained in the pneumococcal vaccine (see Chapter 6 on prevention of infections). Of all the serotypes, type III with its extensive capsule appears to be especially virulent in adults, including the elderly (5).

The incidence and mortality of pneumococcal disease is unquestionably higher in the elderly population (incidence is also high in young children, but mortality is much less than in the elderly group). Table 21.1 shows the frequency and mortality of serious S. pneumoniae infection in young and old adults from recently published reports (6–11). However, it cannot be stated definitively that age alone is the only predisposing factor, since several underlying diseases or conditions that increase the sus-

TABLE 21.1   Serious Pneumococcal Infections in Young and Old Adults

TYPE OF INFECTION	TOTAL ADULT CASES	FREQUENCY (%)		MORTALITY (%)		
		YOUNG	OLD	YOUNG	OLD	REF
All types[a]	285	2.4–7.6[b]	11.6–16.4[b]	NS[c]	NS[c]	6
All types[d]	400	196(49)	204(51)	NS	NS	7
Pneumonia[e]	71	16[e](23)	55[e](77)	3(19)	18(33)	8
Pneumonia[f]	14	1[f](7)	13[f](93)	0	4(31)[f]	9
Bacteremia	289	135[g](47)	154[g](53)	32(24)	57(37)	10
Meningitis	114	41[h](36)	73(64)	13(32)	35(49)	11

[a]Meningitis, empyema, bacteremia, otitis, sinusitis, arthritis, osteomyelitis, facial cellulitis.
[b]Age-specific incidence (cases/100,000 inhabitants): age 20–29 years (2.4), 30–39 (4.4), 40–49 (6.6), 50–59 (7.6); age 60–69 (11.6), 70–79 (16.4), 80 and older (14.1).
[c]Not stated. "Highest in patients older than 50 years."
[d]Meningitis, bacteremia, pneumonia, bone and joint, ear and mastoid, skin, heart valve. Age ranges were 5–59 years and 60 years and older.
[e]Bacteremic cases only. Young adults, age 14–49 years; old adults age 50.
[f]Bactermic cases only. One patient <59 years, and 13 were 59 years or older. Four deaths were aged 63, 65, 68, and 78.
[g]Young adults, age 20–59; old adults, 60 years and older.
[h]Young adults, age 15–50; old adults, 51 years and older.

ceptibility to pneumococcal infections also occur frequently in the elderly. These conditions include chronic lung disease, chronic liver disease, hematologic malignancies (e.g., myeloma), alcoholism, and chronic renal disease.

The major portal of entry for *S. pneumoniae* is the upper and lower respiratory tract.

Group D Streptococci

Group D streptococci include the enterococci (primarily *S. faecalis*) and the nonenterococci (primarily *S. bovis*). Without using the formal Lancefield precipitation reaction, streptococci can be identified as group D by a positive reaction to the bile-esculin hydrolysis test. The ability to grow in 6.5% sodium chloride indicates enterococci (nonenterococci fail to grow in this solution).

ENTEROCOCCI

The enterococci are present as part of the indigenous microflora of the oral cavity, gastrointestinal tract (especially the colon), vagina, endocervix, and urethral meatus (12). Hence, enterococci infections are commonly found in these areas. The pathogen has relatively low virulence, but can cause life-threatening infections (e.g., endocarditis, urosepsis, intraabdominal sepsis) under appropriate circumstances. The prior use of antibiotics is an important factor that permits superinfection to occur with enterococci.

Enterococcal infections occur in two populations: young women and elderly men and women (13–15). It appears that the high incidence in the elderly is primarily due to the associated clinical circumstances (i.e., abdominal surgery, chronic urinary catheters, and antibiotic usage) rather than age-related biologic changes.

S. BOVIS

S. bovis may be part of the normal colonic fecal flora. However, its frequency of isolation appears to increase in patients with a variety of intestinal disorders, particularly colonic carcinoma (16–19). Earlier clinical studies indicated the mouth and genitourinary tract as potential sources for *S. bovis* infection (20,21). The high incidence of *S. bovis* bacteremia in the elderly (mean age 61–73 [refs. 16–21]) most likely is related to the higher frequency of occurrence of gastrointestinal disorders associated with *S. bovis* colonization in this age group.

Group B Streptococci

Group B streptococcus, *S. agalactiae,* can be identified presumptively by beta-hemolysis in blood agar, hydrolysis of sodium hippurate (hippuricase activity), and a negative bile-esculin reaction. The CAMP reaction is positive anaerobically or aerobically for group B streptococci (group A is positive only under anaerobic conditions; group C and G are negative) (22). Formal Lancefield typing confirms the identification of the organism as group B.

Group B streptococcal infection occurs predominantly in neonates, with urogenital tract of women being the reservoir for this organism. However, data on the source for adult infection have been sparse. Nevertheless, it appears group B streptococci is harbored in the pharnyx, upper respiratory tract, or genitourinary tract (23).

Group B streptococcal disease occurs in populations at the two extremes of age, that is, neonates and the elderly. Several reports of group B streptococcal infection in adults indicate that 30 to 80% of cases occur in adults 60 years or older (22,24,25). This age relationship appears to be in large part due to the underlying conditions the elderly patients have, such as diabetes mellitus, malignancy, chronic liver disease, and genitourinary tract disease.

Group G Streptococci

The identification of group G streptococci is confirmed by Lancefield serologic testing. The majority of these organisms are beta-hemolytic on blood agar and are negative for bile-esculin hydrolysis.

Group G streptococci are part of the normal flora of the pharnyx, skin, gastrointestinal tract, and vagina (26). Consequently, these sites are either the primary site of infection or the source of bacteremia.

Recent studies of group G streptococcal infection show that 40 to 60% occur in persons 60 years or older (26,27). As with other streptococcal infections, such underlying conditions as malignancy, chronic liver disease, alcoholism, and diabetes mellitus appear to play an important role in predisposing the elderly to group G streptococcal infections (26–28).

CLINICAL SYNDROMES

S. pneumoniae

PULMONARY

Involvement of the respiratory tract is the most frequent site for pneumococcal infection in the elderly. Pneumonia is the most common pulmonary infection; bronchitis is also quite common. Empyema and lung abscess may complicate S. pneumoniae pneumonia in the elderly. Bacteremia occurs as a complication of pneumococcal pneumonia and permits hematogenous spread of organisms to extrapulmonary sites (29–30).

EXTRAPULMONARY
Meningitis is the most common extrapulmonary infection due to *S. pneumoniae* in the elderly (5,6,10,11). Other sites of involvement include heart valves, bones and joints, and ears.

Group D Streptococci

ENTEROCOCCI
Enterococci are frequent causes of urinary tract infection in the aged, especially in patients with chronic bladder catheters. These pathogens are also isolated from elderly patients with acute cholecystitis as well as from those with intraabdominal sepsis caused by appendicitis, diverticulitis, or abscesses (15).

S. BOVIS
The primary infection associated with *S. bovis* in the elderly is infective endocarditis. Nearly all cases involve infection of the valves of the left side of the heart.

Group B Streptococci

Group B streptococcal infections in the elderly include endocarditis, meningitis, cellulitis, infected decubitus ulcers, septic arthritis, osteomyelitis, urinary tract infection, and pneumonia (23–25,31).

Group G Streptococci

Cutaneous infection (cellulitis) is the most frequent type of infection caused by group G streptococci in the elderly. Other infections include pneumonia, pharyngitis, endocarditis, meningitis, bacteremia (without defined focus), and septic arthritis (26–28,32).

DIAGNOSTIC APPROACH

For all streptococcal infections, blood cultures are essential since bacteremia is a relatively frequent occurrence in the geriatric age group. Gram stain and culture of potentially infected body fluids, purulent drainage, inflamed or necrotic tissue, and biopsy material should be part of the routine diagnostic evaluation for streptococcal infections. Other radiologic studies as well as scans should be obtained when they are clinically indicated.

TREATMENT

S. pneumoniae

The drug of choice for most *S. pneumoniae* infections is penicillin G. The dose of penicillin G administered varies from 2–20 million units a day depending on the type of infection and severity of illness. Other effective agents include ampicillin, oxacillin, nafcillin, antipseudomonas penicillins (e.g., piperacillin), and most cephalosporins. Patients allergic to beta-lactam drugs may be treated with erythromycin, clindamycin, vancomycin, chloramphenicol, or trimethoprim-sulfamethoxazole.

Group G Streptococci

ENTEROCOCCI
Ampicillin is the drug of choice for most enterococcal infections. However, because strains of enterococci may be tolerant to beta-lactam drugs, serious enterococcal infections (e.g., endocarditis) should be treated with combination chemotherapy, that is, ampicillin (12 g a day in six divided doses, given intravenously) plus an aminoglycoside (the dose is dependent on drug and renal function). Penicillin G may be effective against enterococci if given in large doses (e.g., 20–30 million units a day) or if it is combined with an aminoglycoside. Vancomycin is also effective against enterococci. Trimethoprim-sulfamethoxazole may be active against this pathogen, although many strains of enterococci may be resistant to the drug. Imipenem and the quinolones are newer drugs that appear to be effective against enterococci.

S. BOVIS
Penicillin G is the drug of choice. Like *S. pneumoniae, S. bovis* may be treated effectively with a number of other drugs including ampicillin, oxacillin, nafcillin, cephalosporins, chloramphenicol, erythromycin, and clindamycin as well as vancomycin and trimethoprim-sulfamethoxazole. However, for *S. bovis* endocarditis, only bactericidal agents (e.g., beta-lactams) should be used. We would recommend penicillin G, 18–20 million units a day in four to six divided doses.

Group B Streptococci

Group B streptococci are susceptible to penicillin G, ampicillin, cephalosporins, erythromycin, clindamycin, and chloramphenicol as well as vancomycin (23,25,33). Because group B streptococci may show tolerance, it is recommended that serious infections (e.g., endocarditis) be treated with penicillin (18–20 million units a day) plus an aminoglycoside (25).

Group G Streptococci

Group G streptococci are much like group B streptococci in terms of antimicrobial susceptibility. Penicillin G is the drug of choice, but the antipseudomonas penicillins, cephalosporins, vancomycin, and erythromycin are also effective (34). Tolerance may be seen with group G streptococci. Serious infections should be treated with combination therapy of a beta-lactam drug plus an aminoglycoside or rifampin (34).

PREVENTION

S. pneumoniae infection may be prevented effectively by the pneumococcal vaccine (see Chapter 6 on the prevention of infections). Effective methods of preventing group D, B, and G streptococcal infections in the elderly are currently not available.

REFERENCES

1. Ruben FL, Norden CW, Heisler B, et al: An outbreak of *Streptococcus pyogenes* infections in a nursing home. *Ann Intern Med* 101:494–496, 1984.
2. Reid RI, Briggs RS, Seal DV, et al: Virulent *Streptococcus pyogenes:* Outbreak and spread within a geriatric unit. *J Infect* 6:219–225, 1983.
3. Stein DS, Panwalker AP: Group C streptococcal endocarditis: Case report and review of the literature. *Infection* 13:282–285, 1985.
4. Mohr DN, Feist DJ, Washington JA II, et al: Infections due to group C streptococci in man. *Am J Med* 66:450–456, 1979.
5. Austrian R, Gold J: Pneumococcal bacteremia with especial reference to bacteremic pneumococcal pneumonia. *Ann Intern Med* 60:759–776, 1964.
6. Burman LA, Norrby R, Trollfors B: Invasive pneumococcal infections: Incidence, predisposing factors, and prognosis. *Rev Infect Dis* 7:133–142, 1985.
7. Colman G, Hallos G: Systemic disease caused by pneumococci. *J Infect* 7:248–255, 1983.
8. Mufson MA, Oley G, Hughey D: Pneumococcal disease in a medium-sized community in the United States. *JAMA* 248:1486–1489, 1982.
9. Banks RA, George RC, McNicol MW: Pneumococcal pneumonia with bacteraemia. *Br J Dis Chest* 78:352–357, 1984.
10. Grandsen WR, Eykyn S, Phillips I: Pneumococcal bacteraemia: 325 episodes diagnosed at St. Thomas's Hospital. *Br Med J* 290:505–508, 1985.
11. Bohr VB, Rasmussen N, Hansen B, et al: Pneumococcal meningitis: An evaluation of prognostic factors in 164 cases based on mortality and on a study of lasting sequelae. *J Infect* 10:143–157, 1985.
12. Kaye D: Enterococci: Biologic and epidemiologic characteristics and in vitro susceptibility. *Arch Intern Med* 142:2006–2009, 1982.
13. Jawetz E, Sonne M: Penicillin-streptomycin treatment of enterococcal endocarditis. A re-evaluation. *N Engl J Med* 274:710–715, 1966.
14. Mandell GL, Kaye D, Levison ME, et al: Enterococcal endocarditis. An

analysis of 38 patients observed at the New York-Cornell Medical Center. *Arch Intern Med* 125:258–264, 1970.

15. Barrall DT, Kenney PR, Slotman GJ, et al: Enterococcal bacteremia in surgical patients. *Arch Surg* 120:57–63, 1985.

16. Klein RS, Recco RA, Catalano MT, et al: Association of *Streptococcus bovis* with carcinoma of the colon. *N Engl J Med* 297:800–802, 1977.

17. Murray HW, Roberts RB: *Streptococcus bovis* bacteremia and underlying gastrointestinal disease. *Arch Intern Med* 138:1097–1099, 1978.

18. Klein RS, Catalano MT, Edberg SC, et al: *Streptococcus bovis* septicemia and carcinoma of the colon. *Ann Intern Med* 91:560–562, 1979.

19. Reynolds JG, Silva E, McCormack WM: Association of *Streptococcus bovis* bacteremia with bowel disease. *J Clin Microbiol* 17:696–697, 1983.

20. Hoppes WL, Lerner PI: Nonenterococcal group-D streptococcal endocarditis caused by *Streptococcus bovis*. *Ann Intern Med* 81:588–593, 1974.

21. Moellering RC Jr, Watson BK, Kunz LJ: Endocarditis due to group D streptococci. Comparison of disease caused by Streptococcus bovis with that produced by the enterococci. *Am J Med* 57:239–256, 1974.

22. Lerner PI, Gopalakrishna KV, Wolinsky E, et al: Group B streptococcus (*S. agalactiae*) bacteremia in adults: Analysis of 32 cases and review of the literature. *Medicine* 56:457–473, 1977.

23. Bayer AS, Chow AW, Anthony BF, et al: Serious infections in adults due to group B streptococci. Clinical and serotypic characterization. *Am J Med* 61:498–503, 1976.

24. Gallagher PG, Watanakunakorn C: Group B streptococcal bacteremia in a community teaching hospital. *Am J Med* 78:795–800, 1985.

25. Gallagher PG, Watanakunakorn C: Group B streptococcal endocarditis. Report of serious cases and review of the literature, 1962–1985. *Rev Infect Dis* 8:175–188, 1986.

26. Auckenthaler R, Hermans PE, Washington JA II: Group G streptococcal bacteremia. *Rev Infect Dis* 5:196–204, 1983.

27. Vartian C, Lerner PI, Shlaes DM, et al: Infections due to Lancefield group G streptococci. *Medicine* 64:75–88, 1985.

28. Watsky KL, Kollisch N, Densen P: Group G streptococcal bacteremia. The clinical experience at Boston University Medical Center and a critical review of the literature. *Arch Intern Med* 145:58–61, 1985.

29. Esposito AL: Community-acquired bacteremic pneumococcal pneumonia. Effect of age on manifestations and outcome. *Arch Intern Med* 144:945–948, 1984.

30. Murphy TF, Fine BC: Bacteremic pneumococcal pneumonia in the elderly. *Am J Med Sci* 288:114–118, 1984.

31. Pischel K, Weisman MH, Cone RO: Unique features of group B streptococcal arthritis in adults. *Arch Intern Med* 145:97–102, 1985.

32. Venezio FR, Gulbery RM, Westenfelder GO, et al: Group G streptococcal endocarditis and bacteremia. *Am J Med* 81:29–34, 1986.

33. Anthony BF, Concepcion NK: Group B *Streptococcus* in a general hospital. *J Infect Dis* 132:561–568, 1975.

34. Rolston KVI: Group G streptococcal infections. *Arch Intern Med* 146:857–858, 1986.

SUGGESTED READINGS

Burman LA, Norrby R, Trollfors B: Invasive pneumococcal infections: Incidence, predisposing factors, and prognosis. *Rev Infect Dis* 7:133–142, 1985.

Gallagher PG, Watanakunakorn C: Group B streptococcal bacteremia in a community teaching hospital. *Am J Med* 78:795–800, 1985.

Grandsen WR, Eykyn S, Phillips I: Pneumococcal bacteraemia: 325 episodes diagnosed at St. Thomas's Hospital. *Br Med J* 290:505–508, 1985.

Kaye D: Enterococci: Biologic and epidemiologic characteristics and in vitro susceptibility. *Arch Intern Med* 142:2006–2009, 1982.

Klein RS, Catalano MT, Edberg SC, et al: *Streptococcus bovis* septicemia and carcinoma of the colon. *Ann Intern Med* 91:560–562, 1979.

Mandell GL, Kaye D, Levison ME, et al: Enterococcal endocarditis. An analysis of 38 patients observed at the New York-Cornell Medical Center. *Arch Intern Med* 125:258–264, 1970.

Vartian C, Lerner PI, Shlaes DM, et al: Infections due to Lancefield group G streptococci. *Medicine* 64:75–88, 1985.

Chapter 22

Listerial Infections

GENERAL CONSIDERATIONS

Human listeriosis has received little attention as an important clinical entity until the recently reported outbreak of food-borne listerial infections (1–4). *Listeria monocytogenes* has a propensity to infect persons at the extremes of the age spectrum, that is, infants and the aged, as well as individuals with certain underlying diseases (5). Listerial infection in the aging person is primarily a disease of the central nervous system (CNS) with an associated mortality of 30%. Thus, its recognition in the elderly is extremely important.

MICROBIOLOGY, EPIDEMIOLOGY, AND HOST-PARASITE INTERACTION

Listeria monocytogenes is a non-spore-forming, facultatively anaerobic, gram-positive bacillus that is a member of the family Cornybacteriaceae. It has peritricous flagellae, is motile, and has a characteristic tumbling motion in cultures grown at 18–20°C (6). On Gram stain, *L. monocytogenes* has a diphtheroid appearance and may be discarded as a contaminant. Serotyping may be done on *L. monocytogenes* with at least seven serotypes that are identified. Serotypes 1 and 4b are the most common cause of human listerial infections.

This bacterial species is ubiquitous and has been isolated from nonhuman mammals, birds, ticks, and crustaceans as well as from soil, sewage, and stream water (6). Listeriosis in animals has been described primarily in cattle, sheep, and goats. *L. monocytogenes* is occasionally found in feces of healthy asymptomatic adults. However, a human reservoir for *L. monocytogenes* does not appear to be the source for listeriosis. Most likely, ingestion of contaminated foods (especially milk products) is the pathogenetic mechanism for initiating listerial infection (1–4).

L. monocytogenes appears to enter the host via the gastrointestinal tract. Since *L. monocytogenes* is acid sensitive, gastric acidity may be an important defense mechanism (4). Persons that ingest antacids and agents that block gastric acid production (e.g., cimetidine) have been associated with higher frequency of listeriosis (4). Perhaps, the age-associated change of atrophic gastritis may be a contributory factor to the higher incidence of listerial infection in the aged. Once the pathogen enters the gut, it may cause a gastroenteritis and/or enter the bloodstream. Bacteremia then permits the seeding of *L. monocytogenes* to other body sites, especially the CNS.

In humans, listerial infection occurs predominantly in neonates, in the aged, in persons with lymphoreticular or hematologic malignancy, and in those receiving immunosuppressive therapy as well as in individuals with diabetes mellitus and alcoholic cirrhosis (1–4,7–9). Like many other infectious diseases, it is unclear whether age alone and/or age-associated disorders contribute to the higher incidence of listeriosis. Although clinical studies of listeriosis in adults indicate that many of the elderly patients with listeriosis had predisposing underlying conditions (i.e., malignancy, diabetes, cirrhosis, immunosuppression), a significant number of elderly had no obvious coexisting disorders (2,4,10–12). It appears that both infancy and old age as well as some of the previously mentioned predisposing disease states have a higher susceptibility to listerial infections because of their association with altered cell-mediated immunity. Host response and immunity to *L. monocytogenes* infections is based on cell-mediated immune mechanisms (13). Moreover, animal models of *L. monocytogenes* infection confirm the association of declining host response to this pathogen with extremes of age (14).

CLINICAL SYNDROMES

In older adults, listerial infections occur most frequently in the CNS, primarily as meningitis (5). However meningoencephalitis, brain abscess, and necrotizing encephalitis may also occur (11,12,15,16). Primary bacteremia (without an identifiable focus of infection), endocarditis, pleuropulmonary infection, localized abscess, and osteomyelitis are other listerial infections that are described in the elderly (5,12).

DIAGNOSTIC APPROACH

Any elderly patient suspected of having a CNS infection or bacteremia should have *L. monocytogenes* considered as a potential etiologic pathogen. This is especially important in patients suspected of having bacterial meningitis, since (*1*) this organism is frequently not seen on cerebrospinal fluid (CSF) Gram stain (59–76%) (5,10); and (*2*) laboratory isolation of *L. monocytogenes* may be interpreted initially as "diphtheroids" and discarded as a contaminant. Furthermore, listerial meningitis may be associated with a pleocytosis of either polymorphonuclear leukocytes or mononuclear white blood cells. This latter finding may be interpreted incorrectly as an "aseptic," viral, tuberculous, or fungal meningitis.

All patients suspected of listeriosis should have blood cultures obtained. Bacteremia associated with meningitis occurs with extremely high frequency (50–90%) (5,10,15).

TREATMENT

The drug of choice for treating listerial infections is either penicillin G (10–20 million units a day) or ampicillin (6–12 g a day) (17). In cases of CNS infections treated with penicillin G or ampicillin, the results are quite similar. However, strains of *L. monocytogenes* may be inhibited but not killed by these drugs (tolerance) (18), which could have an adverse outcome in patients with meningitis and/or bacteremia. Thus, in severely ill patients with listeriosis, or in patients who fail to respond to single-drug therapy of penicillin G or ampicillin, the addition of an aminoglycoside (e.g., gentamicin, 5 mg/kg a day) or rifampin (600–1,200 mg a day) may be worthwhile (16,17).

Patients who are allergic to penicillin should be treated with either trimethoprim-sulfamethoxazole (trimethoprim, 10–15 mg/kg a day) (19), chloramphenicol (4–6 g a day), or vancomycin (1.5–2.0 g a day). Third-generation cephalosporins are generally ineffective against *L. monocytogenes* (20). Imipenem may be active against this pathogen; however, its role in treating listeriosis has not been defined.

PREVENTION

Other than routine public health measures (i.e., pasteurization and monitoring of milk products), no practical means to prevent listeriosis is currently available.

REFERENCES

1. Schlech WF, Lavigne PM, Bortolussi RA, et al: Epidemic listeriosis: evidence for transmission by food. *N Engl J Med* 308:203–206, 1983.
2. Fleming DW, Cochi SL, MacDonald KL, et al: Pasteurized milk as a vehicle of infection in an outbreak of listeriosis. *N Engl J Med* 312:404–407, 1985.
3. Centers for Disease Control: Listeriosis outbreak associated with Mexican-style cheese—California. *MMWR* 34:357–359, 1985.

4. Ho JL, Shands KN, Friedland G, et al: An outbreak of type 4B *Listeria monocytogenes* infection involving patients from eight Boston hospitals. *Arch Intern Med* 146:520–524, 1986.
5. Nieman RE, Lorber B: Listeriosis in adults: A changing pattern of eight cases and review of the literature, 1968–1978. *Rev Infect Dis* 2:207–227, 1980.
6. Chow AW: Listeriosis, in Yoshikawa TT, Chow AW, Guze LB (eds): *Infectious Diseases. Diagnosis and Management.* New York, John Wiley & Sons, 1980, p 330.
7. Gantz NM, Meyerowitz RL, Medeiros AA, et al: Listeriosis in immunosuppressed patients. A cluster of eight patients. *Am J Med* 58:537–643, 1977.
8. Louria DB, Hensle T, Armstrong D, et al: Listeriosis complicating malignant disease. A new association. *Ann Intern Med* 67:261–280, 1967.
9. Schroter GPJ, Weil R III: *Listeria monocytogenes* infection after renal transplantation. *Arch Intern Med* 137:1395–1399, 1977.
10. Lavetter A, Leedom JM, Mathies AW Jr, et al: Meningitis due to *Listeria monocytogenes.* A review of 25 cases. *N Engl J Med* 285:598–603, 1971.
11. Larrson S, Linell F: Correlations between clinical and postmortem findings in listeriosis. *Scand J Infect Dis* 11:55–58, 1979.
12. Larrson S, Cronberg S, Windblad S: Clinical aspects of 64 cases of juvenile and adult listeriosis in Sweden. *Acta Med Scand* 204:503–508, 1978.
13. Emmerling P, Finger H, Hof H: Cell-mediated resistance to infection with *Listeria monocytogenes* in nude mice. *Infect Immunity* 15:382–385, 1977.
14. Patel PJ: Aging and cellular defense mechanisms: age-related changes in resistance of mice to *Listeria monocytogenes. Infect Immunity* 32:557–562, 1981.
15. Pollock SS, Pollock TM, Harrison MJG: Infection of the central nervous system by *Listeria monocytogenes:* A review of 54 adult and juvenile cases. *Q J Med* 53(No 211):331–340, 1984.
16. Trautmann M, Wagner J, Chahin M, et al: Listeria meningitis: Report of ten recent cases and review of current therapeutic recommendations. *J Infect* 10:107–114, 1985.
17. Tuazon CU, Shamsudden D, Miller H: Antibiotic susceptibility and synergy of clinical isolates of *Listeria monocytogenes. Antimicrob Agents Chemother* 21:525–527, 1982.
18. Wiggins GL, Albritton WL, Feeley JC: Antibiotic susceptibility of clinical isolates of *Listeria monocytogenes. Antimicrob Agents Chemother* 13:854–860, 1978.
19. Spitzer PG, Hammer SM, Karchmer AW: Treatment of *listeria monocytogenes* infection with trimethoprim-sulfamethoxazole: Case report and review of the literature. *Rev Infect Dis* 8:427–430, 1986.
20. Kawaler B, Hof H: Failure of cephalosporins to cure experimental listeriosis. *J Infection* 9:239–243, 1984.

SUGGESTED READINGS

Chow AW: Listeriosis, in Yoshikawa TT, Chow AW, Guze LB (eds): *Infectious Diseases. Diagnosis and Management.* New York, John Wiley & Sons, 1980, p 330.

Nieman RE, Lorber B: Listeriosis in adults: A changing pattern of eight cases and review of the literature, 1968-1978. *Rev Infect Dis* 2:207-227, 1980.

Patel PJ: Aging and cellular defense mechanisms: Age-related changes in resistance of mice to *Listeria monocytogenes. Infect Immunol* 32:557-562, 1981.

Tuazon CU, Shamsudden D, Miller H: Antibiotic susceptibility and synergy of clinical isolates of *Listeria monocytogenes. Antimicrob Agents Chemother* 21: 525-527, 1982.

Chapter 23

Gram-Negative Bacillary Infections

GENERAL CONSIDERATIONS

It was stated in the chapter on sepsis that most cases of bacterial sepsis in adults, including the elderly, are caused by aerobic or facultative anaerobic gram-negative bacilli. This is understandable because many of the most common infections in the aged involve gram-negative bacillary organisms. Additionally, nosocomial infections (which occur in hospitals and nursing homes) are caused primarily by these pathogens, and the elderly are the largest segment of the population who occupy hospital and nursing home beds.

MICROBIOLOGY, EPIDEMIOLOGY, AND HOST PARASITE INTERACTION

The gram-negative bacilli that are clinically relevant to the aged are members of the families Enterobacteriaceae and Pseudomonoadaceae.

The Enterobacteriaceae organisms are aerobic or facultatively anaerobic (they grow under both aerobic and anaerobic conditions) bacilli that ferment glucose and produce gas. They comprise the major aerobic or facultatively anaerobic flora of the colon. They grow well on artificial media; some are motile, and others are nonmotile. Several genera and species are members of the enterobacterial group; some of the more important ones are listed in Table 23.1 (1). It is beyond the scope of this book to discuss the laboratory procedures that are required to identify each species.

TABLE 23.1 Important Members of the Enterobacteriaceae Family

Escherichia coli
Enterobacter sp.
Klebsiella sp.
Serratia marcescens
Proteus sp.
Morganella morganii
Providencia sp.
Salmonella sp.
Shigella sp.
Citrobacter sp.

The family Pseudomonadaceae has many species; however, *Pseudomonas aeruginosa* is the most clinically important pseudomonad in elderly patients. Pseudomonads do not ferment glucose or produce gas from carbohydrates; they oxidate glucose. Most pseudomonads, including *P. aeruginosa,* grow well on most media and can survive in a purely mineral medium that relies on atmospheric carbon dioxide as its carbon source (2,3). In contrast to Enterobacteriaceae organisms, *P. aeruginosa* is an obligate aerobe and does not grow under anaerobic conditions.

Such enterobacterial organisms as *Escherichia coli, Klebsiella* sp., *Proteus* sp., and *Enterobacter* sp. are found as part of the normal colonic flora. These enteric organisms also colonize the perineal region, vagina, and cervix. *P aeruginosa* is a free-living organism and is often found in sewage, natural water, spoiled foods, and plants. It is usually not part of the normal body flora; only 4 to 12% of the normal population are fecal carriers of *P. aeruginosa* (4). However, immunosuppression or antimicrobial therapy can increase the fecal carriage rate.

Both Enterobacteriaceae organisms and *P. aeruginosa* have cell walls containing lipopolysaccharides called *endotoxin.* Endotoxin has a variety of biologic properties and is responsible for the physiologic changes associated with gram-negative bacillary sepsis or shock (see Chapter 18 on sepsis).

Host defense against gram-negative bacilli depends primarily on the availability of functional polymorphonuclear neutrophils (PMNs). Consequently, severely neutropenic patients (e.g., elderly patients receiving cancer chemotherapy) are at great risk for severe gram-negative bacillary infections. Aging appears to be a risk factor to gram-negative bacillary infections, although it is not clear whether age-related chronic disorders are the major influencing factors. Debilitation, hospitalization, invasive diagnostic and therapeutic procedures, immunosuppression, and chronic antibiotic administration, all factors more common to the elderly, increase the susceptibility to gram-negative bacillary infection. (See Chapter 2 on predisposing factors to infection for additional discussion on this topic.)

CLINICAL SYNDROMES

Enterobacteriaceae

Because the organisms of the Enterobacteriaceae family are part of the fecal flora, they are ubiquitous. Thus, these pathogens can infect any organ or tissue (5–7). Table 23.2 lists the most common sites of infections by enterobacterial organisms in the elderly, as well as other associated factors that contribute to these infections.

Pseudomonas aeruginosa

Like Enterobacteriaceae organisms, *P. aeruginosa* has the capacity to infect any organ or tissue. Table 23.3 summarizes the more important sites that are infected by *P. aeruginosa* in elderly patients. Important associated risk factors are also listed in the table (3,4,8).

DIAGNOSTIC APPROACH

Certainly in the elderly, if bacterial infection is suspected, gram-negative bacilli must always be considered as a potential pathogen. All patients

TABLE 23.2   Common Sites of Infection
by Enterobacteriaceae Organisms in the Elderly

SITE	ASSOCIATED FACTORS
Urinary tract	Chronic bladder catheters, prostatic disease, stones, dysfunctional bladder, previous antibiotics
Prostate	Urethral catheterization
Gallbladder	Gallstones
Colon	Diverticulosis, cancer, surgery
Appendix	—
Skin	Chronic pressure, poor vascularity, trauma
Bone and joint	Trauma, previous joint disease
Lungs	Aspiration, intubation, tracheostomy
Central nervous system	Cranial trauma or surgery
Vascular	Chronic intravenous catheter
Prosthetic	Heart valves, shunts, joints
Blood	Leukopenia[a], immunosuppression[a], chronic underlying diseases[a]

[a]These factors may also increase the risk to infections for the urinary tract, lungs, and central nervous system.

TABLE 23.3 Common Sites of Infection
by *Pseudomonas aeruginosa* in the Elderly

SITE	ASSOCIATED FACTORS
Urinary tract	Chronic bladder catheters, multiple previous antibiotics
Skin	Burns
Lungs	Intubation, tracheostomy, leukopenia, immunosuppression, chronic underlying diseases, multiple previous antibiotics
Central nervous system (CNS)	Leukopenia, immunosuppression, CNS surgery
Vascular	Chronic intravenous catheters
External ear	Diabetes mellitus
Blood	Leukopenia, immunosuppression, leukemia

should have a minimum of two sets of blood cultures obtained immediately. Fluid, drainage, or pus from the primary site of infection should be Gram stained immediately and sent for culture. Detection of endotoxin in body fluids that are normally sterile (e.g., cerebrospinal fluid) is presumptive evidence of gram-negative bacillary infection. The limulus lysate gelation test is a commercially available test that is extremely sensitive and specific for detecting endotoxin from body fluids except blood (9). Reliable serologic tests for gram-negative bacilli are not available.

Radiologic tests and radionuclide scans should be obtained as clinically indicated. Catheters, both intravenous and bladder, should be removed and the tips sent for culture. Similarly, most infected prosthetic devices require removal, and these should be cultured appropriately for gram-negative bacilli (as well as for other bacteria).

TREATMENT

Bacteremia, or sepsis, is always a significant risk in any elderly patient with a gram-negative bacillary infection. Thus, the first and most important aspect of managing gram-negative bacillary infections is to determine whether sepsis, with or without shock, is present and to begin treatment immediately to stabilize the cardiovascular and hemodynamic status of the patient. (See Chapter 18 on sepsis.)

The approach to antimicrobial therapy depends on the answers to several important questions:

1. How sick is the patient, that is, is the patient septic and/or hypotensive?

2. Where is the primary site of infection?
3. Is the infection community-acquired, or did it occur in a hospital or nursing home?
4. What associated diseases or conditions are present that might influence outcome (e.g., leukopenia, immunosuppression)?
5. Does the patient have renal dysfunction or a history of significant drug allergies (e.g., penicillin)?
6. Has the patient been on antibiotics recently?

If empiric antimicrobial therapy is deemed appropriate or necessary, the reader is referred to Table 18.3 for antibiotic recommendations for urinary tract infections, pneumonia, and intraabdominal infections. Also, the specific chapters that describe the various sites of infections should be reviewed for drug regimens and doses.

After culture and sensitivity data become available, the antibiotic regimen should be changed by the clinician based on the clinical status of the patient, the patient's response, and the site of infection.

PREVENTION

The prevention of gram-negative bacillary infection is difficult. However, such measures as restricting hospitalization, limiting invasive procedures, and avoiding unnecessary use of antibiotics can reduce the incidence of these infections. Whether an effective vaccine can be developed against gram-negative organisms is unknown.

REFERENCES

1. Yoshikawa TT: *Enterobacteriaceae* infections, in Yoshikawa TT, Chow AW, Guze LB (eds): *Infectious Diseases. Diagnosis and Management.* New York, John Wiley & Sons, 1980, p 351.
2. Yoshikawa TT: *Pseudomonas* infections, in Yoshikawa TT, Chow AW, Guze LB (eds): *Infectious Diseases. Diagnosis and Management.* New York, John Wiley & Sons, 1980, p 366.
3. Gould IM, Wise R: *Pseudomonas aeruginosa:* Clinical manifestations and management. *Lancet* 2:1224–1227, 1985.
4. Bodey GP, Bolivar R, Fainstein V, et al: Infections caused by *Pseudomonas aeruginosa. Rev Infect Dis* 5:279–321, 1983.
5. Bouza E, Garcia de la Torre M, Erice A, et al: Enterobacter bacteremia. An analysis of 50 episodes. *Arch Intern Med* 145:1024–1027, 1985.
6. Drelichman V, Bond JD: Bacteremia due to *Citrobacter diversus* and *Citrobacter freundii.* Incidence, risk factors, and clinical outcome. *Arch Intern Med* 145:1808–1810, 1985.
7. Garcia de la Torre, M, Romero-Vivas J, Martinez-Beltran J, et al: *Klebsiella* bacteremia: An analysis of 100 episodes. *Rev Infect Dis* 7:143–150, 1985.

8. Bodey GP, Jadeja L, Elting J: *Pseudomonas* bacteremia: Retrospective analysis of 410 episodes. *Arch Intern Med* 145:1621–1629, 1985.
9. Gardi A, Arpagaus GR: Improved microtechniques for endotoxin assay by the *Limulus* amebocyte lysate test. *Analytic Biochem* 109:382–385, 1980.

SUGGESTED READINGS

Gould IM, Wise R: *Pseudomonas aeruginosa:* Clinical manifestations and management. *Lancet* 2:1224–1227, 1985.
Yoshikawa TT: *Enterobacteriaceae* infections, in Yoshikawa TT, Chow AW, Guze LB (eds): *Infectious Diseases. Diagnosis and Management.* New York, John Wiley & Sons, 1980, p 351.

Chapter 24

Legionella Infections

GENERAL CONSIDERATIONS

Since the first description of Legionnaires' disease that affected 182 persons who attended the Fifty-eighth Annual Convention of the Pennsylvania Chapter of the American Legion (1), this infecious disease has been described in several different populations. One group that is particularly susceptible to Legionnaires' disease is the aging population. Because the aged are prone to respiratory infections (and Legionnaires' disease is primarily a pneumonia), it is incumbent on clinicians caring for the elderly to consider Legionnaires' disease in the differential diagnosis of an older patient with pulmonary complaints.

MICROBIOLOGY, EPIDEMIOLOGY, AND HOST PARASITE INTERACTION

Infections caused by *Legionella* organisms have been termed *legionellosis.* Table 24.1 summarizes the *Legionella* species currently described in the literature (2,4–10). The discussion in this chapter focuses on *L. pneumophila,* which causes Legionnaires' disease and has six serotypes (i.e., 1–6) (2). Since the original description of Legionnaires' disease, it has been discovered that *L. pneumophila* may cause other clinical syndromes (3).

Legionella species are fastidious, strictly aerobic gram-negative bacilli. However, they are difficult to visualize with Gram stain and thus require special staining methods such as the Gimenez stain or Dieterle silver impregnation stain (11). The organisms do not grow on commonly used

TABLE 24.1 *Legionella* Organisms

CURRENT NOMENCLATURE	OTHER NAMES
Legionella pneumophila (serotypes 1-6)	Legionnaires' organisms, agent of Legionnaires' disease
Legionella micdadei	Pittsburg pneumonia agent, TATLOCK, HEBA
Legionella bozemanii	WIGA, ALLO$_1$, ALLO$_2$, GA-PH
Legionella dumoffii	ALLO$_4$, NY-23, TEX-KL
Legionella gormanii	LS-13
Legionella jordanii	BL-540
Legionella longbeachae	Long Beach 4
Legionella wadsworthii	Wadsworth 81-716A

bacteriologic media. *L. pneumophila* may grow in Mueller-Hinton agar supplemented with IsoViteX and 1% hemoglobin as well as in special chemically defined medium (12,13). However, as *L. pneumophila* is a potential laboratory pathogen, only specialized laboratories should attempt bacterial culture of this organism. Identification of specific species of *Legionella* can be done by DNA studies and direct immunofluorescent testing.

L. pneumophila is an organism commonly found in water, which has been isolated both from domestic tap water and potable water (14-16). Transmission appears to be by aerobic spread with inhalation of contaminated aerosols from faucets, showers, potable hot water, air conditioners, and so on. The organism then invades the respiratory tract.

Cases of Legionnaires' disease may be sporadic or occur as outbreaks. The infection occurs in both the community and institutions (nosocomial). Predisposing factors for Legionnaires' disease include malignancy, immunosuppression, renal failure, chronic pulmonary disease, diabetes mellitus, and cardiac disease (2). Although the elderly are also at risk for nosocomial Legionnaires' disease (16), the majority of patients with nosocomial *L. pneumophila* appear to be younger and have more severe underlying diseases, such as, malignancy, renal failure, or immunosuppression (17-19). In contrast, community-acquired cases appear to occur in older patients, and the associated underlying diseases are primarily those that commonly occur in the aged (e.g., cardiovascular disease, pulmonary disease, diabetes mellitus) (17). Thus, the impact of these age-related diseases on the susceptibility to Legionnaires' disease is unclear.

The major host defense mechanism against *L. pneumophila* appears to be cell-mediated immunity (20). *L. pneumophila* actively replicates intracellularly within resident alveolar macrophages. However, when macrophages become activated by various lymphokines, bacterial growth is inhibited (21). Perhaps, the relative vulnerability of cellular immunity to aging may be a factor in the increased suscpetibility of the elderly to *Legionella* infections.

CLINICAL SYNDROMES

L. pneumophila causes Legionnaires' disease, a severe, multisystem disease with pneumonia as the major or prominent feature (3). This syndrome attacks people over the age of 50, as well as those with the previously described predisposing factors. Initial symptoms may be nonspecific, including anorexia, malaise, lethargy, and headache. Gastrointestinal symptoms, especially diarrhea (50% of cases), is a unique feature of this pneumonic illness. A nonproductive cough occurs initially, which later becomes productive of blood-streaked sputum in 30% of patients and purulent sputum in 50% of patients. Most patients experience fever, and relative bradycardia is found in 60 to 70% of cases. Change in mental status occurs frequently in the elderly; some patients may exhibit overt neurologic manifestations suggestive of an encephalopathy (22). However, meningitis or focal encephalitis is unusual. The pulmonary involvement ranges from patchy unilobular or lobar pneumonia to multilobar disease as well as pleural effusion. Occasionally empyema or rarely lung abscess develop.

In addition to Legionnaires' disease, *L. pneumophila* causes a different syndrome called Pontiac fever. It has a very high attack rate (95–100% compared to 15–20% for Legionnaires' disease), a short incubation period of 1 to 2 days (2–10 days for Legionnaires' disease), multisystemic involvement without pneumonia, and complete recovery in all patients (3). There is no predilection for any age group or sex in Pontiac fever.

DIAGNOSTIC APPROACH

Direct fluorescent antibody examination of sputum, lung tissue, pleural fluid, pus, or other tissue is the most rapid method of diagnosis of Legionnaires' disease (23). The test has a sensitivity of 70% and a specificity of 95% for sputum samples (2). Occasional cross-reactions occur with rare strains of *Pseudomonas fluorescens, Bacterioides fragilis,* and other *Pseudomonas* species (2).

The serologic test for this infection is the most widely used method of diagnosis. The indirect fluorescent antibody (IFA) test confirms the diagnosis if there is at least a fourfold (at least to 1:128) rise in serum specimens taken during the acute and convalescent periods of illness. However, many patients may not show a titer change until 4 to 8 weeks after the onset of illness. Moreover, cross-reactions may occur in patients with tularemia, *B. fragilis* bacteremia, and leptospirosis (2).

A culture of specimens for *L. pneumophila* also confirms the diagnosis of Legionnaires' disease. Growth occurs in about 2 to 7 days.

TREATMENT

The treatment of choice for Legionnaires' disease is erythromycin. The penicillins, cephalosporins, aminoglycosides, vancomycin, and clindamycin are ineffective against this infection. In seriously ill elderly patients with Legionnaires' disease, intravenous erythromycin should be given in a dose of 4 g a day in four divided doses. For less serious illness, a dose of 2 g a day is generally sufficient. After a clinical response, the drug can be administered orally. Therapy should be for at least 3 weeks (2).

An alternative but significantly less effective drug is doxycycline. An initial dose of 200 mg is given intravenously, followed by 100 mg 12 hours later, and then 100 mg a day. If the patient is moderately ill, rifampin, 1,200 mg a day should also be added to the doxycycline (2).

PREVENTION

When a case of Legionnaires' disease is diagnosed, a search for other possible cases should be initiated. Environmental sampling, especially water or water-associated equipment or devices, may be indicated. Hyperchlorination of water sources (if water is contaminated) may be required.

REFERENCES

1. Fraser DW, Tsai TR, Orenstein W, et al: Legionnaires' Disease. Description of an epidemic of pneumonia. *N Engl J Med* 297:1189–1197, 1977.
2. Meyer RD: Legionella infections: A review of five years of research. *Rev Infect Dis* 5:258–278, 1983.
3. Shands KN, Fraser DW: Legionnaires' Disease. *Disease-a-Month* 27:5–39, 1980.
4. Edelstein PH, Brenner DJ, Moss CW, et al: *Legionella wadsworthii* species nova: A cause of human pneumonia. *Ann Intern Med* 97:809–813, 1982.
5. Rudin JE, Wing EJ: A comparative study of *Legionella micdadei* and other nosocomially acquired pneumonias. *Chest* 86:675–680, 1984.
6. Thomason BM, Harris PP, Hicklin MD, et al: A *Legionella*-like bacterium related to WIGA in a fatal case of pneumonia. *Ann Intern Med* 91:673–676, 1979.
7. Lewallen KR, McKinney RM, Brenner DJ, et al: A newly identified bacterium phenotypically resembling but genetically distinct from *Legionella pneumophila:* An isolate in a case of pneumonia. *Ann Intern Med* 91:831–834, 1979.
8. Morris GK, Steigerwalt A, Feeleg JC, et al: *Legionella pneumophila* sp. nov. *J Clin Microbiol* 12:718–721, 1980.

9. Cherry WB, Gorman GW, Orrison LH, et al: *Legionella jordanis:* A new species of *Legionella* isolated from water and sewage. *J Clin Microbiol* 15: 290–297, 1982.
10. McKinney RM, Porshen RK, Edelstein PH, et al: *Legionella longbeachae* species nova, another etiologic agent of human pneumonia. *Ann Intern Med* 94:739–743, 1981.
11. Chandler FW, Hicklin MD, Blackman JA: Demonstration of the agent of Legionnaires' Disease on tissue. *N Engl J Med* 297:1213–1220, 1977.
12. Feeley JC, Gorman GW, Weaver RE, et al: Primary isolation media for Legionnaires' Disease bacterium. *J Clin Microbiol* 8:320–335, 1978.
13. Warren WJ, Miller RD: Growth of Legionnaires Disease bacterium (*Legionella pneumophila*) in chemically defined medium. *J Clin Microbiol* 10: 50–55, 1979.
14. Arnow PM, Chow T, Weil D, et al: Legionnaires' Disease caused by aerosolized tap water from respiratory devices. *J Infect Dis* 146:460–467, 1982.
15. Stout J, Yu VL, Vickers RM, et al: Ubiquitousness of *Legionella pneumophila* in the water supply of a hospital with endemic Legionnaire's Disease. *N Engl J Med* 306:466–468, 1982.
16. Neill MA, Gorman GW, Gibert C, et al: Noscomial legionellosis, Paris, France. Evidence for transmission by potable water. *Am J Med* 78:581–588, 1985.
17. Helms CM, Viner JP, Weisenburger DP, et al: Sporadic Legionnaires' Disease: Clinical observations in 87 nosocomial and community-acquired cases. *Am J Med Sci* 288:2–12, 1984.
18. Cordonnier C, Farcet J-P, Desforges L, et al: Legionnaires' Disease and hairy-cell leukemia. An unfortuitous association? *Arch Intern Med* 144:2373–2375, 1984.
19. Kugler JW, Armitage JO, Helms CM, et al: Nosocomial Legionnaires' Disease. Occurrence in recipients of bone marrow transplants. *Am J Med* 74: 281–288, 1983.
20. Horwitz MA: Cell-mediated immunity in Legionnaires' Disease. *J Clin Invest* 71:1686–1697, 1983.
21. Horwitz MA, Silverstein MC: Activated human monocytes inhibit the intracellular multiplication of Legionnaires' disease bacteria. *J Exp Med* 154: 1618–1635, 1981.
22. Johnson JD, Raff MJ, Van Arsdall JA: Neurologic manifestations of Legionnaires' Disease. *Medicine* 63:303–310, 1984.
23. Broome CV, Cherry WB, Winn WC Jr, et al: Rapid diagnosis of Legionnaires' disease by direct immunofluorescent staining. *Am J Intern Med* 90:1–4, 1979.

SUGGESTED READINGS

Helms CM, Viner JP, Weisenburger DP, et al: Sporadic Legionnaires' Disease: Clinical observations in 87 nosocomial and community-acquired cases. *Am J Med Sci* 288:2–12, 1984.

Horwitz MA: Cell-mediated immunity in Legionnaires' Disease. *J Clin Invest* 71:1686–1697, 1983.

Meyer RD: Legionella infections: A review of five years of research. *Rev Infect Dis* 5:258–278, 1983.

Shands KN, Fraser DW: Legionnaires' Disease. *Disease-a-Month* 27:5–39, 1980.

Index